Elsevier would like to acknowledge the Traditional Custodians of the lands and waters on which we live and work. We acknowledge that Aboriginal and Torres Strait Islander peoples have continuously passed on knowledge for millennia, using resources from the land and waters to nurture and promote healthy communities, and we pay our respects to Elders past and present.

Contexts of Nursing

AN INTRODUCTION

SEVENTH EDITION

EDITED BY

DEBRA JACKSON
ANN BONNER
JACQUELINE BLOOMFIELD
JOHN DALY

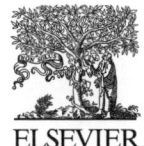

ELSEVIER

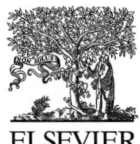

Elsevier Australia. ACN 001 002 357
(a division of Reed International Books Australia Pty Ltd)
475 Victoria Avenue, Chatswood, NSW 2067

Copyright 2026 Elsevier Australia. All rights reserved, including those for text and data mining, AI training, and similar technologies.

Publisher's note: *Elsevier* takes a neutral position with respect to territorial disputes or jurisdictional claims in its published content, including in maps and institutional affiliations.

1st edition © 2000; 2nd edition © 2006; 3rd edition © 2010; 4th edition © 2014; 5th edition © 2017; 6th © edition 2021 Elsevier Australia

All rights reserved. No part of this publication may be reproduced or transmitted in any form or by any means, electronic or mechanical, including photocopying, recording, or any information storage and retrieval system, without permission in writing from the publisher. Details on how to seek permission, further information about the Publisher's permissions policies and our arrangements with organizations such as the Copyright Clearance Center and the Copyright Licensing Agency, can be found at our website: www.elsevier.com/permissions.

This book and the individual contributions contained in it are protected under copyright by the Publisher (other than as may be noted herein).

ISBN: 978-0-7295-4500-6

Notice

Practitioners and researchers must always rely on their own experience and knowledge in evaluating and using any information, methods, compounds or experiments described herein. Because of rapid advances in the medical sciences, in particular, independent verification of diagnoses and drug dosages should be made. To the fullest extent of the law, no responsibility is assumed by Elsevier, authors, editors or contributors for any injury and/or damage to persons or property as a matter of products liability, negligence or otherwise, or from any use or operation of any methods, products, instructions, or ideas contained in the material herein.

National Library of Australia Cataloguing-in-Publication Data

 A catalogue record for this book is available from the National Library of Australia

---

Content Strategist: Elizabeth Coady
Content Project Manager: Fariha Nadeem
Edited by Lynn Watts
Proofread by Annabel Adair
Cover Designer: Gopalakrishnan Venkatraman
Index by Innodata
Typeset by GW Tech

Printed in Kuan Press, Malaysia

Last digit is the print number: 9   8   7   6   5   4   3   2   1

CONTENTS

Contributors	vii
Reviewers	xi
Preface	xiii

1. **Presenting nursing ... a career for life** — 1
   Debra Jackson, Jacqueline Bloomfield, Ann Bonner and John Daly

2. **Visioning the future by knowing the past** — 9
   Madonna Grehan

3. **Ethics in nursing** — 33
   Megan-Jane Johnstone

4. **An introduction to legal aspects of nursing practice** — 45
   Jayne Hewitt

5. **Cultural safety in nursing and midwifery** — 61
   Rakime Elmir and Zoe Tipa

6. **Key concepts informing nursing: caring, compassion and emotional competence** — 75
   Jacqueline Bloomfield

7. **Patient perspectives and person-centred care in nursing** — 87
   Horas Wong and Georgia Tobiano

8. **Nursing and the quest for care quality and patient safety** — 103
   Brigid Gillespie and Debra Jackson

9. **Becoming a critical thinker** — 117
   Marion Tower

10. **Power and politics in nursing** — 135
    Sharon Brownie and Letitia Del Fabbro

11. **Reflective practice: the importance and ways of reflection in nursing** — 153
    Kim Usher

12. **Interprofessional learning and working** — 167
    Ann Bonner and Jacqueline Bloomfield

13	Engaging with social media: opportunities and challenges for nursing professionals *Matthew Barton, Michael Todorovic and Jessica Stokes-Parish*	179
14	Using digital health to enhance patient care and clinical quality *Debra Jackson, Rikki Jones and Kim Usher*	197
15	Social justice, health disparities and equity in nursing *Denise Wilson, Stephen Neville and Lynore Geia*	213
16	Nursing and family violence *Denise Wilson and Debra Jackson*	229
17	Rural and remote nursing *Marie Hutchinson and Leah East*	243
18	Primary healthcare and nursing *Elizabeth Halcomb*	257
19	Simulation learning in nursing *Kerry Reid-Searl, Melanie Barlow, Danny Sidwell and Colleen Ryan*	267
20	Preparing for and making meaning of clinical placement *Lynda Hughes and Sandra Johnston*	289
21	Research in nursing *Thomas Buckley and Andrea P. Marshall*	305
22	Becoming a nurse leader *Patricia M. Davidson and Kelly Lewer*	321
23	Nursing and the environment *Kim Usher and Naomi Tutticci*	339
24	Global health and nursing *Michele Rumsey*	357
	Glossary	377
	Index	391

CONTRIBUTORS

Melanie Barlow RN, BN, MN (ICU), GradDip(Crit care), GradCertEd(Leadership & Management), PhD

    Associate Professor, Australian Catholic University, Brisbane, QLD, Australia

Matthew Barton RN, MN, BMedSci(Hons), PhD, GradCert HigherEd, FHEA

    Senior Lecturer, School of Nursing and Midwifery, Griffith University, Gold Coast Campus, QLD, Australia

Jacqueline Bloomfield RN, BN, MN, PGDip(Midwifery), PGDip(Professional Healthcare Education), PhD, SFHEA

    Professor of Nursing Education, The University of Sydney, Susan Wakil School of Nursing and Midwifery, The University of Sydney, NSW, Australia

Ann Bonner BAppSc(Nurs), RN, MA, MACN, PhD

    Professor and Head of School of Nursing and Midwifery, Griffith University, QLD; Kidney Health Service, Metro North Health, QLD, Australia

Sharon Brownie RN, RM, BEd, MEd Admin, MHthSMgt, MAppMgtN, GAICD, FCNA, FACHSM, DocBusAdmin, PhD

    Professor Health Workforce Development and Director of Health Strategy and Partnerships, Swinburne University of Technology, Hawthorn, VIC, Australia

Thomas Buckley RN, BSC(Hons), MN, PhD, Cert(ICU), Cert(HPol)

    Associate Professor, Susan Wakil School of Nursing and Midwifery, The University of Sydney, NSW, Australia

John Daly RN, PhD, DrNurs(Hons), FACN, FAAN, FFNMRCSI

    Emeritus Professor, University of Western Sydney; Emeritus Professor, University of Technology, Sydney; Honorary Professor, University of Wollongong, NSW, Australia

Patricia M. Davidson RN, MED, PhD

    Vice Chancellor's Fellow, University of New South Wales, Sydney, NSW, Australia

Letitia Del Fabbro RN, BN, BHlthSc(Hons), GradDipA(Aboriginal Studies), MPH, FPHAA, SFHEA

    Lecturer, Griffith University, School of Nursing and Midwifery, Gold Coast Campus, QLD, Australia

Leah East RN, BN(Hons), PhD, GradCertAP

    Professor in Nursing, University of Southern Queensland, School of Nursing and Midwifery, Centre of Health Research, Toowoomba Campus, QLD, Australia

Rakime Elmir RM, RN, BN(Hons), Grad Cert Clinical Teaching, PhD

    Associate Professor of Nursing and Midwifery, Western Sydney University, School of Nursing and Midwifery, Sydney, NSW, Australia

Lynore Geia RM, RN, MP&TM, BN, PhD

    Professor of Nursing and Midwifery, Edith Cowan University, Joondalup, WA, Australia

Brigid Gillespie RN, PhD, FACORN

    Professor and Director, NHMRC Centre of Research Excellence in Wiser Wounds, Griffith University; Gold Coast Health, Gold Coast, QLD, Australia

Madonna Grehan RN, Midwife, GradDipHlthEth, PhD
Honorary Fellow, Department of Nursing, School of Health Sciences, The University of Melbourne, VIC, Australia

Elizabeth Halcomb RN, BN(Hons) GradCertHE, GradCertICNurs, PhD, FACN
Professor of Primary Health Care Nursing, School of Nursing, University of Wollongong, NSW, Australia

Jayne Hewitt RN, BN, LLB, LLM, PhD
Senior Lecturer, Griffith University, School of Nursing and Midwifery, Gold Coast Campus, QLD, Australia

Lynda Hughes RN, PhD, SFHEA
Program Director, School of Nursing and Midwifery, Brisbane South (Nathan), Griffith University, QLD, Australia

Marie Hutchinson RN, MN, BapSci, Grad Dip HA, MHSc, PhD
Professor of Nursing, Southern Cross University, Coffs Harbour Campus, NSW, Australia

Debra Jackson AO, RN, CommNsgCert, DipAppSci(Nsg), BHlthSc(Nsg), MN(Ed), PhD, FCNA, SFHEA
Professor of Nursing, Sydney Nursing School, The University of Sydney, NSW, Australia

Sandra Johnston RN, MBA, PhD
Associate Professor, School of Nursing, Queensland University of Technology, QLD, Australia

Megan-Jane Johnstone AO, PhD, BA, RN
Adjunct Professor, School of Nursing and Midwifery, La Trobe University, Melbourne, VIC, Australia

Rikki Jones RN, BN, PhD
Professor in Nursing, University of New England, Armidale Campus, Armidale, NSW, Australia

Kelly Lewer BN, MEd, PhD
Lecturer, School of Nursing, University of Wollongong, Wollongong, NSW, Australia

Andrea P. Marshall PhD
Professor of Intensive Care Nursing, School of Nursing and Midwifery, Griffith University and Nursing and Midwifery Education and Research Unit, Gold Coast Health, Southport, QLD, Australia

Stephen Neville RN, PhD, FCNA(NZ)
Professor and Head of Discipline – Nursing, University of the Sunshine Coast, QLD, Australia

Kerry Reid-Searl RN, RM, MClin Ed, BHlth Sc, PhD
Professor of Nursing, University of Tasmania, Australia

Michele Rumsey RN, PhD
Professor and Director WHO Collaborating Centre Nursing, Midwifery and Health Development, Faculty of Health, University of Technology Sydney, NSW, Australia

Colleen Ryan RN, MHPE, PhD
Head of Professional Practice/Senior Lecturer, CQUniversity, School of Nursing, Midwifery and Social Sciences, Brisbane, QLD, Australia

Danny Sidwell RN, MAdvancedPrac, HProfEd, MEdProfSt Res
Senior Lecturer in Nursing, University of Tasmania (Hobart Campus), TAS, Australia

Jessica Stokes-Parish RN, BNurs, MN, PhD, GradCertSciComm, AFANZAHPE

Assistant Professor Medicine, Faculty of Health Sciences and Medicine, Bond University, Varsity Campus, QLD, Australia

Zoe Tipa RN, BHSc(Nursing), MPhil, PhD

Chief Nurse, Office of the Chief Nurse, Whānau Āwhina Plunket, Wellington, New Zealand (Aotearoa)

Georgia Tobiano BN(Hons), PhD, Senior Research Fellow, NHMRC CRE in Wiser Wound Care

MHIQ, Parklands, WA, Australia

Michael Todorovic BBioMolSci(Hons), PhD

Associate Professor, Health Science and Medicine, Bond University, QLD, Australia

Marion Tower RN, BN(Hons), MN, PhD, GAICD, SFHEA

Associate Professor, School of Nursing and Midwifery, Nathan Campus, Griffith University, QLD, Australia

Naomi Tutticci BN, RN, Master Ed Studies, GradCert Academic Practice, PhD

Senior Lecturer, School of Nursing and Midwifery, Brisbane South Campus, Griffith University, QLD, Australia

Kim Usher AM RN, BA, DipHSc(Nsg), MNSt, PhD

Executive Dean, Faculty of Medicine and Health, Elm Avenue, University of New England, Armidale, NSW, Australia

Denise Wilson RN, MA(Hons), PhD, FCA(NZ), FRSNZ, FAAN

Associate Dean Māori Advancement/Professor Māori Health, Auckland University of Technology, Auckland, New Zealand (Aotearoa)

Horas Wong RN, BN(Hon), MPH, MA, PhD

Senior Lecturer in Nursing (Social Sciences), Susan Wakil School of Nursing and Midwifery, The University of Sydney, NSW, Australia

REVIEWERS

Faye Davenport BA, RN, MN, MEd

Senior Lecturer – Nursing Education, Nurse Education Team, Universal College of Learning, Palmerston North, New Zealand

Aaron Grogan NP, RN, BN, GC Emerg, MNP, MBA, PhD Cand

Program Lead – Master of Nurse Practitioner (MNP), School of Nursing, Midwifery and Social Work, The University of Queensland, Brisbane, QLD,ld 4072 Australia

Benjamin Hay BN, RN, PGCert Crit Care, PGCert Uni Teaching, MN, PhD

Senior Lecturer and 2nd Year Academic Advisor School of Nursing & Midwifery, The University of Notre Dame Australia, Fremantle Campus, Perth, WA

Adjunct Research Consultant – SCGOPHCG – Centre for Nursing Research (CNR), Sir Charles Gairdner Hospital (SCGH), Nedlands, Perth, WA, Australia

Patricia Jones RN, CertIVTAE, GradCertNursingGP, GradCertVET, MAClinLead, FHEA

Program Convenor Diploma of Health Care, Griffith College, Gold Coast, QLD, Australia

Kate Lowe MN (Management), GC (Higher Education), GC (Paed Nursing), LLB, GradDipLaw, BN

Lecturer in Nursing, School of Nursing, Midwifery and Paramedicine (NSW), Australian Catholic University, Australia

PREFACE

We are delighted to present the seventh edition of *Contexts of Nursing*. We hope this edition proves to be a valuable and insightful resource for you, the reader. As with previous versions, this book serves as an introduction to the theoretical foundations, language and scholarship of nursing and healthcare. Since the publication of the first edition, our primary goal has been to offer comprehensive coverage of key concepts that shape contemporary nursing practice.

The concept of 'contexts' remains central to this edition, reflecting our perspective that nursing knowledge is like a woven fabric, interlacing theoretical strands to form a comprehensive whole. With this in mind, we have incorporated several new threads into this latest edition, addressing contemporary challenges that impact nursing practice.

In response to extensive consultation with nursing professionals, we have included new chapters on critical issues such as family violence, patient safety, simulation learning, patient perspectives and person-centred care and nursing and the environment. These additions reflect the evolving healthcare landscape and the necessity for nurses to be equipped with knowledge and skills relevant to these contemporary challenges and concerns.

This book is a collection of diverse perspectives, and as such, the chapters vary in their approach and presentation. We believe that engaging with a range of viewpoints—including those that may challenge existing beliefs—enriches learning and supports critical thinking. As nursing continues to evolve both locally in Australia and New Zealand (Aotearoa), and on a global scale, exposure to differing perspectives prepares students for the dynamic nature of the profession.

Throughout this edition, we continue to emphasise accessibility and pedagogical strength, maintaining the use of reflective questions and exercises to foster critical thinking and deeper learning. We have also introduced new strategies to encourage personal reflection, embedding them at key points in each chapter. This approach allows readers to pause, absorb and engage more meaningfully with the material. Additionally, case studies and real-world stories further contextualise key topics, helping to bridge the gap between theoretical concepts and practical application.

We extend our sincere gratitude to Elizabeth Coady, Fariha Nadeem and the dedicated team at Elsevier for their continuing support and enthusiasm throughout the development of this edition. Above all, we thank our contributors, who have once again embraced the challenge of producing engaging, scholarly and thought-provoking content to inspire reflection, discussion and growth within the nursing community.

Debra Jackson AO
Ann Bonner
Jacqueline Bloomfield
John Daly
May, 2025

CHAPTER 1

PRESENTING NURSING ... A CAREER FOR LIFE

Debra Jackson, Jacqueline Bloomfield, Ann Bonner and John Daly

KEY WORDS

career
critical perspectives
lifelong learning
nursing
nursing stereotypes

LEARNING OBJECTIVES

After reading this chapter, readers should be able to:

- list some of the myths, legends and stereotypes that surround nursing
- arrive at a personal beginning definition of nursing
- understand their passion for nursing
- discuss some of the choices that a nursing degree offers for graduates
- describe the meaning of the term 'professional conduct'.

Why nursing?

Nursing is a unique and wonderful career choice. It is a curious mix of technology and myth, of science and art, of reality and fiction. It blends the concrete and the abstract. It combines thinking and doing, 'being with' and 'doing for'. Nurses have privileged access to people's homes and share some of the most precious and highly intimate moments in people's lives—moments that remain hidden from most other people and professions. Nurses witness birth and death, and just about everything in between. Nurses share in people's most difficult moments of suffering and pain, and also bear witness to times of great joy and happiness. Because of the special place in society that nurses hold, nurses enjoy a high level of community trust. Indeed, in Australia and New Zealand (Aotearoa), nurses continually rank very highly in surveys of public confidence and trust.

In this opening chapter, we aim to share what captured us and created our passion and enthusiasm for the wonderful career that is nursing—the passion and enthusiasm that has sustained and carried us successfully through our nursing careers. We also introduce you to some of the ideas of interest to nurses and nursing, many of which are discussed in more detail in subsequent chapters of this book.

> ### REFLECTION
> What are the main reasons you have chosen a career in nursing?

Nursing: myths, legends and stereotypes

Philosophically, nursing has gone through a number of historical transitions. Asceticism, arising from our origins in religion and the army, then romanticism, followed by humanism. Perhaps more than any other professional group, nursing and nurses are the subject of myth and popular belief; there are also many fictionalised (or romantic) connotations. Certain of these myths and beliefs are almost folkloric, yet they strongly influence the ways in which nurses are perceived by the general public and also in the ways that nurses see themselves. Through the media, nursing is often portrayed as a dramatic, exciting, glamorous and romantic activity, with nurses frequently represented in the role of handmaiden/helper to medical doctors.

Nursing is endlessly fascinating to many people, and this is reflected in the number of documentaries and reality shows, fictional television dramas, novels and movies that feature nursing and nurses as a major component. A recent Australian study examining the representation of nurses in a reality show highlighted that while nurses were a major part of the show (with 19/54 characters being nurses), they tended to be represented as background actors, and the medical role was privileged (Hayward 2023). So, while the representation of nurses is not always accurate, or realistic, there is not the same level of entertainment interest in bank workers or bus drivers or beauty therapists, or even other health professionals such as pharmacists or dietitians, for example.

Nursing is ripe with imagery. Many of the images associated with nurses are seemingly at odds with one another, yet all may be conjured up by the word 'nurse'. Images of selflessness, kindness, compassion and dedication, hard work, long hours, submission and low pay are among the things that come to mind for some people when they think of nurses. But though nursing practice has current or historical elements of all these things, there is so much more to nurses than these portray.

The recent global COVID-19 pandemic revealed the importance and centrality of nurses and nursing to public health, and this was shown across all areas from intensive care through to primary care environments, and everything in between. Throughout the pandemic, nurses all over the world worked in conditions of incredible stress in difficult conditions and very rapidly changing environments (Anderson et al 2023, Yang et al 2022). Nurses were subject to widespread redeployment into different areas and new roles, such as medical hotel quarantine roles (Jefferies et al 2023, Veerapen & McKeown 2021). Student nurses also experienced massive and rapid disruption as a result of the pandemic (Griscti et al 2023, Usher et al 2023). Despite the unprecedented challenges presented by the pandemic, nurses made an enormous contribution across multiple areas. In addition to providing the direct care of patients affected by COVID-19, nurses were active in the vaccination effort (Burden et al 2021), and nurses developed and implemented new ways of working (Endacott et al 2022). Nurses led the development of many life-saving initiatives such as immunisation centres and infection control procedures. Nurse researchers all over the world remained very active, publishing large amounts of literature to contribute to knowledge that could inform future pandemic responses (Jackson 2022).

The actions and service of nurses during the COVID-19 pandemic is only the latest chapter in nursing history. Throughout nursing history, there are many stories of the fortitude, bravery and courage shown by Australian, New Zealand (Aotearoa) and global nurses in wartime and other times of community hardship. Chapter 2 in this book provides a comprehensive overview of nursing history to extend the reader's understanding of the rich and varied history of nursing.

Nursing and nurses are subject to various entrenched stereotypes (Girvin 2015, Girvin et al 2016), and some of these are at least partly derived from the myth that surrounds nursing. In what has become an important and classic work, Kalisch et al (1983) identified some major ways that nursing and nurses were stereotyped, and though this work was undertaken in the United States more than two decades ago, it still remains relevant to nurses today. The media and popular literature also tend to present nurses as having stereotyped personal characteristics such as youthfulness, femaleness, purity and naivety, altruism and idealism, compliance and diminutive stature and 'good character' (Fealy et al 2015).

REFLECTION

Consider the popular stereotypes of nurses. How many can you identify? Do any describe you? Did any of these stereotypes influence your decision to become a nurse?

Co-existing with the romantic myths and stereotypes surrounding nurses is the reality of nursing. This reality is that nurses become acquainted with the visceral and raw aspects of humanity that are usually hidden from the world, because of the illness, the incapacity, the frailty, the disability or other needs of those who are the recipients of nursing care. The practice of nursing provides opportunities for human connectedness and growth that few other careers can offer. Values of humanism in nursing are enacted and embodied through the commitment to compassion and respectful relationships that are sensitive to the belief systems and cultural practices of others.

It is important to recognise that the concept of 'nurse' is socially constructed, and that nurses may want to believe in their power and control, but the broader societal context situates nurses in a much more fragile position. Nurses and nursing practice exist within a healthcare system, bound by authority and power that generally nurses do not have control over. Some of the effects of this on nursing can be found later in this book, in Chapter 10.

How to define nursing?

The urge to define nursing has attracted the attention of nurse scholars for many years. While defining a nurse is relatively simple, as you will see as you read further in this chapter, nursing itself has proved somewhat more challenging to define. There is a wide variation internationally in the definitions of nursing roles. Though you can probably describe what you think nursing is, the nature and breadth of activities that comprise nursing have contributed to the difficulties associated with defining nursing. Some definitions centre on the functions of a nurse, rather than offering an intrinsic definition of nursing. In a now historical piece of writing which has endured, Henderson produced such a definition of nursing:

> The unique function of the nurse is to assist the individual, sick or well, in the performance of those activities contributing to health or its recovery (or to a peaceful death) that he [sic] would perform unaided if he [sic] had the necessary strength, will or knowledge. And to do this in such a way as to help him [sic] gain independence as rapidly as possible.
>
> (Henderson 1964)

Though many people may feel they have a clear view of what a nurse is and what a nurse does, nursing is complex. The complexities associated with defining nursing mean that some definitions may seem cumbersome and quite ambiguous. But remember that this is more a reflection of the complex nature of nursing than any lack of clarity on behalf of those who have proffered a definition. The International Council of Nurses (ICN), a coalition of nurses' associations that represents nurses in more than 120 countries, has captured some of the complexities in its definition:

> Nursing encompasses autonomous and collaborative care of individuals of all ages, families, groups and communities, sick or well and in all settings. Nursing includes the promotion of health, prevention of illness, and the care of ill, disabled and dying people. Advocacy, promotion of a safe environment, research, participation in shaping health policy and in patient and health systems management, and education are also key nursing roles.
>
> (International Council of Nurses [ICN] n.d.)

REFLECTION

1. Why do you think nursing has proved difficult to define?
2. How is nursing defined in your own jurisdiction? Consider this definition in relation to one from another jurisdiction, region or country and consider any differences or similarities.

Choosing nursing

We have accumulated more than 100 years of being a nurse between us, and none of us have any regrets about choosing nursing. Our careers have taken us in many exciting and rewarding directions and to work in many different contexts and regions. A degree in nursing provides a foundation for lifelong learning. It is the entry requirement to a fulfilling career, to a range of postgraduate courses in areas as diverse as paediatrics, midwifery, emergency nursing, disaster nursing, flight nursing, cancer care, community nursing, women's health, nurse education, nursing research and healthcare administration. Age and experience are valued in nursing.

Nursing has long been viewed as an appropriate career choice for females, but males also form a significant (and increasing) part of the nursing workforce. The most current figures in Australia indicate that 11.9% of the Australian nursing workforce is male (NMBA 2024). In New Zealand

(Aotearoa), the number of men in the nursing workforce is 9% (Guy et al 2022). Recent research has highlighted a lack of awareness of nursing as a career choice for men (Guy et al 2022), and men in nursing experiencing some forms of stigma and misconceptions, though there is some evidence that this is improving (Ramjan et al 2023).

A career in nursing offers continuing potential for achievement, growth and development. It has also traditionally been a profession that attracted people motivated by altruism and the desire to make a difference to people suffering because of illness, injury, disability and disadvantage. Indeed, this is still a significant motivator for people who choose nursing today. Since the 1970s the profession of nursing has made stronger claims for a focus on health promotion and primary healthcare, and this now has greater emphasis in the construction of nursing knowledge and in the conceptualisation of practice due to the ageing of the population, the increase in chronic disease, and the pressures on the healthcare system. But further to that, there was an overriding quest for understanding and caring for people.

Nursing is not just one thing and over the past couple of decades, nurses' roles and career structures have grown and developed, meaning that nursing can be (and is), a career for life. Unlike many other professions and career choices in which people experience increasing difficulty in obtaining work as they get older, nurses can remain productively employed until retirement, and even post-retirement. Career interruption because of family responsibilities (or other reasons) can be extremely disadvantaging in some professions, but many nurses have effectively blended very successful careers with raising families. Nursing opens many doors. Internationally, Australian and New Zealand (Aotearoa) registered nurses are well respected and can gain registration and practise nursing in many other countries.

Nursing: what sustains us?

One of the things that has sustained us all through our own careers is the ability to continue to effect positive change in nursing. As nurses, educators and researchers we have been able to identify areas for change, help generate the knowledge needed to inform that change and then participate in the implementation and evaluation of that change. Nurses work in climates of continual change, and over the years of our own nursing careers we have witnessed many developments—from how students are prepared for registration as nurses, through to alterations in the environment in which nurses work. Nursing curricula and nurse education have changed enormously over the years, and today's nursing students have a comprehensive and well-rounded education with an awareness of social determinants of health and the need to recognise culture as central to human experience (Jackson 2023). Another major difference is the increased realisation of the importance of research; the importance of both generating and drawing on robust evidence to underpin our practice as professional nurses. As students of nursing, you will hear and learn a lot about evidence and its role in shaping practice. In Chapter 21 you will be able to learn more about research evidence and its relevance to, and use for, nursing.

Nursing is an incredibly rewarding and gratifying career. However, as with all professions that work closely with people experiencing crises and challenges, there is increasing awareness of the need for support and deliberate self-care. This is essential as people working in professions with high emotional involvement, who work long hours and work in situations of pressure are at risk of experiencing negative sequelae, such as burnout. Over the past couple of decades, healthcare organisations have developed an increased awareness of the need to adequately support staff, and so most now have a range of services for staff, including counselling and other services. Nurse wellbeing has become an active area for nurse researchers, who provide evidence that can help healthcare organisations to enhance retention by providing more positive work environments for nurses (see, e.g., Poghosyan et al 2022, Teoh et al 2022). An increased awareness of the links between nurse wellbeing and staff retention means that more and more organisations are paying more attention to quality leadership, and strategies such as self-rostering to assist nurses to better manage work as well as their other (personal) responsibilities.

> ### REFLECTION
> 1. What has been your experience, so far, of nursing?
> 2. What motivated you to become a nurse?
> 3. What now sustains you?

Professional regulation and conduct

Nurses are expected to be people of integrity who conduct themselves with a high level of personal honour, accountability and veracity. It is important that members of the public feel safe in hospitals and believe themselves to be in trustworthy and competent hands. If people do not feel safe, they would not be able to feel secure in leaving their loved ones in the care of nurses and healthcare facilities. Nursing authorities in Australia, New Zealand (Aotearoa) and many other countries act to ensure the safety of the public by holding nurses accountable for their actions and making nurses answerable for their behaviour and any complaints that are made against them. To gain initial registration as a nurse, nursing applicants need to demonstrate they are competent and of good character, and this must be maintained throughout professional life.

> ### REFLECTION
> What do you see as essential personal qualities for nurses?
>
> Nurses are answerable to registering authorities that have the power to question nurses and suspend or remove them from the register. These same authorities can also place conditions on registration, restricting practice or, in certain circumstances, requiring a nurse to participate in educational programs. The conduct of nurses is also guided by various codes that inform professional conduct. Though these vary depending on country, they are remarkably similar in substance. This is because the values of nursing cross national and international boundaries. It is an interesting exercise to use the internet and search for the Code of Conduct that governs nurses in your location.

> **REFLECTION**
> What are some examples of good and poor professional conduct? If you have worked in a clinical setting, or been on a clinical placement, can you think of some from your own practice experience?

CONCLUSION

Nursing attracts people from all walks of life. Many readers of this text will be entering nursing as school leavers, but others will be mature-age students who come to nursing with a variety of life experiences. Welcome to the profession of nursing, and congratulations on making a choice that will open many doors for you and provide you with a career for life. You may find it challenging and, possibly, not quite what you expected. But go with your passion and believe in yourself—because you can create your life. The road you have chosen is not an easy one, but you need to believe in yourself, as we do, to succeed. We take this opportunity to wish you as satisfying a career in nursing as we have had.

Recommended readings

Endacott R, Pearce S, Rae P et al 2022 How COVID-19 has affected staffing models in intensive care: a qualitative study examining alternative staffing models (SEISMIC). Journal of Advanced Nursing 78:1075–1088 https://doi.org/10.1111/jan.15081

Jackson D 2022 Reflections on nursing research focusing on the COVID-19 pandemic. Journal of Advanced Nursing 78:e84–e86 https://doi.org/10.1111/jan.15281

Jefferies D, Ramjan L M, Stanbrook T et al 2023 'Their tenacity to just keep going': Nurses' experiences in medical hotel quarantine during the COVID-19 pandemic. Journal of Advanced Nursing 79:4280–4291 https://doi.org/10.1111/jan.15758

References

Anderson H, Scantlebury A, Galda P et al 2023 The well-being of nurses working in general practice during the COVID-19 pandemic: A qualitative study (The GenCo Study). Journal of Advanced Nursing 00:118 https://doi.org/10.1111/jan.15919

Burden S, Henshall C, Oshikanlu R 2021 Harnessing the nursing contribution to COVID-19 mass vaccination programmes: addressing hesitancy and promoting confidence. Journal of Advanced Nursing 77:e16–e20 https://doi.org/10.1111/jan.14854

Endacott R, Pearce S, Rae P et al 2022 How COVID-19 has affected staffing models in intensive care: a qualitative study examining alternative staffing models (SEISMIC). Journal of Advanced Nursing 7:1075–108 https://doi.org/10.1111/jan.15081

Fealy G M, Hallett C E, Dietz S M (eds) 2015 Histories of nursing practice. Manchester University Press

Girvin J 2015 I despair at the public's perception of nurses as selfless or sexed up. The Guardian, 14 September

Girvin J, Jackson D, Hutchinson M 2016 Contemporary public perceptions of nursing: a systematic review and narrative synthesis of the international research evidence. Journal of Nursing Management 24(8):994–1006

Griscti O, Sammut R, Camilleri L et al 2023 The impact of COVID-19 on nursing students' lives and online learning: a cross-sectional survey. Journal of Advanced Nursing 00:1–11 https://doi.org/10.1111/jan.15979

Guy M, Hughes K-A, Ferris-Day P 2022 Lack of awareness of nursing as a career choice for men: a qualitative descriptive study. Journal of Advanced Nursing 78:4190–4198 https://doi.org/10.1111/jan.15402

Hayward B A 2023 Nurses are background actors in medical reality television: a character network analysis and call for authentic action. Journal of Advanced Nursing 79:3035–3046 https://doi.org/10.1111/jan.15583

Henderson V 1964 The nature of nursing. American Journal of Nursing 64:63

The International Council of Nurses (ICN) n.d. Online. Available: http://www.icn.ch/who-we-are/ Accessed 22 Jan 2025

Jackson D 2022 Reflections on nursing research focusing on the COVID-19 pandemic. Journal of Advanced Nursing 78:e84–e86 https://doi.org/10.1111/jan.15281

Jackson D 2023 Perpetuating the whiteness of nursing: enculturation and nurse education. In: Lipsombe M (ed) Routledge handbook of philosophy and nursing. Routledge, London, Ch 38

Jefferies D, Ramjan L M, Stanbrook T et al 2023 'Their tenacity to just keep going': Nurses' experiences in medical hotel quarantine during the COVID-19 pandemic. Journal of Advanced Nursing 79:4280–4291 https://doi.org/10.1111/jan.15758

Kalisch P, Kalisch B, Scobey M 1983 Images of nurses on television. Springer Publishing, New York

Nursing and Midwifery Board of Australia (2024) Annual report summary 2023/24. Australian Health Practitioner Regulation Agency (AHPRA). https://www.nursingmidwiferyboard.gov.au/News/Annual-report.aspx

Poghosyan L, Kueakomoldej S, Liu J et al 2022 Advanced practice nurse work environments and job satisfaction and intent to leave: six-state cross sectional and observational study. Journal of Advanced Nursing 78:2460–2471 https://doi.org/10.1111/jan.15176

Ramjan L M, Maneze D, Salamonson Y et al 2023 Undergraduate nursing students challenge misconceptions towards men in nursing: a mixed-method study. Journal of Advanced Nursing 00:1–14 https://doi.org/10.1111/jan.15914

Teoh K-H, Kinman G, Harriss A et al 2022 Recommendations to support the mental wellbeing of nurses and midwives in the United Kingdom: a Delphi study. Journal of Advanced Nursing 78:3048–3060 https://doi.org/10.1111/jan.15359

Usher K, Jackson D, Massey D 2023 The mental health impact of COVID-19 on pre-registration nursing students in Australia: findings from a national cross-sectional study. Journal of Advanced Nursing 79:581–592 https://doi.org/10.1111/jan.15478

Veerapen J D, McKeown E 2021 Exploration of the views and experiences of research healthcare professionals during their redeployment to clinical roles during the COVID-19 pandemic. Journal of Advanced Nursing 77:4862–4875 https://doi.org/10.1111/jan.14998

Yang B-J, Yen C-W, Lin S-J et al 2022 Emergency nurses' burnout levels as the mediator of the relationship between stress and posttraumatic stress disorder symptoms during COVID-19 pandemic. Journal of Advanced Nursing 78:2861–2871 https://doi.org/10.1111/jan.15214

CHAPTER 2

VISIONING THE FUTURE BY KNOWING THE PAST

Madonna Grehan

KEY WORDS
education
history
hospitals
midwifery
nursing
regulation

LEARNING OBJECTIVES

After reading this chapter, readers should be able to:

- understand the benefits of having a knowledge of the history of nursing
- develop a critical understanding of received accounts of the history of nursing
- identify the lineage of nursing and its occupational relatives
- identify significant events that have influenced the evolution of nursing in Australia and New Zealand (Aotearoa)
- describe aspects in nursing and midwifery that warrant historical research.

INTRODUCTION

This chapter offers a snapshot of the vast history of nursing. It considers the antecedents of contemporary nursing and examines the formations of care in Australia and New Zealand (Aotearoa) that established patterns of care provision. It considers some of the historical influences on nursing, milestones in the evolution of nursing, and it raises the relationship between history and professional identity. The chapter concludes with remarks on what history can tell us about the future of nursing.

Disclaimer: Aboriginal and Torres Strait Islander people are warned that this chapter may contain images of deceased people.

History and its relevance to nursing

History, heritage, tradition and the past are concepts that may be familiar to most of us, but what is their relevance to nursing? This chapter explains why having an understanding of the history of nursing is useful for all nurses, whether working in practice, education, administration or the policy arena. An Australian historian, Graeme Davison (2000), argues that, among other things:

> History ... tells us who we are, gives us an imaginative and sympathetic insight into the lives of others, encourages a critical attitude to question social and political change, and equips us to participate in a political community.
>
> (Davison 2000:263)

Learning about our history can help us to understand how things have come to be, why some things change and others do not, or are difficult to change (Davison 2000). Applied to nursing and healthcare, history can illuminate the background to issues in the contemporary field, many of which are not new (Connolly 2004, Fairman & Lynaugh 1998, Lewensen 2004, Nelson 1997, 2004). For example, perennial issues in the Australian nursing and midwifery field include shortages of nurses and midwives, problems with educating nurses, and regulating nursing practice (Grehan 2009a). Further, Australian historian Sioban Nelson argues that history can help us to understand the extent of the impact of nursing on healthcare and society (Nelson 2000).

History can offer insights into present circumstances. Nursing's pivotal role in the 1918–1919 influenza pandemic was echoed in the recent COVID-19 pandemic. History can illustrate what the future might bring, although clearly it is impossible to be certain about the future. But if we have a sophisticated understanding of nursing's development, understand what has influenced that development and the longstanding issues it has faced, it may be possible to devise novel responses to these issues. How, then, can nurses learn about the history of nursing?

TRADITIONAL VIEWS OF NURSING'S HISTORY

In the early twentieth century, nurse luminaries in the United States of America (Nutting & Dock 1907) and Britain (Tooley 1906) recorded the triumphs of the nursing profession. Histories of Australian nursing (Walsh 1955, Webster 1942) and New Zealand (Aotearoa) nursing (Maclean 1932) reiterated the profession's celebratory achievements. The premise of these conventional accounts was simple: the care of the sick and of childbearing women was unskilled work of low status until so-called Nightingale nurses, worldwide, transformed bedside attendance from an age of darkness into one of light, from ignorance into science, from an occupation into a profession. Popular culture aided these accounts through stories of prominent nurses, such as Florence Nightingale, whose role in the Crimean War (1853–1856) was lauded in books and films. Likewise, the life of Elizabeth Kenny and her pioneering of physical therapies for poliomyelitis featured in a 1946 movie, *Sister Kenny*.

Celebratory histories are known as conventional or 'received' history. They offer simplistic explanations of complex episodes and events without context and analysis. They leave out aspects of history that do not 'fit' a narrative of the progress of nursing. In recent decades, more enlightened views of the history of nursing have emerged through the discipline of critical history.

AN ENLIGHTENED VIEW OF THE HISTORY OF NURSING

Scholars of nursing's history in Australia (Godden 2006, Nelson 2000, Strachan 2001), New Zealand (Aotearoa) (Sargison 2001, Wood 1992, 2008, 2022) and elsewhere (Connolly 2004, D'Antonio 1999,

Helmstadter & Godden 2011, MacPherson 1996, Nelson & Rafferty 2010, Rafferty et al 1997) use the tools of critical history to reappraise conventional narratives. Critical history does not mean 'judgmental'. Rather, critical history rejects long-held assumptions, such as the idea that history is about progress or that complex events can be explained simply. A critical historical acknowledges that nursing is a fundamental part of the society that it serves, within political and social contexts (Connolly 2004).

Critical history is characterised by a measured and effective analysis that can address omissions in received histories, such as the contributions of Aboriginal and Torres Strait Islander nurses. Indigenous women like Sadie Corner (Fig. 2.1) and Lowitja (Lois) O'Donohue had to overcome considerable odds to train as nurses and midwives and forge a place in Australia's white healthcare system. Examining the roles of Indigenous nurses in Australia and New Zealand (Aotearoa) entails consideration of politics, race, social attitudes and geography and a critical analysis of colonisation and assimilation practices. The story of Indigenous nurses is just one of many fascinating and instructive episodes in Australian and New Zealand (Aotearoa) nursing history worthy of critical inquiry.

Modern nursing's antecedents

As Nelson (2000) puts it, the act of nursing is as old as the human race itself. This longevity makes it impossible to say when nursing started to identify its 'roots'. An alternative is to examine nursing's evolution from a contemporary standpoint, the present. If we accept that nursing in the twenty-first century is 'modern', we can look to the antecedents that have evolved to produce nursing as we know it today.

In the twenty-first century, a large proportion of healthcare is provided in what historians call the 'modern' hospital. The idea of the 'modern' hospital emerged in the Western world in the late nineteenth century, a time when medicine was developing a sophisticated understanding of disease and illness, applying germ theory and experimenting with novel treatments such as vaccinations and surgery (Rosenberg 1987). Received accounts of medical history held that the modern hospital was an innovation that replaced disorder with order and hierarchical systems of caregiving. These histories praised the emergence of modern nursing, with its own hierarchical structures, as parallel to this medical innovation (Nelson 2000). Yet the hospital, as a place for delivering systematised care, was not a 'new' concept. Rather, the modern hospital constituted new ways of doing 'old' things, in which structures and standards were modified or replicated but evangelised by

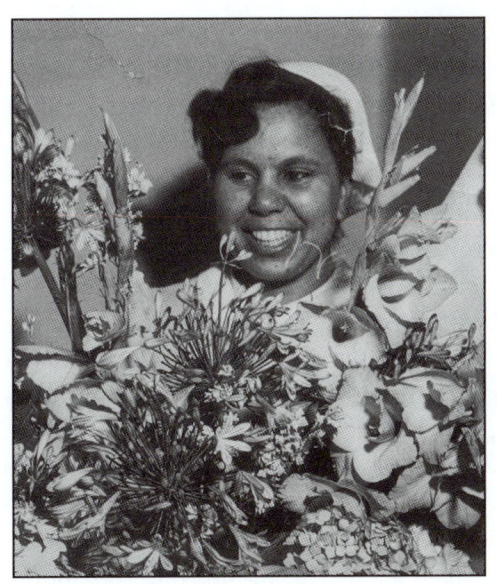

FIGURE 2.1
Sadie Corner

Source: Salvation Army Australia, Southern Territory Archives and Museum, Melbourne and Sadie Canning, née Corner.

their proponents as pioneering. The forebears of modern nursing, similarly, can be found in these older ways of care provision (Nelson 2000).

Pre-modern nursing

The historical antecedents of modern nursing lie with the care of the sick poor as strangers, provided by religious orders as 'an integral part of Christian practice' (Nelson 2000:3). In the early Christian era and beyond, these religious groups emulated the work of Jesus Christ in tending to the people as his flock by providing care in hospices (early forms of hospitals), feeding the poor, tending the infirm and applying palliative treatments. One group of nurses who has sustained this philosophy of care for centuries is the Catholic order of women, the Sisters of Charity of St Vincent de Paul (Nelson 2000), mentioned later in this chapter.

The care of the sick poor as a charitable endeavour was also practised by Protestant organisations in the nineteenth century. In England, for example, women such as Elizabeth Fry, Jane Shaw Stewart, Agnes Jones and Sister Dora (Agnes Pattison) formed nursing 'sisterhoods' that delivered nursing care to the poor (Summers 1989). Research by Carol Helmstadter and Judith Godden (2011) has established that during the first half of the nineteenth century some hospitals in London contracted out their nursing to sisterhoods. In Australia, philanthropically minded Christian people imitated these conventions, organising care provision to the poor who were judged as deserving of it (Grehan 2009a). This judgmental approach had a foundational influence on the development of care provision in Australia and New Zealand (Aotearoa).

Healthcare in early Australia and New Zealand (Aotearoa)

As the British Empire expanded in the eighteenth century, its customs and conventions of caregiving were replicated in the newly claimed colonies of Australia (Grehan 2004) and New Zealand (Aotearoa) (Sargison 2001). Early care was performed in challenging environments without modern-day technologies of sanitation, in circumstances where water was obtained from a nearby stream or a stagnant pond, where 'watching' the patient at night was done by candlelight and where help in the form of a doctor or educated nurse was several days' travel away by horse or on foot (Grehan 2009b).

At the convict settlements of Sydney and Hobart Town, Australia's colonial administrations established general hospitals and government asylums. In the 1790s, the New South Wales (NSW) government appointed wives of convicts to act as midwives in specific geographic locations and female factories (Grehan 2009a). From the 1840s in Australia and in New Zealand (Aotearoa) (Sargison 2001), institutions emerged to cater for the indigent. Known as 'voluntary' or 'charity' hospitals, their work was funded by subscription; in return for their financial support, subscribers were able to recommend individuals for hospital treatment (McCalman 1998) and earn heavenly rewards. As colonists expanded the white frontier, local communities constructed hospitals, following industrial catastrophes such as mining and transport accidents (Collins 1999).

In the mid-nineteenth century, the predominant medical theory was miasmatism. Miasmas were understood to be noxious vapours arising from filthy conditions, suppurating wounds, ill-ventilated rooms, cesspits, cemeteries and even the 'menstrual discharge of the nurse' (Grehan 2009a:160). Miasmatic vapours were believed to result from certain disease states, such as smallpox, tuberculosis and forms of cancer. People with these conditions were excluded from admission to hospitals and pregnant women, likewise, were not admitted to general hospitals because of a perceived risk from miasmas (Grehan 2009a). As a result, maternity hospitals, called lying-in institutions, were established geographically separate from general hospitals, mirroring practice in England, Scotland and Ireland (McCalman 1998).

INSTITUTIONAL NURSES

Government hospitals and charitable institutions in the colonial world were hierarchical places. What a nurse was expected to do when working depended on the type of establishment where she was employed, and on what basis she was employed—that is, as a head nurse, assistant nurse or pupil nurse. Smaller hospitals were operated by a married couple who attended to the patients, cooked their food and did the laundry (Collins & Kippen 2003). Asylums (Monk 2008) and other establishments, particularly in rural areas (Collins & Kippen 2003), employed men and women as attendants for male and female patients, respectively. In every instance, nursing in the mid-nineteenth century was extremely hard work for little reward: a mixture of bedside attendance and household tasks.

The predominance of miasmatic theory translated into concerns about the sick person's environment as potentially harbouring disease. To maintain the purest environment possible in the sick room and minimise these harmful vapours, hospitals and institutions employed 'sanitary' science, an extensive regimen of cleaning and ventilation practices. Nursing included scrubbing floors, brushing carpets, dusting, polishing brassware and furniture, washing the patients, providing nourishment for those who could not do it for themselves, making and applying poultices and other remedies (Nelson 2000). With hospitals unsewered until the late nineteenth century, it was the nurses' job to dispose of bodily wastes such as blood, faeces, urine and sputum, stored in buckets at the end of wards and the nurses' job to empty the buckets into outdoor cesspits (Templeton 1969). Nurses had to clean and fumigate straw mattresses, known as palliasses, in special airing rooms, and carry soiled linen to the laundry for washing (McCalman 1998). In some hospitals, nurses slept at the end of wards so that they could attend the patients throughout the night when called (Grehan 2009a).

Unsurprisingly, attracting new recruits was always difficult. Not only was the work hard and the pay poor, but hospital managements could also be unsympathetic employers. If a nurse became unwell, she usually had to resign to recover her health. On top of that, hospital nursing did not enjoy a lofty status in society. Newspapers reported nurses being drunk on duty, being cruel to patients or being ignorant (Grehan 2004). Institutions such as the Women's Hospital in Melbourne attempted to weed out potential troublemakers, and those unlikely to succeed, at the start. Applicants for training had to provide a testimonial from a minister of religion or medical practitioner, vouching for the nurse's character. And the same attitude applied to the patients. They were vetted to ensure that each was respectable and deserving of the hospital's charity (McCalman 1998). Hospital histories are well recorded, although these institutions accommodated only a small proportion of the population. Most people experienced care at their home, which was sometimes a tent or hut (Grehan 2009a).

Care provided in the community

In colonial Australia a range of people worked at bedsides; among them were doctors, nurses, midwives, herbalists, oculists, druggists and dentists (Grehan 2009a). Similarly in New Zealand (Aotearoa), a range of people practised (Sargison 2001). Who the patient chose depended on who was available, what the purchaser expected of his or her care, and what the patient was willing to pay. In the cities and in rural areas, local women attended births and cases of sickness as a neighbourly gesture (Grehan 2009a). Some women combined tending to the sick, preparing the dead for burial and acting as midwife with running the local postal service (Forth et al 1998).

Nursing and midwifery at bedsides were easy to adopt as paid work. No restrictions applied to the field so anyone could take it up and name their price. And bedside work was portable. A proportion of women held formal qualifications from theoretical and practical education schemes available in Britain or Europe (Grehan 2009a). Some learned their craft by apprenticeship, while others attended public lectures given by medical doctors. Other women had their own experience of childbearing and rearing to rely on; others had no experience whatsoever. 'Handywomen' was a derogatory term applied to women who attended others for payment. It implied they had no education or training for their work but did it simply for the money. For the patient, selecting an attendant for a birth or case of sickness could be a gamble, without guarantees of qualifications or skill (Grehan 2009c).

A study by historian Glenda Strachan (2001) of all births registered in an isolated rural district of the Colony of NSW, during the years 1856–1896, confirms this diversity of female maternity attendants. In South Australia, nursing historian Joan Durdin (1991) cites the example of Mrs Elizabeth Knight, a well-respected midwife in the Mount Gambier region who took up the work at the age of 70 after the death of her husband. Likewise in New Zealand (Aotearoa), Sargison (2001) reports numerous women and men who fulfilled the role of attendant on the sick and childbearing women. But critics of this unregulated and haphazard arrangement of care provision were vocal. Perceptions prevailed that colonial nurses were unsuited to the important duty of bedside attendance.

Worldwide calls to reform nursing

Disapproval of nurses working in domiciliary and institutional settings was fuelled in part by the writings of author and social commentator Charles Dickens. His serialised novel *The Life and Adventures of Martin Chuzzlewit* (1843) opened a window on the realm of private nursing through two fictitious but infamous London characters, Sarah Gamp and her friend Betsy Prig. Mrs Gamp, styling herself as a nurse and midwife, was available for all the important milestones in life: attending at births, tending to the sick and laying out of the dead. Betsy Prig was a hospital nurse by day and moonlighted as a 'private' nurse in people's homes at night, where they were too tired to care. Dickens' narrative, combined with graphic pen and ink sketches, depicted the two 'nurses' as ignorant, unrefined and untrustworthy. The descriptor 'Gamp' came to symbolise all that was perceived to be wrong with female nurses and nursing throughout the English-speaking world (Grehan 2004).

A welcome human solution to the perceived problem of colonial Gamps appeared in the 1850s, in the form of Miss Florence Nightingale, celebrated for her work in the Crimean War. When a public subscription campaign raised money for a memorial to Nightingale, she asked that the memorial be an institution for the training of nurses and hospital attendants. It became the 'Nightingale Fund for Nursing'. The Fund's enduring message was that nursing needed role models, educated 'ladies' of good character who could demonstrate to less educated nurses how to behave (Baly 1987). New Zealand (Aotearoa) sent at least £1000 to the Fund (*New Zealand Spectator and Cook's Strait Guardian*, 1856) and the Colony of Victoria sent £150, the latter expecting that nurses would soon be trained 'properly' (*Argus*, 10 July 1856).

The Nightingale Fund established two training schools in London. At St Thomas' Hospital nurses were trained for general work in public hospitals and infirmaries, and although Nightingale's name was attached to the school at St Thomas', in practical terms she had little to do with its operation (Godden 2006). At King's College Hospital women undertook training in midwifery nursing sponsored by local communities who wanted nurses for the poor, but this school closed after only 5 years. Nightingale had far greater influence on the nursing world through her multiple publications: on nurses, midwives, training, caregiving, disease, hospital design and sanitary science, all of which were embraced (Grehan 2009a).

Why did Nightingale's ideas gain such traction? Miasmatic theory dictated that ill-health and disease were problems of filth, literally and metaphorically, that could be solved with the application of sanitary science. As Bashford (1998) argues, female unmarried nurses were positioned as the ideal agents to fulfil sanitary science's objectives, sweeping a new broom through institutions and in the process elevating nursing as a respectable vocational calling.

Other confluent forces hastened reforms in nursing and reinforced what was a feminisation of the workforce. With the emergence of the modern hospital came new treatments and surgical operations that required a team of staff to guarantee success (Helmstadter & Godden 2011, Rosenberg 1987). The nurses providing pre-operative and postoperative care needed to be literate, cooperative, diligent and consistent. At the Women's Hospital in Melbourne, for example, nurses caring for gynaecology patients needed to be able to observe changes in the patient's physical condition, apply new technologies of care such as the thermometer, use a watch to count pulsations (Grehan 2004) and deliver regimens of nutrition and pharmacological agents such as poultices, fomentations and champagne enemas. To produce the nurses that they needed, hospitals in Australia (Grehan 2009a) and New Zealand (Aotearoa) (Sargison 2001) in the last quarter of the nineteenth century introduced their own training schemes for pupil nurses.

INSTITUTIONAL TRAINING SCHEMES

Nurse 'training' schemes in nineteenth-century hospitals were far less sophisticated than the term suggests. Training involved on-the-job learning, combined with lectures by medical practitioners and sometimes senior nurses, which pupils attended only if they could be freed from their ward work (Mitchell 1977). Up to the turn of the twentieth century at least, nurse training was organised around an institution's associated medical specialty. Inevitably, the result was an idiosyncratic training. For instance, an eye and ear hospital's training scheme produced nurses who dealt with eye and ear problems; children's hospitals produced nurses expert in children's afflictions; lying-in hospitals produced nurses for maternity and gynaecological care and so on. Training in Australia was so specific to each hospital's needs that the nurse's skills were not always transferable to another hospital environment (Trembath & Hellier 1987).

Often hard up for funds, some hospitals hired out pupils to nurse private patients in the home. It meant a pupil nurse could spend a substantial portion of her training time away from the hospital, without any supervision or teaching (Templeton 1969). The variability in training schemes also meant that the product of training, a 'trained' nurse, was fluid. Coupled with the plurality of attendants working in the community, it is little wonder that ideas of compulsory, uniform training, proof of claimed qualifications and superior senior nurses of impeccable character who could raise standards in nursing were enthusiastically welcomed in the colonies.

In 1868, NSW welcomed a cohort of so-called Nightingale nurses, superintended by Miss Lucy Osburn (Fig. 2.2) who was engaged to improve conditions at the Sydney Hospital. Received histories of Australian nursing celebrate this milestone as breaking new ground, but Godden's (2006) research on Osburn shows that the Sydney Hospital was not ill-managed at all by the matron preceding Osburn, Bathsheba Ghost.

Unsurprisingly, other Nightingale-associated events have enjoyed prominence in nursing history. In Australia's southern colony of Tasmania, three 'Nightingale' nurses were welcomed in 1885, reportedly to institute necessary urgent reforms at Hobart's General Hospital. Recent research shows that the success of the three was overstated (Grehan 2015). Two of the nurses later worked in colonial Victoria and again were celebrated as instituting urgent and necessary reforms (Grehan 2004). In New Zealand (Aotearoa), received history similarly records accounts of neglect and wretchedness in hospitals that were subsequently transformed under the watch of reputable nurses with Nightingale connections. French (2001) notes Mary Lyons, Mrs Bernard Moore and Annie Crisp among these women, the latter credited with overhauling nursing at the Auckland Hospital and establishing its nurse training school. Crisp, awarded a Royal Red Cross in 1883, was a military nurse feted for her work in Africa (Masters 1993).

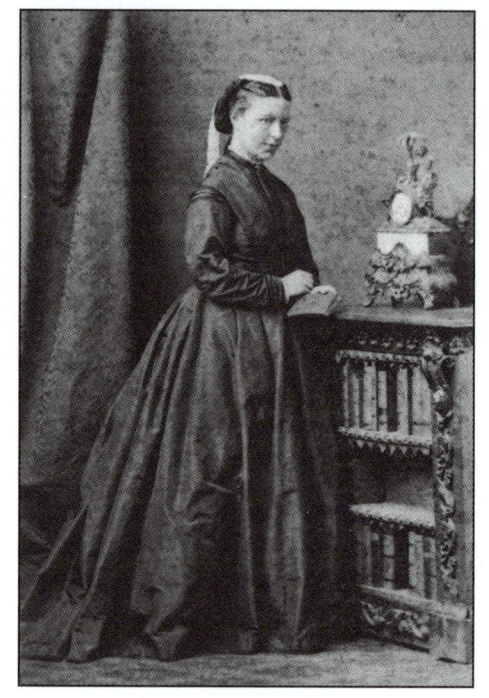

FIGURE 2.2
Lucy Osburn

Source: South Eastern Sydney and Illawarra Area Health Service, NSW Government.

So the story goes, under the steady eye of these superior nurses, hospitals around Australia (Grehan 2004) and New Zealand (Aotearoa) (Hill 1982) adopted the so-called Nightingale scheme of nurse training, with its two categories of pupil. 'Lady' probationers were reputedly of higher social standing. They paid for their training, were exempt from menial work and were expected to supervise their subordinates. 'Regular' probationers were the subordinates who instead of paying for pupillage trained for a longer time; they did household work and scrubbing and were expected to model the example set by their superiors. Received history declares that the Nightingale model was universally embraced and transformed the healthcare landscape (Grehan 2009a). Was this what really happened?

In fact, research by Godden (2006) and Grehan (2009a, 2015) shows that the evolution of nurse training in Australian institutions was a complex process. Monk's (2015) work on bedside employees in colonial Victoria's government asylums shows that male warders and attendants opposed undertaking education as part of their employment conditions. Female asylum nurses in the same institutions were more amenable to attending lectures on nursing beginning in the 1890s. There is no doubt that some hospitals gradually modernised training, but the process was difficult and expensive. Change was achieved incrementally. There was no miraculous shift from old to new models of training. When changes were introduced, no one individual, or group of individuals, was responsible for those developments, despite what received history would have us believe. Not only that, as Nelson (2000) argues, reforms in nursing and hospitals did not occur in isolation but were just one element in a wave of lasting social change that swept throughout the English-speaking world in the late nineteenth century.

From the haphazard world of nineteenth-century nursing and midwifery, our discussion now moves to the twentieth century, to consider some of the factors that have shaped nursing and midwifery practice as we know them today.

Some historical influences on nursing

Nursing, like other professions and occupations, exists as part of the society it serves. And while nursing has been shaped by the profession itself to an extent, it has been subject to external factors well beyond its control. Some of the major influences on nursing are obvious. Perhaps the most consistent is the healthcare environment, constantly evolving technologies of care, from the thermometer to all sorts of instruments that deliver measurements of clinical status, to practices such as fluid replacement, asepsis and infection control. Often driven by developments in medicine, these changes impact on nursing at the bedside.

New ideas about health, wellbeing and illness have impacted on nursing education and practice, the concept of person-centred care to name one of them (Grehan 2009a). Less obvious influences are the political, economic and social climates in which nursing is practised. Historically in Australia, a pivotal external influence on nursing is the three tiers of government that hold differing responsibilities for aspects of healthcare provision. World financial conditions may impact on hospital funding availability, with flow-on effects for how nurses and nursing is funded within hospital budgets applied by the states. Changes of government mean that the policy platform can change rapidly with effects on the clinical arena (Grehan 2008).

Using the tools of critical history, it is possible to examine external factors and trends, momentous and less momentous events, to understand how these have shaped nursing as we know it today. Earlier in this chapter we discussed mounting pressure in the last decade of the nineteenth century to raise standards in nursing and midwifery attendance (Grehan 2009a). How governments in New Zealand (Aotearoa) and Australia responded to these calls stemmed from the respective structures of those governments. The entirety of New Zealand (Aotearoa) was one colony with a small population, and the government instituted statutory regulation for nursing seamlessly (Maclean 1932). By contrast, when Australia's six colonies became states at Federation in 1901, each state apart from Tasmania resisted regulating nursing. Governments in Australia saw nursing as difficult to define and they argued that healthcare was largely a private matter. Thus, in Australia, disagreement persisted on how to run hospitals, how to teach nurses, what to teach nurses and even what constituted a nurse. Arguments prevailed over the length of training, what it should consist of, and whether training was beneficial at all (Grehan 2009a). In the absence of regulation by government, sectors in the Australian nursing fraternity opted for voluntary professional self-regulation.

Voluntary regulation

Efforts to introduce voluntary professional regulation for nurses and midwives in Australia mirrored those in Britain where a British Nurses' Association was established in late 1887 (Grehan 2009a). Voluntary regulation by professional association was designed to do what legislation might have done: set standards in education and training, admit people who met those standards, and maintain publicly accessible registers so that the public could differentiate trained nurses from untrained people.

A Victoria Trained Nurses' Association formed in 1886 as a professional organisation of private nurses in the city of Melbourne, but it lasted for only 2 years. In 1891, Tasmanian nurses sought to form a professional association, but without a critical mass, they turned to Victoria where a Nurses' Association of Australasia was founded in Melbourne in 1892. It also failed to flourish, but momentum was gathering (Grehan 2004). In 1899, nurses and doctors formed the Australasian Trained Nurses' Association (ATNA) based in NSW and in 1901, the Victorian Trained Nurses' Association formed. Awarded Royal Charter in 1904, the Victorian organisation added Royal to its name (RVTNA) (Trembath & Hellier 1987).

These two nursing organisations have been judged as having marginal impact (Trembath & Hellier 1987) because nurses and midwives did not need to be registered with them to obtain employment. Even so, these organisations deserve some credit. Both laid the foundations for statutory regulation which came later. With the support of the medical profession, both forced larger hospitals to institute uniform curricula, examinations and certification, which gradually came to be accepted as the norm. When legislation was introduced for nursing and midwifery, at different times in different states and territories of Australia, the ATNA's and the RVTNA's systems for assessing qualifications and skills informed aspects of registration (Grehan 2009a).

While voluntary regulation preceded statutory regulation in all states and territories of Australia, in New Zealand (Aotearoa) the reverse occurred. Compulsory registration for nurses and midwives was in place in New Zealand (Aotearoa) by 1904. Voluntary regulation by professional association for 'private' nurses followed in 1909 when the New Zealand Trained Nurses' Association formed in response to developments in the international nursing arena (Sargison 2001). The International Council of Nurses (ICN), founded in 1899, was a network of national nurses' associations, consisting of organisations that were governed by nurses alone, not doctors (Grehan 2009a). The New Zealand Trained Nurses' Association was a national organisation which met that criterion so New Zealand (Aotearoa) became a member of the ICN almost 30 years ahead of Australia. Australia meanwhile founded two colleges of nursing, one in NSW and one in Victoria. In 2011 these colleges, the Royal College of Nursing Australia and the College of Nursing based in NSW, overcame long-held differences and united as a national college, the Australian College of Nursing (Grehan 2012). Away from the colleges, a range of industrial organisations advocated for nurses' and midwives' employment conditions (McCoppin & Gardner 1994).

Statutory regulation

As we have noted, New Zealand's (Aotearoa's) pathway to government regulation of nursing and midwifery was uncomplicated. New Zealand (Aotearoa) appointed a Scots-born, English-trained nurse, Mrs Grace Neill, to assist in developing its legislative framework. Regulation for all nurses applied in New Zealand (Aotearoa) from 1901, and a *Midwives Registration Act* was passed in 1904 (French 2001). By contrast, when the six colonies in Australia became states, the 1901 Australian Constitution protected their capacity to regulate aspects of commerce, trade and legal matters (Macintyre 1986). This included the regulation of occupations and professions. Consequently, statutes and subordinate regulations pertaining to nursing and midwifery varied considerably across Australia, with reciprocity of registration between the states a major obstacle for nurses who sought employment opportunities across state borders. Tasmania introduced the first statutory regulation in Australia for nurses practising midwifery, in 1901. By the mid-1920s, legislation governing midwifery and nursing practice applied in all states (Grehan 2009a).

Externally to the profession, the development of trade agreements and the globalisation of workforces have forced change in the regulation of nurses and midwives as healthcare practitioners. In 1992, the Australian and New Zealand (Aotearoa) national governments signed a *Mutual Recognition Agreement*, extending it in 1997 to include the Australian state governments under the *Trans-Tasman Mutual Recognition Act 1997* (Cth) and in New Zealand (Aotearoa) as the *Trans-Tasman Mutual Recognition Act 1997*. Designed to 'promote economic integration and increased trade', these agreements have enabled the reciprocal recognition of most occupational qualifications in New Zealand (Aotearoa) and Australia, including nurses and midwives. Within Australia, a national registration system for all nurses and midwives was introduced in July 2010, making qualifications within the nation portable across the country (Grehan 2012).

An accurate perspective of the history of nursing requires us to look beyond the profession itself, to the political landscape, to societal shifts in understanding of health and illness, and to issues of gender and power. Tumultuous events, also, have had a lasting influence on nursing, stimulating the profession's aspirations. Some of these are considered next.

Milestones in Australian and New Zealand (Aotearoa) nursing

Even in the relatively short history of nursing in New Zealand (Aotearoa) and Australia, significant events have had lasting effects on the profession. Here we concentrate on two particular milestones in the history of nursing: the role of war and the development of nursing education with the eventual transfer to the tertiary setting. It is their context and their sequelae that are of interest in historical terms.

WAR

The role of nurses in nineteenth-century military conflicts, from Nightingale's well-publicised role in Crimea to women's contributions during the American Civil War (1861–1865), attracted the admiration of the public worldwide. As Nelson argues 'the successes of the war nurses stimulated a shift in public perceptions of the role of the nurse' because, in the organised arena of tending the war wounded, 'nursing came to be seen as a useful profession' and a rather more lofty exercise than simply nursing the poor (Nelson 2000:148).

The Second Anglo-Boer War, World Wars I and II

By the turn of the twentieth century, nurses believed their profession could make a useful contribution through military service. During the Second Anglo-Boer War (1899–1902), nurses from the Australian colonies and from New Zealand (Aotearoa) volunteered (Speirs 2010). In late 1899 a group of NSW nurses formed the first Army Nursing Service Reserve in Australia. Fourteen were dispatched to South Africa, employed and paid for by the NSW government, the only colony to do so. With financial support contributed by public subscription campaigns, others joined the British Imperial service. A number of nurses volunteered as private citizens. New Zealand (Aotearoa) nurses likewise joined the call, supported by public subscription (Wood 2022). In World War I (1914–1918), New Zealand-trained nurses served in stationary hospitals, trains, hospital ships and other locations (Dahl 2009). Of the estimated 550 New Zealand (Aotearoa) nurses who served, 10 died when the *Marquette*, a British transport ship carrying medical corps personnel, was torpedoed in the Aegean Sea (Maclean 1923). More than 2500 nurses served with the Australian Army Nursing Service (AANS) in the Middle East, in the south of Europe, France, England and India on land and sea (Harris 2010).

New Zealander and Australian nurses volunteered again during World War II (1939–1945), serving in North Africa, the Middle East, the south of Europe and across the Pacific. In Australia, nurses were members of the AANS, the Royal Australian Air Force Nursing Service or the Royal Australian Naval Nursing Service (Harris 2007). New Zealand (Aotearoa) recognised serving nurses as officers by 1942 (Clendon 1997) and in 1943 Australia awarded nurses military rankings, formally placing women in charge of men at a time when no comparable positions were open to women in civilian life (Milligan & Foley 1993).

Two particular events in World War II involving Australian nurses drew attention to the ordinary women who risked their lives as military nurses.

The sinking of the Vyner Brooke and the Bangka Island massacre

In February 1942, members of the AANS were serving in military hospitals in Singapore when the city was invaded by Japanese forces. The nurses were ordered to evacuate, along with civilians. One group boarded the *Empire Star* with more than 2100 others. A second group of 65 nurses was among 200 passengers on a small coastal steamer, the *Vyner Brooke*. As the ships navigated the Malacca Straits, Japanese bombers attacked them from the air. Two nurses on the *Empire Star* shielded wounded soldiers with their own bodies (Shaw 2010).

Survivors of the *Vyner Brooke*'s bombardment and sinking swam to Radji Beach on the Indonesian Island of Bangka, landing in two groups on different parts of the coast. One group, including 31 nurses, was taken as prisoners of war. Japanese soldiers discovered a second party of service personnel and civilians 2 days later and separated the men and women. At Radji Beach, the Japanese soldiers ordered the nurses to march into the sea where they were shot. Vivian Bullwinkel, then aged 26, was the only survivor of this war crime. After hiding for 12 days in the jungle with a severely wounded British soldier, Bullwinkel surrendered to the Japanese army, and was reunited with the other party of nurses. Until the end of the war, this group of women remained secret prisoners of war. News of the Bangka Island massacre did not reach Australia until well after hostilities had ceased in 1945 (Jeffrey 1954).

The sinking of the Australian Hospital Ship Centaur

A second incident occurred in May 1943, just off the Queensland coast, north east of Brisbane. The 2/3rd Australian Hospital Ship, *Centaur*, was on its second journey from Sydney to New Guinea to collect injured servicemen. The *Centaur* carried 332 non-combatant personnel: the ship's crew, members of a field ambulance unit, and the ship's medical team, including 12 AANS sisters (Milligan & Foley 1993). At 4.10 a.m., the *Centaur* was torpedoed by a Japanese submarine without warning, caught fire and sank. Only 64 of those on board survived. They spent the next 36 hours awaiting rescue. The only nurse to survive, Ellen Savage (Fig. 2.3), took charge of rationing food and attended to the injured. This was despite Savage's own injuries: a fractured palate, nose and ribs, as well as perforated ear drums, burns and severe bruising. Her courage and bravery in these circumstances was recognised with the award of the George Medal, Australia's civilian equivalent to the Victoria Cross (Milligan & Foley 1993).

The sinking of the *Centaur* was judged to be a war crime because hospital ships had the protection of the Geneva and Hague Conventions (Milligan & Foley 1993). In a propaganda campaign, the Australian government encouraged Australians to avenge the nurses' deaths by supporting the war effort. Subsequently, the Australian public gave generously to various war nurses' memorials, including the Centaur Memorial Fund for Nurses in Queensland and the War Nurses Memorial Centre in Melbourne (Williams 1991).

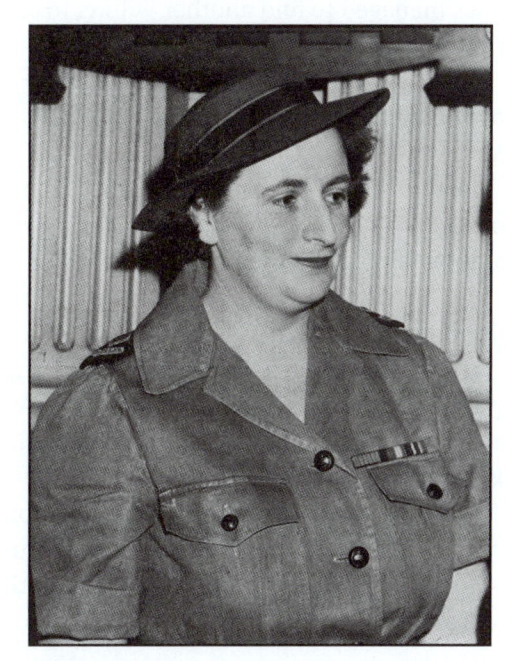

FIGURE 2.3
Ellen Savage GM
Source: AWM 61952.

On the home front

The duration of World Wars I and II had substantial impacts on nursing and midwifery, certainly in Australia. In World War I, acute shortages resulted in every area of nursing when nurses joined up (Harris 2007). Some hospitals attempted to overcome the shortage by extending nursing training from 3 to 4 years, but this had an unintended effect of discouraging young women from applying for training places. In Victoria, a new category of nurse, the 'war emergency nurse', was introduced in 1915 when there were no fully trained nurses available. After the war there were disputes about whether these nurses should be allowed to continue as trained nurses (Grehan 2009a). Chronic shortages prevailed in rural areas. In the 5 years before World War I, a Bush Nursing scheme was formulated in Australia to provide healthcare, particularly maternity care, to Australians in rural and remote areas. Bush Nurses had to hold qualifications in midwifery and general nursing, but this strict policy had to be relaxed during the war when the scheme could not attract nurses with both certificates (Grehan 2009a). New Zealand (Aotearoa) established a Rural Nursing Service in the 1930s, which incorporated 'back-blocks' nursing, district nursing and Māori nursing (Wood 2022).

In World War II, out of an estimated 13,000 trained nurses working in Australia, around 4000 volunteered. Shortages became so dire that the Australian government recognised nursing's importance to national stability and security (Nelson & Rabach 2002), designating it a protected industry. From 1942 until 1945, the movement of nurses and midwives was controlled by the Manpower Directorate, a federal authority. Any nurse who wanted to work or train interstate required the permission of the Directorate to do so. But it was possible to circumvent the restrictions. Some nurses managed to find another willing to exchange places, and contacted the Manpower Directorate for permission (Grehan 2009a).

Adjustment to civilian life after the war was difficult for some service nurses, particularly so for those who had occupied positions of authority in the military. For instance, Colonel Annie Sage was Matron-in-Chief of the AANS from 1943 until 1947. Back in civilian roles, Sage was unable to reach the heights of leadership that were tacit in her military position. Her aspirations to elevate Australian nursing into a more professional sphere were dashed at the Women's Hospital in Melbourne by civilian doctors who vigorously objected to her authority and her ideas (Nelson & Rabach 2002).

War service was a rare opportunity for Australian and New Zealand (Aotearoa) nurses in the military to mix with their international counterparts. Military service opened nurses' eyes to alternative ways of learning, teaching and practising their profession. Most understood that developing and expanding education was critical to the growth of nursing, yet opportunities for nurses to undertake postgraduate education were extremely limited. New Zealand (Aotearoa) was ahead of Australia in this, offering postgraduate education in 1928 (Wood 2022) whereas Australia's modest efforts began in the 1930s (Grehan 2022). In the post-World War II period, nurses in Australia harnessed the support of the public to establish memorial 'centres' where the profession could grow. The centres were designed to be places for education, recreation and accommodation, with memorialising embedded in advancing the profession. Our discussion now turns to the theme of education.

DEVELOPING EDUCATION

The apprenticeship model of training nurses on the job was the mainstay of institutional nursing education in New Zealand (Aotearoa) and Australia throughout the nineteenth and twentieth centuries. Learning by apprenticeship meant that service provision came first and education a poor second (Trembath & Hellier 1987). In Australia, having the triple certificates of general nursing, midwifery and infant welfare nursing was the pinnacle of possibility up to the 1930s. Nurses who wanted formal qualifications in teaching, hospital administration, dietetics or sanitation had to enrol at American universities, at the Royal College of Nursing in England (Smith 1999) or in New Zealand (Aotearoa) at the Wellington Hospital in conjunction with Victoria University (Sargison 2001).

As discussed earlier in this chapter, nursing's two professional organisations in Australia, the ATNA based in NSW and RVTNA in Victoria, did not see eye to eye, even though a national college of nursing was an aspiration of both. In Victoria, the RVTNA changed its constitution and metamorphosed into the Royal Victorian College of Nursing (RVCN), which offered postgraduate courses in teaching, administration and industrial nursing from the mid-1930s. In May 1949, NSW established a college, offering postgraduate education programs with support from professional groups in that state (Smith 1999) and in the same year, a College of Nursing Australia, based in Victoria, was established.

Despite their differences, both entities shared the philosophy that beginning practitioners needed a broad-based education delivered in the tertiary sector, rather than learning on the job in hospitals. A principles-based foundational degree in general nursing was expected to produce nurses ready to practise in a range of clinical areas with specialisation to follow through postgraduate studies. Momentum gathered to realise that goal (Lusk et al 2001). In 1977, after continued lobbying from the profession, the NSW state government transferred nursing education from the health portfolio to education, a move that enabled the state's Colleges of Advanced Education to assume responsibility for pre-registration nurse education. Other states and territories followed. In 1984, under an Australian federal government plan, nursing as a pathway in tertiary education became a reality (McCoppin & Gardner 1994). Midwifery education transferred to the tertiary sector in the early 1990s. Apprenticeship schemes in psychiatric nursing were phased out in the mid-1980s with mental health nursing a postgraduate specialty following a bachelor's degree in nursing. This change was confluent with deinstitutionalisation, whereby large psychiatric institutions closed, and care was transferred to community-based services. Collectively, these shifts in Australia ended 140 years of nurses learning by apprenticeship. In New Zealand (Aotearoa) pilot programs of diploma-based education in technical institutes were underway from 1973. After sustained agitation an undergraduate degree program was adopted in the mid-1990s as the only pre-registration pathway to study nursing (Lusk et al 2001). An important difference in New Zealand's (Aotearoa's) midwifery education is discussed in the next section.

Streams of specialisation

Much of our discussion has focused on the 'general' nature of nursing, but an important element in this history are the specialisms that have developed within clinical practice. Some specialisms emerged within the institutions that catered for medical specialties, such as eye and ear hospitals producing eye and ear nurses, orthopaedic hospitals and so on. Prebble and Bryder (2008) point out that in New Zealand (Aotearoa) psychiatric nursing, formerly called mental nursing, had its foundations in asylums. These were geographically and philosophically distant from other hospitals' nurse training schemes and developed their own schemes, as was the case in Australia (Monk 2008).

Some specialisms emerged in tandem with rapid developments in medicine but not always because of medicine itself. One example, associated with a specific body of nursing knowledge, is the development of the intensive care nursing unit in the 1960s (Fairman & Lynaugh 1998). Maxine Dahl (2009), a historian of Australian military nursing, argues that Royal Australian Air Force air evacuation nurses established the specialty of flight nursing and retrieval, during military service in World War II and the Korean War (1950–1953), with those practices later adopted by hospitals.

Numerous specialisms within nursing sometimes reflect the location of care and the population receiving care. Community health, neonatal intensive care, occupational health and school nursing are examples. Other specialisms are connected with a disease or its consequences, such as diabetes care, movement disorders, infection control, women's health, adolescent health, cancer nursing, stomal therapy, paediatrics, health promotion and palliative care, all of which have emerged since the 1970s. Their evolution as specialisations in nursing and healthcare will make for fascinating historical inquiry in the future. Another area of historical interest is the relationship between history and professional identity, discussed next.

History and identity

Earlier in this chapter, we noted that history can tell us about our identity as individuals and as members of a recognised profession. According to received histories, nursing's identity is a 'modern' and foundational entity with many branches. For the greater part of the nineteenth and twentieth centuries in Australia, maternity attendance in hospitals was called midwifery 'nursing'; that is, a practice that involved the nursing of women during birth. As the concept of general nursing solidified in the 1890s, midwifery was positioned as a specialist branch of the practice of nursing

(Grehan 2009a). Since the 1980s, in New Zealand (Aotearoa) and Australia, that status of midwifery as a branch of nursing has been disputed, part of a worldwide movement aimed at professionalising midwifery. This movement has sought to have midwifery recognised as a profession in its own right, separate and distinct from nursing (Australian College of Midwives Incorporated Victorian Branch 1999).

New Zealand's (Aotearoa's) government prioritised midwifery when it placed nursing and midwifery under separate legislation in 1990 (Grehan 2009a). A Bachelor of Midwifery (BM) was introduced and is now the only pathway to becoming a midwife in New Zealand (Aotearoa). Emulating the New Zealand (Aotearoa) model, in 2001 several Australian universities introduced the BM, while midwifery education in Australia can still be pursued at postgraduate diploma level and a 'double' degree in nursing and midwifery is available. This development raises the relationship between a profession, its identity and its history.

THE IDENTITY OF MIDWIFERY, NOT 'NURSING'

For proponents of the BM, the main distinction between nursing and midwifery is that midwifery involves care in a natural healthy episode in the female life cycle, while nursing involves the care of the sick (Fahy 1998). Advocates of this distinction argue that midwifery has a unique history and identity, vastly different from that of nursing (Grehan 2009a). 'Identity' histories, sometimes categorised as 'revisionist' histories, have been popular since the 1960s when second-wave feminism and the movement in social change critiqued existing historical narratives as a march of progress (Davison 2000). Revisionist history aimed to give 'voice' to groups whose contributions had been ignored in received interpretations of history, such as women, African Americans, ethnic and other minority groups (Davison 2000).

Yet focusing on identity in this way is no less problematic than received history is. Without doubt, revisionist history can acknowledge those whose voices have been ignored previously, but its very aim of righting wrongs or locating origins that resonate with the present raises concerns. Revisionist history can be crafted so that it 'fits' with an author's view of the world (Davison 2000, Ulrich 2002). These interpretations can be invested with nostalgia and lack critical and effective analysis of evidence, yet masquerade as history (Ulrich 2002).

Two histories of midwifery, produced during the revival of midwifery in the 1990s, illustrate the effects of an uncritical approach to examining professional identity. The first is an oral history of midwifery in England; the second is a study of South Australian midwifery. Leap and Hunter, the authors of the English study, declare in their introduction that: 'We expected to uncover a treasure chest of forgotten skills: experience that would enhance midwifery practice and inspire the midwives of today' (Leap & Hunter 1993:xi). In the Australian text, Annette Summers examines the 'historical terrain which led to the demise of the community midwife, whose lost autonomy is lamented by the midwife of the 1990s' (Summers 1995:1).

The authors of these texts searched for forgotten skills and lost autonomy; concepts likely to resonate with contemporary midwifery's professional aspirations to distinguish itself from nursing (Grehan 2009a). In setting out to locate a preconceived history, these inquiries mimic histories of celebrating Nightingale-style nurses and their mythical transformation of healthcare. Leap and Hunter, for example, found no evidence to suggest that handywomen were dealing out 'death and destruction' to pregnant women or that handywomen midwives were involved in performing abortions (Leap & Hunter 1993:22).

Their conclusion runs counter to ample documentary evidence in England confirming that some untrained women, as well as trained midwives, were ill-equipped (as were many doctors) for even the most common of complications in labour, such as haemorrhage. Ample evidence exists of female midwives in England and elsewhere facilitating what were then crimes of abortion and infanticide (Grehan 2009a). Likewise, Summers locates midwifery's 'lost' autonomy in South Australian midwifery at a time before the profession of nursing eclipsed this 'ancient' form of women's practice. This work ignores extensive documentary evidence of midwives' roles in abortion and infanticide in Australia, and evidence that some women lacked basic skills at bedsides (Grehan 2009a). It is no surprise that these authors, for the most part, find the history they set out to, because neither inquiry applies the self-consciousness of critical history.

Applying criticism of these revisionist histories is not to suggest that independent midwifery was not extinguished, nor is it to suggest that medicine and nursing did not wish to institute control over midwifery as it was practised by women. But history, even misinformed history, can have an impact on the fundamentals of a professional identity and be influential in making special claims for status and privilege on that basis. Thus, it is critical for nurses and midwives to be conscious of how all of the histories of nursing have been constructed, and to understand the motivations of those who write them. For those willing to investigate the history of nursing from the perspective of critical history, the rewards are great. In the next section, we raise some aspects of New Zealand's (Aotearoa's) and Australia's nursing and healthcare history, which are worthy of critical inquiry.

RELIGIOUS NURSES

Based on existing interpretations, we can be forgiven for believing that no skilled nurses worked in Australia or New Zealand (Aotearoa) in the nineteenth century. The powerful and longstanding narrative that only ignorant and incompetent nurses were in practice until 'Nightingale' nurses replaced them in 1868 has endured. Yet research shows that there were many with qualifications and considerable skills. Aside from midwives whose claimed training and qualifications have been confirmed (Grehan 2009a), the Catholic Sisters of Charity have a long history of care provision in Australia. As early as 1838, five religious Sisters from Dublin were providing care in Sydney. Of these five, one had trained as a nurse, and another had been sent to Paris to gain nursing experience (MacGinley 2002). These Sisters visited 'the sick poor in their own homes' as well as Parramatta's female factory (MacGinley 2002:72). In 1857, the Sisters of Charity opened the first St Vincent's Hospital in Australia, at Sydney's Potts Point. Since that time, the St Vincent's network has expanded substantially, with their hospitals providing a considerable proportion of public health services.

The St John of God Catholic Sisters cared for people with leprosy in isolated settlements in Western Australia and the Northern Territory (Robson 2022). The Sisters of the People, associated with the Methodist Church, tended the indigent in cities (Grehan 2008). In New Zealand (Aotearoa), too, Christian-based sisterhoods and other organisations tended the sick and dying, one of them being Sibylla Maude, a committed Anglican and trained nurse who established a district nursing service in the South Island of New Zealand (Aotearoa) in 1896 (Sargison 2001), which continues today. The role of religious or faith organisations in nursing and nurse training is one of the most interesting and challenging topics in Australia's and New Zealand's (Aotearoa's) nursing history because it encompasses aspects of colonisation. Two Christian religious groups with enormous influence on Australian nursing are the Presbyterian Church and the Salvation Army, for their pioneering of nursing provision to remote communities in Australia.

The Australian Inland Mission

The Australian Inland Mission (AIM), an offshoot of the Presbyterian Church, provided charitable assistance to rural and remote communities. In the early twentieth century, with others, the Reverend John Flynn, of the Flying Doctor fame, established AIM centres in extremely isolated territory and staffed them with duos of a trained nurse and helper (Cockrill 1999). In the AIM's early years, the nurses were deaconesses of the Presbyterian Church, and in this sense could evangelise on health and faith. In AIM centres, the nurses attended patients, conducted Sunday School and offered spiritual comfort to people in their communities (Cockrill 1999).

Working in isolation, AIM nurses faced all kinds of challenges, particularly before the introduction of pedal radio. Not all AIM nurses were trained in midwifery nursing, yet they were expected to attend births. Some were able to undertake brief midwifery 'training' to gain a degree of experience, one of whom was Mary Ann Bett, a deaconess and nursing sister recruited to the AIM centre at Oodnadatta in South Australia in 1909. In preparation for that appointment, Bett gained experience in the midwifery department at the Women's Hospital in Melbourne (Women's Hospital Board of Management Meeting Minutes 1909). Sister Jean Finlayson (pictured in Fig. 2.4 on a mode of desert transport) also worked at the AIM's Oodnadatta centre. In 1915, she was inaugural trained nurse at the Northern Territory's Alice Springs AIM Centre and later at the Alice Springs Hospital (Cockrill 1999).

Aboriginal nurses

Mainstream hospitals were reluctant to accept Indigenous women as pupil nurses, at least until the mid-1950s, whereas the Salvation Army, a Christian organisation with a network of hospitals around Australia, did accept Indigenous pupils from missions. Miss Sadie Corner (see Fig. 2.1) moved from Mount Margaret Mission in Western Australia to train at Bethesda, a Salvation Army hospital in Melbourne with a recognised nurse training school (Grehan 2008).

Corner was first a nurses' aide, then she trained as a general nurse, and later as a midwife. Miss Corner is believed to be the first Aboriginal woman to work as a trained nurse and hospital matron in Western Australia. As Mrs Canning, Sadie was awarded an MBE (Member of the British Empire) and a Queen's Jubilee Medal for her contribution to the health of the community of Leonora and surrounding district (Australian Legal Information Institute 2000).

Lowitja (Lois) O'Donohue CBE, AM, DSG from South Australia was 2 years old when she was removed from the care of her mother and sent to the

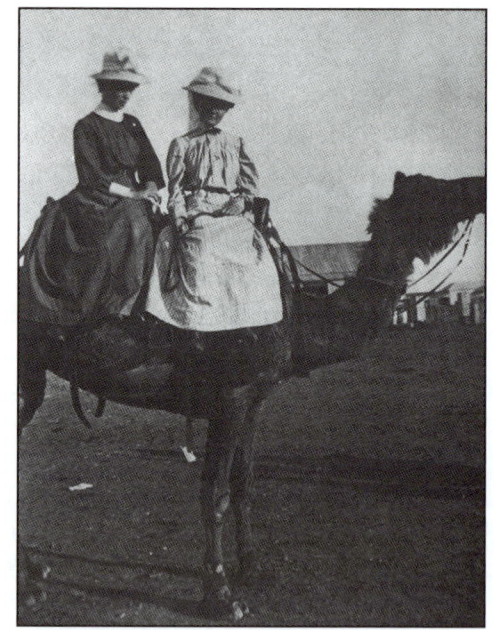

FIGURE 2.4

Jean Finlayson (right) and fellow deaconess at Alice Springs c1915

Source: Adelaide House Museum and Alice Springs Uniting Church.

United Aborigines Mission, the Colebrook Home, in Quorn. O'Donohue's initial application for nurse training at the Royal Adelaide Hospital was rejected because she was of Aboriginal descent. O'Donohue fought the decision and in 1954 Royal Adelaide admitted her to general nurse training. She worked in Adelaide as a charge sister and later spent time in India with a missionary society, before taking up positions in national Aboriginal affairs (State Library of South Australia 2001).

Research by Odette Best (2015), an Indigenous nurse from Queensland, is extending knowledge about Australian Aboriginal women with training in nursing and midwifery. Best has described a 'Native Nurses Training Scheme', which existed on three of Queensland's mission stations in the 1940s, devised because white trained nurses were not attracted to work with Aboriginal people. Best's research has also uncovered several Aboriginal women who undertook hospital-based midwifery training well before the 1950s, including May Yarrowick who graduated from Sydney's Crown Street Women's Hospital in 1906.

The New Zealand (Aotearoa) experience was somewhat different. Scholarships for Māori women to train as nurses were available in 1898 and by 1905 the training took 3 years (Bryder 2015, Wood 1992). The government then introduced a Native Health nursing scheme designed to improve the health of Māori populations living in isolated areas. Trained Māori nurses and midwives were to be offered positions first, and then white (Pākehā) nurses if those places could not be filled. Bryder (2015) reports that the work was challenging for both Māori and white nurses who dealt with difficult clinical problems and had little support.

This emerging scholarship demonstrates a nexus between faith organisations and nurse training programs for Indigenous women. The colonial and post-colonial history of faith nursing is worthy of further research, as is the pivotal role of faith organisations in buttressing the rural and remote nursing workforces in Australia and New Zealand (Aotearoa). Equally, governments' forays into devising and implementing training schemes as public health measures are worthy of critical inquiry.

The future

At the beginning of this chapter, we proposed that sometimes history can offer insights into the future. It is impossible, of course, to tell what the future will bring. An understanding of history may indicate what is *unlikely* to happen, rather than what *will* happen, simply because history never repeats in exactly the same way (Davison 2000). When considered over a sweep of time, history can reveal consistencies and patterns that emphasise the perennial nature of fundamental challenges.

Perhaps the most striking consistency in the history of nursing is the problem of attracting people to study nursing and retaining their services in nursing. Nursing has been affected by chronic and acute shortages of personnel since Europeans arrived in the colonies. Chronic shortages have prompted reforms in education and training. During wartime in Australia, acute shortages provoked government intervention to control the supply and movement of nurses (Grehan 2009a). Shortages have led governments to recruit nurses from other countries, and new tiers of care attendant have emerged, such as nursing aides, enrolled nurses and personal care attendants. Workforce supply is an enduring problem in nursing. and it is likely that solutions proposed in the future will be new iterations of old ideas: changing education programs, creating new categories of nurse, or adjusting the public's expectations of what a nurse is and what a nurse does. Governments will continue to bolster the nursing workforces in New Zealand (Aotearoa) and Australia through skilled migration schemes and inviting retired nurses to return to work, as occurred during the recent COVID-19 pandemic.

It is even feasible that governments may manage nursing shortages by invoking controls over the profession, just as Australia's Directorate of Manpower did during World War II. Circumstances where this is foreseeable are public health emergencies such as pandemics.

A second trend that is likely to continue into the future is the shift in locus of care. In the late nineteenth century the primary domain for care changed from the home to the modern hospital. Today, the pattern is reversed with patients receiving sophisticated treatments in the community that previously were only available in hospitals. As costs for inpatient health services balloon, the trend to home-based care is likely to continue. An area where the trend from hospital to community-based care is likely to escalate is aged care, as people live longer and are encouraged to 'age in place', which for most means their home.

Trends guaranteed to characterise nursing in the future are the role of technologies of care and changing understandings of life, death, health and illness. As philosophies and technologies evolve, nurses in practice will need ongoing education to stay up to date. Technology is generally recognised as beneficial, yet attracts criticism too. Since the introduction of the thermometer in the nineteenth century, technologies of care of all kinds have been blamed for producing a 'mechanistic' nurse, one focused on technologies at the expense of delivering basic care needs. These concerns are likely to persist given technology's dominance in the scope of nursing practice. Another guarantee is that arguments about professional identities will continue and possibly strengthen. The movement to separate midwifery from nursing might encourage other branches of nursing to pursue a similar path. Psychiatric nursing had its foundations in asylums, geographically and philosophically separate from general hospitals and general nurse training schemes. Yet structural service and educational reforms later positioned psychiatric nursing as a postgraduate specialty of nursing. Just as contemporary midwifery has advanced regulatory independence from nursing based on its historical differences, so may psychiatric nursing draw on its history to argue its separation from nursing.

CONCLUSION

This brief overview of the history of nursing in Australia and New Zealand (Aotearoa) has considered just some aspects of nursing history: women combining nursing with their evangelical missionary work, Aboriginal women as nurses, migrant nurses and aspects of nursing practice—that is, doing, organising, planning and implementing the care of others. More historical inquiry may illuminate the background to contentious areas in the history of nursing, such as nursing's relationships with Indigenous Australians and nursing's contribution to colonisation in healthcare terms. Research on the impact of world events and globalisation on nursing may provide clues about how to deal with workforce shortages. What is important for nurses and nursing is to accept its history 'warts and all', celebrating ordinariness alongside triumphs (Nelson 1997:234) and recognising less celebratory episodes. The pursuit of critical history, without judgment, will provide a realistic vision of the history of nursing in the Australian and New Zealand (Aotearoa) context, one that factually illuminates the richness and complexity of that history.

REFLECTIVE QUESTIONS

1. How does knowing about the history of nursing help nurses to understand the profession's place within healthcare systems today?
2. What have been some of the major historical influences on nursing and midwifery?
3. What new questions could be asked about the history of nursing?

Recommended readings

Helmstadter C, Godden J Nursing before Nightingale 1815–1899. Ashgate, Farnham, 2016
Nelson S 1998 How do we write a nursing history of disease? Health and History 1 (1):43–47
Nelson S 2001 Say little, do much: nurses, nuns, and hospitals in the nineteenth century. University of Pennsylvania Press, Pennsylvania
Nelson S 2002 The fork in the road: nursing history versus the history of nursing? Nursing History Review 10:175–188
Nelson S, Rafferty A M 2010 Notes on Nightingale: the legacy and influence of a nursing icon. Cornell University Press, Ithaca, New York
Sweet H, Hawkins S (eds) 2015 Colonial caring: a history of colonial and post-colonial nursing. Manchester University Press, Manchester

References

Argus, 10 July 1856, Melbourne
Australian College of Midwives Incorporated (ACMI) Victorian Branch 1999 Reforming midwifery: a discussion paper on the introduction of Bachelor of Midwifery Programs into Victoria. ACMI Victorian Branch, Melbourne
Australian Legal Information Institute 2000 Council for Aboriginal Reconciliation archives, Members of Council 1991–2000. Online. Available: www.austlii.edu.au/au/other/IndigLRes/car/2000/16/appendices04.htm 23 February 2024
Baly M 1987 The Nightingale nurses: the myth and reality. In: Maggs C (ed) Nursing history: the state of the art. Croom Helm, New Hampshire, pp 33–59
Bashford A 1998 Purity and pollution: gender, embodiment and Victorian medicine. St Martin's Press, New York
Best O 2015 Training the 'natives' as nurses in Australia: so what went wrong? In: Sweet H, Hawkins S (eds) Colonial caring: a history of colonial and post-colonial nursing. Manchester University Press, Manchester, pp 104–125
Bryder L 2015 'They do what you wish; they like you; you the good nurse!': colonialism and native health nursing in New Zealand, 1900–40. In: Sweet H, Hawkins S (eds) Colonial caring: a history of colonial and post-colonial nursing. Manchester University Press, Manchester, pp 84–103
Clendon J 1997 New Zealand military nurses fight for recognition World War One–Two. Nursing Praxis in New Zealand Journal of Professional Nursing (1)24–28
Cockrill P 1999 Healing the heart: 60 years of Alice Springs Hospital 1939–1999. Alice Springs Hospital's 60th anniversary reunion organising committee. Alice Springs
Collins Y 1999 The provision of hospital care in country Victoria 1840s to 1940s. Unpublished PhD thesis. Department of History of Philosophy and Science, University of Melbourne, Melbourne
Collins Y, Kippen S 2003 The 'Sairey Gamps' of Victorian nursing? Tales of drunk and disorderly wardsmen in Victorian hospitals between the 1850s and the 1880s. Health and History 5(1):42–64
Connolly C 2004 Beyond social history: new approaches to understanding the state of and the state in nursing history. Nursing History Review 12(3):5–24

Dahl M 2009 Air evacuation in war: the role of RAAF nurses undertaking air evacuation of casualties between 1943–1953. Unpublished PhD thesis. Institute of Health and Biomedical Innovation, Queensland University of Technology, Brisbane

D'Antonio P 1999 Revisiting and rethinking the rewriting of nursing history. Bulletin of the History of Medicine 73(2):268–290

Davison G 2000 The use and abuse of Australian history. Allen & Unwin, Sydney, p 263

Dickens C 1843 The life and adventures of Martin Chuzzlewit. Chapman and Hall, London

Durdin J 1991 They became nurses: a history of nursing in South Australia 1836–1980. Allen & Unwin, Sydney

Fahy K 1998 Being a midwife or doing midwifery? Australian College of Midwives Incorporated Journal 11(2):11–16

Fairman J, Lynaugh J E 1998 Critical care nursing: a history. University of Pennsylvania Press, Pennsylvania

Forth G, Critchett J, Yule P (eds) 1998 The biographical dictionary of the Western District of Victoria. Hyland House, Melbourne

French P 2001 A study of the regulation of nursing in New Zealand. Victoria University of Wellington Graduate School of Nursing and Midwifery Monograph Series 2/2001, Wellington

Godden J 2006 Lucy Osburn, a lady displaced: Florence Nightingale's envoy to Australia. University of Sydney Press, Sydney

Grehan M 2004 From the sphere of Sarah Gampism: the professionalisation of nursing and midwifery in the colony of Victoria. Nursing Inquiry 11(3):192–201

Grehan M 2008 A historical perspective of community nursing in Australia. In: Kralik D, Van Loon A, Community health care nursing in Australia. Blackwell's, Oxford, pp 1–16

Grehan M 2009a Professional aspirations and consumer expectations: nurses, midwives and women's health. Unpublished PhD thesis, School of Nursing and Social Work, The University of Melbourne, Melbourne

Grehan M 2009b A most difficult and protracted labour case: midwives, medical men and coronial investigations into maternal deaths in nineteenth century colonial Victoria. Provenance, Journal of Public Record Office Victoria 8:63–74

Grehan M 2009c. Heroes or villains? Midwives, nurses, and maternity care in mid-nineteenth century Australia. Traffic [Parkville], 11 https://link.gale.com/apps/doc/A214458324/AONE?u=anon,a3d81ef5&sid=googleScholar&xid=4e3d5ff4

Grehan M 2012 Realising unity: the Australian College of Nursing's long gestation. Connections Royal College of Nursing, Australia 15(2):2–3

Grehan M 2015 Typhoid epidemic 1885–1887, Tasmania, Australia. In: Mann Wall B, Keeling A (eds) Nurses and disasters: global historical case studies. Springer Publishing, New York, pp 1–36

Grehan M 2020 'Eliminating the drudge work': campaigning for university-based nursing education in Australia, 1920-1935, Quality Advancement in Nursing Education, Special History of Education issue, September 2020. Online. Available: https://doi.org/10.17483/2368-6669.1254

Harris K 2007 Not just 'routine nursing': the roles and skills of the Australian Army Nursing Service during World War I. Unpublished PhD thesis, History Department, University of Melbourne

Harris K 2010 More than bombs and bandages: Australian Army Nurses at work in World War. I Big Sky Publishing, Newport, New South Wales

Helmstadter C, Godden J 2011 Nursing before Nightingale 1815–1899. Ashgate, Farnham

Hill A 1982 The history of midwifery from 1840–1979: with specific reference to the training and education of student midwives. Unpublished MA thesis, Department of Education, University of Auckland

Jeffrey B 1954 White Coolies: a graphic record of survival in World War Two. Angus & Robertson, Sydney

Leap N, Hunter B 1993 The midwife's tale: an oral history from handywoman to professional midwife. Scarlett Press, London, p xi

Lewensen S 2004 Integrating nursing history into the curriculum. Journal of Professional Nursing 20(6):374–380

Lusk B, Russell R L, Rodgers J, Willson-Barnett J 2001 Pre-registration nursing in Australia, New Zealand, the United Kingdom and the United States of America. Journal of Nursing Education 40(5):197–202

McCalman J 1998 Sex and suffering: women's health and a women's hospital. Melbourne University Press, Melbourne

McCoppin B, Gardner H 1994 Tradition and reality: nursing and politics in Australia. Churchill Livingstone, Melbourne

MacGinley M R 2002 A dynamic of hope: institutes of women religious in Australia, 2nd edn. Crossing Press for the Institute of Religious Studies, Sydney

Macintyre S 1986 A concise history of Australia: Vol. 4, 1901–41. The succeeding age. Cambridge University Press, Cambridge

Maclean H 1923 New Zealand Army nurses. In: Drew Lt H T B The war effort of New Zealand. Whitcombe and Tombs, Auckland, pp 87–104

Maclean H 1932 Nursing in New Zealand: history and reminiscences. Tolan Printing, Wellington

MacPherson K 1996 Bedside matters: the transformation of Canadian nursing 1900–1990. Oxford University Press, Toronto

Masters D 1993 Annie Alice Crisp RRC Lady Superintendent of Auckland Hospital. Auckland Waikato Historical Journal April (62):36–37

Milligan C S, Foley J C H 1993 Australian hospital ship Centaur: the myth of immunity. Nairana Publications, Brisbane

Mitchell A 1977 The hospital south of the Yarra: a history of the Alfred Hospital Melbourne from foundation to the nineteen-forties. Alfred Hospital, Melbourne

Monk L 2008 Attending madness: at work in the Australian colonial asylum. Rodopi, Amsterdam

Monk L 2015 A duty to learn: attendant training in Victoria, Australia, 1880–1907. In: Borsay A, Dale P (eds) Mental health nursing: the working lives of paid carers in the nineteenth and twentieth centuries. Manchester University Press, Manchester, pp 54–74

Nelson S 1997 Reading nursing history. Nursing Inquiry 4:229–236

Nelson S 2000 A genealogy of the care of the sick: nursing, holism and pious practice. Nursing Praxis International, Hants, England, p 148

Nelson S 2004 History v Youthful Folly. Nursing Inquiry 11(3):129

Nelson S, Rabach J 2002 Military experience: the new age of Australian nursing and other failures. Health and History 4(1):79–87

Nelson S, Rafferty A M 2010 Notes on Nightingale: the legacy and influence of a nursing icon. Cornell University Press, Ithaca, New York

New Zealand Spectator and Cook's Strait Guardian, 14 May 1856: 3

Nutting M A, Dock L L 1907 A history of nursing, Vol. 1. Putnam, New York

Prebble K, Bryder L 2008 Gender and class tensions between psychiatric nurses and the general nursing profession in mid-twentieth century New Zealand. Contemporary Nurse 30(2):181–195

Rafferty A M, Robinson J, Elkan R (eds) 1997 Nursing history and the politics of welfare. Routledge, London, pp 192–207

Robson C 2022 Missionary women, leprosy and Indigenous Australians 1936–1986. Palgrave MacMillan, Cham

Rosenberg C E 1987 The care of strangers: the rise of America's hospital system. Johns Hopkins University Press, Baltimore

Sargison P A 2001 Essentially women's work: a history of general nursing in New Zealand 1830–1930. Unpublished PhD thesis, History Department, University of Otago, Dunedin

Shaw I 2010 On Radji Beach: the story of the Australian nurses after the fall of Singapore. Pan MacMillan, Sydney

Smith R 1999 In pursuit of excellence: a history of the Royal College of Nursing, Australia. Oxford University Press, Melbourne

Speirs K 2010 Nursing in the Boer War: the Nurses Database. Online. Available: https://britisharmynurses.com/wiki/index.php?title=The_Boer_War 23 February 2024

State Library of South Australia 2001 Lowitja O'Donohue: elder of our nation. In: Women and politics in South Australia: the Aboriginal voice. Online. Available: https://women-and-politics.collections.slsa.sa.gov.au/ 23 February 2024

Strachan G 2001 Present at the birth: 'handywomen' and neighbours in rural New South Wales 1850–1900. Labour History 81:13–27

Summers A 1989 The mysterious demise of Sarah Gamp: the domiciliary nurse and her detractors c. 1830–1860. Victorian Studies 32(2):365–386

Summers A D 1995 For I have ever so much more faith in her ability as a nurse: the eclipse of the community midwife in South Australia, 1836–1942. Unpublished PhD thesis, History Department, Flinders University

Templeton J 1969 Prince Henry's: the evolution of a Melbourne hospital. Robertson and Mullens, Melbourne

Tooley S 1906 A history of nursing in the British Empire. SH Bousfield, London

Trans-Tasman Mutual Recognition Act 1997 (Cth). Online. Available: https://www.legislation.gov.au/Details/C2019C00116 23 February 2024

Trans-Tasman Mutual Recognition Act 1997 (NZ). Online. Available: https://www.legislation.govt.nz/act/public/1997/0060/latest/whole.html 23 February 2024

Trembath R, Hellier D 1987 All care and responsibility: a history of nursing in Victoria 1850–1934. Florence Nightingale Committee, Australia, Victorian Branch, Melbourne

Ulrich L T 2002 The age of homespun: objects and stories in the creation of an American myth. Random House, New York

Walsh A 1955 Life in her hands: the Matron Walsh story told to Ruth Allen. Georgian House, Melbourne

Webster M E 1942 The history of trained nursing in Victoria. Typescript copy. Royal Women's Hospital Archives, Melbourne, Unaccessioned

Williams J 1991 Victoria's living memorial: history of the Nurses Memorial Centre 1948–1990. Nurses Memorial Centre, Melbourne

Women's Hospital Board of Management Meeting Minutes 1909 Royal Women's Hospital Archives Melbourne, unpublished, Accession No. RWHA 1991/6/26

Wood P J 1992 Efficient preachers of the gospel of health: the 1898 scheme for educating Māori nurses. Nursing Praxis in New Zealand Journal of Professional Nursing 7(1):12–21

Wood P J 2008 Professional, practice and political issues in the history of New Zealand's rural and remote 'backblocks' nursing: the case of Mokau 1910–1940. Contemporary Nurse 30(2):168–180

Wood PJ 2022 New Zealand nurses: caring for our people 1880–1950. Otago University Press, Dunedin

CHAPTER 3

ETHICS IN NURSING

Megan-Jane Johnstone

KEY WORDS

deepfakes (digital forgeries)
ethical and unethical professional conduct
ethics
humanitarian concerns
moral wisdom
nursing ethics
professional responsibility
whole-of-world/whole-of-society scenarios

LEARNING OBJECTIVES

After reading this chapter, readers should be able to:
- clarify the relationship between professional ethics and nursing ethics
- define ethical and unethical professional conduct in nursing
- consider the role and responsibilities of the nursing profession in responding to the ethical issues posed by existing and emerging challenging contexts in which they will be working.

INTRODUCTION

Ethics in nursing has never been more important than it is today. Faced with competing values, beliefs and viewpoints in the workplace and society generally, deciding the 'right' moral course to take in given situations has become increasingly difficult for nurses. To help overcome this difficulty and to enable them to promote the wellbeing of patients through the delivery of *good nursing care*—the ultimate goal of nursing—it is essential that nurses have at least a working knowledge and understanding of nursing ethics and its application in everyday practice. To this end, in the discussion to follow, attention will be given to clarifying the nature and importance of professional ethics and its relationship to nursing ethics; defining ethical and unethical professional conduct; considering the kinds of 'everyday' ethical issues nurses may face; and, finally, to identifying a range of local and global challenges that will test the moral wisdom of nurses and the capacity of the nursing profession as a whole to respond to the challenges posed in morally just ways.

Professional ethics

Ethical standards and exemplary ethical conduct constitute the hallmarks of a profession. Professions operate under strict ethical standards and members who violate those standards are subject to disciplinary measures. Nursing as a profession is no exception in this regard. Upon entering the nursing profession, members are expected to uphold the most stringent standards of ethical professional conduct and can expect to be held to account and to be disciplined if and when they fail to uphold those standards, even if a violation occurs unintentionally. These expectations derive from the potential vulnerability of people requiring and receiving nursing care and the special obligation that nurses have to protect patients from harm when working in a professional capacity. In order to understand why members of the nursing profession must adhere to exemplary standards of ethical professional conduct it is helpful to outline briefly the nature of nursing ethics and then to define what constitutes ethical professional conduct and unethical professional conduct in a nursing context.

Nursing ethics

Nursing ethics (to be distinguished from medical ethics) can be defined broadly as 'the examination of all kinds of ethical and bioethical issues from the perspective of nursing theory and practice' (Johnstone 2023a:15). In turn, these issues rest on a fundamental understanding of the foundational concepts of nursing: person, culture, care, health, healing, environment and nursing itself (i.e. what it is and what its end and purpose are). Unlike other approaches to ethics (e.g. medical ethics, bioethics), nursing ethics recognises the 'distinctive voices that are nurses'. As a starting point for systematic ethical inquiry, nursing ethics emphasises the importance of nurses' *actual experiences* as opposed to hypothetical examples or the experiences of members from other disciplines, which are not always relevant to nursing or to advancing moral wisdom in the practice of nursing.

Ethics functions by providing an authoritative action guide on how to think about, understand, examine and judge how best to 'be moral' and live the moral life. When applied in professional practice contexts, ethics functions in two key ways:

- by *ascribing* moral values to things (e.g. 'it is wrong to cause harm to patients')
- by prompting us to consider and reconsider *what* we have judged to be 'right' and 'wrong' as well as the *justifications* we have used to support and defend those judgments (e.g. 'this action is morally wrong *because* it violates the moral principle of 'do no harm').

Authoritative action guides to ethical decision making and conduct are found in the principles and rules expressed in commonly accepted theories of ethics; for example, utilitarianism, human rights theory, moral rights theory, ethical principlism and virtue ethics (Table 3.1). All of these have informed the development of nursing ethics and have been comprehensively discussed in the nursing literature and expressed variously in nursing codes of ethics (Johnstone 2023a).

Some nurses might think it unnecessary to appeal to 'high-brow' theoretical approaches (e.g. human rights, moral rights, ethical principlism, virtue ethics, etc.) in their practice, preferring instead to draw on their own personal moral values, beliefs and experiences when dealing with ethical issues. While such a stance might serve them well when caring for their own loved ones who share their values and beliefs, its application in a professional context is limited—especially when caring

TABLE 3.1
Common theories of ethics*

MORAL THEORY	EXPLANATORY NOTE
Utilitarianism	A moral theory that positions the general welfare and interests of people *as a whole* above that of the individual; classically advocates achievement of 'the greatest good for the greatest number'
Human rights	A special entitlement or interest that all people are believed to have simply by virtue of being human—e.g. the right to an education, to freedom of thought, etc.
Moral rights	A special entitlement or vital interest that an entity has, and which ought to be protected for moral reasons—for example, the right to be respected, fair treatment, privacy, confidentiality, etc.
Ethical principlism	A system of conduct guiding principles that specify some types of actions are either required, prohibited or permitted. Ethical principles commonly appealed to include: • autonomy—respect others as self-determining choosers • beneficence—do good • non-maleficence—do no harm • justice—be fair and equitable
Virtue ethics (also called character ethics)	The quality or practice of 'moral excellence'; examples include altruism, caring, compassion, courage, diligence, empathy, kindness, trustworthiness

*Further discussion on these theoretical perspectives can be found in Johnstone 2023a, Chapter 3 'Moral theory and the ethical practice of nursing'; see also Beauchamp and Childress 2019 Principles of biomedical ethics, 8th edn. Oxford University Press, New York

for people whose culture and lifeways are unfamiliar to them. Not only might a reliance on personal ethics lead to moral mistakes being made, but also, worse, to errors of moral judgment that result in morally harmful and even catastrophic outcomes.

REFLECTION
How would you apply nursing ethics in practice? Give an example involving patient care.

Ethical and unethical professional conduct

As stated in the opening paragraph to this chapter, exemplary ethical conduct is an important hallmark of a profession. But, what is exemplary ethical conduct?

Exemplary or prototypical ethical professional conduct can be broadly defined as conduct or behaviour that complies with the agreed and expected ethical standards of a profession. Because the ethical standards of a profession tend to require a level of behaviour and demeanour that is above that ordinarily expected of lay people or 'the ordinary person on the street', they are also deemed to be 'ideal', 'archetypal' and, hence, 'exemplary'. By this view, ethical professional conduct in nursing can be defined as conduct by a nurse that complies with the agreed ethical standards of the nursing profession and, by virtue of being characteristic of the ideals that the nursing profession 'professes', is both exemplary and 'right'.

The exemplary ethical standards that registered nurses are expected to uphold are contained in various formal codes and guidelines relevant to the profession and practice of nursing. In Australia, the standards pertaining to moral conduct expected of registered nurses are contained in the International Council of Nurses' (ICN's) 2021 *Code of Ethics for Nurses*. It should be noted that the ICN *Code of Ethics for Nurses* was formally adopted by Australian nursing organisations in 2018 and superseded the Nursing and Midwifery Board of Australia's (NMBA's) *Code of Ethics for Nurses in Australia* (NMBA 2008), which is now redundant (Johnstone 2023a:7–8). The ICN Code is to be read, interpreted and applied in conjunction with the NMBA's *Registered Nurse Standards for Practice* (NMBA 2016). In New Zealand (Aotearoa), the specific standards pertaining to moral conduct expected of registered nurses are given in the Nursing Council of New Zealand's (NCNZ's) *Code of Conduct for Nurses* (NCNZ 2012) and *Competencies for Registered Nurses* (NCNZ 2016) and the New Zealand Nurses Organisation's (NZNO's) *Guideline—Code of Ethics* (NZNO 2019).

These and related standards/guidelines work by setting the 'ethical baseline' against which a nurse's conduct can be measured and evaluated. Thus, if a nurse engages in conduct that breaches the agreed standards of the profession (fails literally to 'measure up' to the standards in question) this may be deemed as unethical professional conduct. This may result in a notification being made, in the case of Australian nurses, to the Australian Health Practitioner Regulation Agency (Ahpra) and, in the case of New Zealand (Aotearoa) nurses, to the NCNZ. If a notification is received by Ahpra, the nurse may be investigated by the NMBA (which works in partnership with Ahpra) to ensure that the necessary action is taken to protect the public. Likewise in the case of notifications received by the NCNZ, which also has regulatory authority to investigate a nurse's conduct.

Unethical professional conduct is more complex than a mere failure to comply with agreed ethical standards, however. Unethical professional conduct may be more comprehensively defined as an umbrella term that incorporates the following three related although distinct notions: 1) unethical conduct; 2) moral incompetence; and 3) moral impairment (Johnstone 2023a). Here, *unethical conduct* may be defined as 'any act involving the deliberate violation of accepted or agreed ethical standards' and can encompass both 'moral turpitude' and 'moral delinquency' (Johnstone 2023a:5). *Moral turpitude* refers to 'conduct that is considered contrary to community standards of justice, honesty or good morals' (The Free Legal Dictionary n.d.; see also Wikipedia contributors 2023). *Moral delinquency*, in turn, refers to any act involving moral negligence or a dereliction of moral duty. In professional contexts, moral delinquency entails a deliberate or careless violation of agreed standards of ethical professional conduct.

Moral incompetence (analogous to clinical incompetence) pertains to a person's lack of requisite moral knowledge, skills, 'right attitude' and soundness of moral judgments (Johnstone 2023a, see also Johnstone 2023b). *Moral impairment* meanwhile is generally distinguished from moral incompetence. Unlike moral incompetence (attributable to a lack of moral knowledge, skills), moral impairment entails a disorder, for example, psychopathy, that interferes with a person's social and moral reasoning and hence capacity to behave ethically. More specifically, because of their impaired moral reasoning, they are unable to engage in the competent discharge of their moral duties and responsibilities towards others. Accepting the notion of moral impairment (a notion which has received little attention in the nursing literature), a nurse could be judged morally impaired when, because of their disorder, they are unable to practise nursing in an ethically just and morally accountable manner (Johnstone 2023a).

REFLECTION
If you observed a nurse engaging in unethical professional conduct towards a patient, how would you respond?

'EVERYDAY' ETHICAL ISSUES IN NURSING

It is important to understand that ethical issues in nursing and healthcare contexts do not only involve the so-called 'big' or 'exotic' issues (e.g. abortion, euthanasia); they also involve fundamental questions about the nature and quality of professional–client relationships. This includes examining the more fundamental day-to-day practical ethical concerns relating to the precise impact that nurses' decisions and actions (or non-actions) have on the lives and welfare of other human beings, and the capacity of nurses to do harm to others while acting in a professional capacity.

The kinds of ethical issues faced by nurses today are as complex as they are varied. While in the past attention has tended to be focused on the better known bioethical issues such as abortion, euthanasia, organ transplantation, reproductive technology, genetic engineering and the like, over the past four decades there has been a significant shift in attention towards examining the other kinds of ethical issues faced by nurses. These issues include:

- 'everyday' practical ethical issues faced by nurses
- a genuine *nursing* perspective on common mainstream bioethical issues, and
- (the otherwise neglected) broader social justice issues associated with promoting the welfare, wellbeing and significant moral interests of highly vulnerable, stigmatised and marginalised groups of people (see, e.g. 'Ethics, dehumanisation and vulnerable populations' in Johnstone 2023a:106–138).

The nursing ethics literature has borrowed heavily from bioethics to shape nursing ethics discourse. As a result, the nursing ethics literature does not always represent or reflect the reality of the 'everyday' problems that nurses face.

What talking with nurses often reveals is that it is not the so-called paramount ('exotic') bioethical issues (such as abortion, euthanasia, organ transplantation, reproductive technology, etc.) that trouble them, but the more fundamental issues of:

- how to help a patient in distress in the 'here and now'
- how to stop 'things going bad for a patient'
- how to best support a relative or chosen carer during times of distress and when the 'system' appears to be against them
- how to make things 'less traumatic' for someone who is suffering
- how to reduce the anxiety and vulnerability of the people being cared for
- where nurses can get help for their own distress, and
- how to make a difference in contexts where indifference to the moral interests of others is manifest (Johnstone 2023a:84).

The above and other related concerns are all issues worthy of attention and consideration within and outside of the nursing profession. They are also issues that deserve to be recognised as being an integral part of a sound moral framework and approach that might be appropriately described as 'nursing ethics'.

> ### REFLECTION
> What do you think are the most pressing ethical issues facing nurses today? And what do you think will be among the biggest ethical challenges facing nurses in the future?

FUTURE ETHICAL CHALLENGES

Over the past century nursing ethics as a field of systematic inquiry has developed in impressive ways. Initially concerned only with polite commentaries in the early nursing journals, nursing ethics is now the subject of a vast body of scholarly literature and is widely recognised as a distinct field of inquiry and practice in its own right (Johnstone 2015a, 2015b, 2015c). The substantive and ever-expanding body of work by scholars in the field informs the ongoing advancement of the ethical standards and practice of the nursing profession, and continues to identify and foster understanding of the complex array of ethical issues faced by nurses in their day-to-day practice. Despite its historical progress, as was predicted over 120 years ago, the project of 'nursing ethics' is not yet complete and, when considered in its broadest sense, is unlikely to be completed in any one lifetime (Dock 1900). This is because, as contemporary contexts change, so too must nursing ethics change and continue to develop if it is to remain compelling and relevant as a discipline and guide to ethical nursing conduct.

There is recognition internationally that healthcare services around the world are facing a range of complex challenges, the immediate and future impact of which cannot be ignored. Included among the list of challenges identified are the:

- growth and increasing diversity of populations with a complex mix of chronic and acute diseases and associated burdens ('burden of disease')
- impact of diverse healthcare needs on resources—including infrastructure, supplies, knowledge, skills and information
- disparities and inequalities in health (particularly among the poor, Indigenous, immigrant and refugee populations)
- changing needs and expectations of people in regard to their health and healthcare
- projected unprecedented financial constraints on healthcare that are unlikely to lessen in the immediate future and challenges posed by associated demands for the equitable allocation and distribution of resources
- global shortage of nurses (according to the ICN [2020] the world could be short of up to 13 million nurses by the year 2030)
- ongoing challenges of leadership and governance, and operationalising responsible innovations in health (Lehoux et al 2019).

In addition to the above challenges, there are several 'whole-of-world' and 'whole-of-society' scenarios that also need to be taken into consideration and which, likewise, stand to have a profound impact on healthcare systems and the people requiring and needing access to them. Notable among the whole-of-world/society scenarios facing people (now and in the future) are the predicted and already occurring negative health impacts of:

- *climate change*, described by the World Health Organization (WHO) as the most significant health threat facing humanity and one that is posing an unprecedented challenge to health systems worldwide (WHO 2020, 2023a)
- *viral disease pandemics* (whereby surges of emerging and re-emerging diseases pose significant public health challenges for which the world needs to be prepared) (Lucero-Prisno et al 2023)
- *antimicrobial resistance* (regarded by WHO as 'one of the top global public health and development threats'—noting that drug resistant infections are difficult to treat and make certain medical procedures such as surgery and chemotherapy riskier) (WHO 2023b)
- *artificial intelligence (AI)* (particularly generative AI) and the ethics of and regulatory considerations for its use in healthcare (WHO 2023c)
- *political conflict and military attacks* on hospitals and healthcare services (attacks on hospitals and ambulances during war have caused death and mayhem, and the decimation of hospitals, which should be safe havens) (Johnstone 2023c, 2023d).

These challenges, individually and collectively, risk contributing to and compounding inequalities in health and healthcare locally and globally—particularly among vulnerable populations. These challenges, when combined with the rise and increasing sophistication of deepfake news and disinformation, pose significant threats to and stand to undermine the WHO's compelling global goal of 'health for all' (WHO 2023d). As the impact of these scenarios is felt around the world, people's health security will also shift as will the social protections they will need and come to expect in order to safeguard this (Gama 2016, Qiu et al 2018, Sazgarnejad & Takian 2022).

The above scenarios are already reshaping the moral landscape in which nursing and healthcare is practised. In light of the changes that are occurring, the most pressing ethical issues that nurses and their co-workers are likely to face in the future will not be of the conventional kind more commonly associated with the big 'exotic' issues of bioethics (e.g. abortion, euthanasia, end-of-life care, reproductive technology, informed consent, etc.). Rather, they will be issues that extend far beyond the parameters of the 'bricks and mortar' walls of hospitals to encompass much broader social justice and humanitarian concerns. Notable among these concerns will be a range of issues generated by the continual unfolding of 'whole-of-world'/'whole-of-society' scenarios and the often soul-destroying moral choices that will need to be made about the rationing, restrictions and responsibilities associated with the provision of healthcare and the 'tragic trade-offs' that will sometimes need to be made in the changing contexts over which nurses will often have little control (Johnstone 2023a:309).

WHAT CAN NURSES DO?

As healthcare providers, nurses have a fundamental role to play in helping to guide a just and humanitarian response to the ethical issues that existing and emerging 'whole-of-world'/'whole-of-society' scenarios inevitably give rise to. To this end, nurses need to think more broadly and creatively about ethics in general and to rethink the conventional (bio)ethical frameworks they have used in the past to ascertain and justify what is 'the right thing to do' in given situations. On this point, engaging with the relatively new discipline of public health ethics offers a way forward. Of particular note is the emergence of robust debate on the development of concepts thought vital to public health ethics but which, to date, have largely been neglected, notably: *membership* (encompassing people's 'equal rights of membership and reciprocal recognition in communities of health justice'); *solidarity* (encompassing a 'cultural sense of obligation and mutual aid in a world of common vulnerability'); and *place* or '*habitus*' (encompassing 'the schemata of human thinking, the patterns and defaults of human lives and behavior, the underlying assumptions and meanings that make certain types of behavior seem appropriate under the circumstances') (Jennings 2015, 2019, Jennings & Dawson 2015).

A second strategy is for nurses to form alliances with other health professional groups and to collectively 'speak out' on matters that are an affront to the ethical standing and humanitarian values of the professional groups involved. A third and largely overlooked strategy is for nurses to develop their media literacy so as to be able to detect and combat deepfake (digital forgeries) and disinformation about healthcare issues. The harmful impact of disinformation and the promulgation of medical conspiracy theories became apparent during the COVID-19 pandemic (Johnstone 2023a:310–313), highlighting the importance of media literacy as an ethical issue for the nursing profession and the professional responsibility of nurses to ensure they are reliably informed in their day-to-day practice.

STORY

During the COVID pandemic, conspiracy theories proliferated about the origins of the virus, its nature, mode of transmission, virulence, its treatment (e.g. injecting bleach versus vaccination), and even whether there was a pandemic at all—views which needlessly cost lives. Referring to the disinformation about COVID and the damage it caused to public health objectives, cybersecurity strategists Mansted and Smith (2020:2) note, in 'our digitally connected world, separating fact from fiction and genuine opinion from geopolitical jostling is increasingly difficult', pointing out that we need to get used to the idea that 'seeing (and hearing) no longer means simply believing'.

Reflective questions

1. What is your understanding of deepfake (digital forgeries) and its role in spreading disinformation about the challenges outlined in this chapter?
2. Do you know how to identify fake digital images and fake videos?
3. To what extent do you regard the problem of deepfake and disinformation as an ethical issue of significance for the nursing profession? What ethical issues does it raise?

In contemplating these questions, learn how to identify fake information by visiting the Australian Broadcasting Corporation (ABC) *Fact Check Essential#3: Spotting fake images + videos* at: https://games.abc.net.au/education/interactive-lessons/fake-images-videos/.

Nursing is fundamentally concerned with caring about fellow human beings. It is our job to provide comfort and care for those who are wounded, distressed and suffering. In addition to our professional obligations, we also have a civic responsibility to help make the world a better place within which to live and work. In the end, what we, as nurses, do about the social justice and humanitarian issues we encounter will reflect what kind of profession we are; and what we think ought to be done about the social justice and humanitarian issues we encounter will ultimately reflect what kind of profession we think we ought to be. It is hoped that by reflecting on the moral challenges that lie ahead, nurses will cultivate new insights and new moral wisdom about the ethical issues they will face both now and in the future, and become inspired to be much more than mere 'morally passive bystanders' in the world of human affairs and to take a stand on the things that really matter.

CONCLUSION

This chapter has sought to clarify the nature and importance of professional ethics in nursing and to identify some of the moral challenges that will confront nurses in the future. It is important to understand, however, that ethics neither emerges from nor operates in a cultural or contextual vacuum, and that its processes (thinking, reasoning, doing) are vulnerable to all sorts of corrupting influences, including politics, prejudice and personal needs. These influences can result in decision making that is arbitrary, biased, capricious, self-interested and precariously based on personal preferences. It is for this reason that proper 'checks and balances' need to be in place that, in turn, are supported by an appropriate infrastructure (policies, processes and procedures).

Whether nursing ethics is 'up to the task' of guiding sound ethical decision making in the healthcare contexts of the future will depend ultimately on its capacity to:

- offer moral insight
- foster moral wisdom
- inform 'good policy'
- provide 'real' solutions to complex problems
- warrant principled dissent against questionable policies, decisions and actions by others
- enable foresight
- guide the prevention of future problems (preventive ethics)
- redress the harm caused by past problems (restorative ethics) (Johnstone 2023a).

There are numerous complexities involved in building the capacity of nurses and nursing ethics to meet the inherent challenges that nurses can and do face during the course of their work. In order to meet these challenges responsibly and effectively, nurses have a professional obligation to advance their knowledge and understanding of what they can do to ensure that their decisions and actions are morally justified and will achieve their intended moral outcomes. Fulfilling this obligation will enable nurses to achieve the best possible position from which to practise and lead as ethical professionals.

REFLECTIVE QUESTIONS

1. Nurses are faced with ethical issues every day. In your view, what are the most pertinent and pressing ethical issues facing nurses today? How might nurses best deal with these issues?
2. How, if at all, might the study of nursing ethics assist nurses to practise nursing in a morally wise, insightful, just, effective and responsible manner?
3. What should nurses do if they witness an instance of unethical professional conduct by either a nurse or other health professional? How would you assess that the conduct in question was, in fact, unethical? Would you report the matter to an appropriate authority? How would you approach this responsibility?
4. In your view what are some standout 'whole-of-world'/'whole-of-society' issues at the present time? To what extent do these issues warrant the nursing profession's attention and action? What would you be willing to do? On what grounds would you justify your actions or non-actions as the case may be?

Recommended readings

Beauchamp T, Childress J 2019 Principles of biomedical ethics, 8th edn. Oxford University Press, New York
Johnstone M 2023 Bioethics: a nursing perspective, 8th edn. Elsevier, Sydney.
Nursing Ethics (e-journal https://journals.sagepub.com/home/nej)

References

Dock L L 1900 Ethics—or a code of ethics? In: Dock L L Short papers on nursing subjects. M Louise Longeway, New York, pp 37–57
Gama E 2016 Health insecurity and social protection: pathways, gaps, and their implications on health outcomes and poverty. International Journal of Health Policy and Management 5(3):183–187
International Council of Nurses (ICN) 2021 The ICN code of ethics for nurses. ICN, Geneva
Jennings B 2015 Relational liberty revisited: membership, solidarity and a public health ethics of place. Public Health Ethics 8(1):7–17
Jennings B 2019 Relational ethics for public health: interpreting solidarity and care. Health Care Analysis 27:4–12
Jennings B, Dawson A 2015 Solidarity in the moral imagination of bioethics. Hastings Center Report 45(5):31–38
Johnstone M (ed) 2015a Nursing ethics, volume I: developing theoretical foundations for nursing ethics. Sage, Oxford
Johnstone M (ed) 2015b Nursing ethics, volume II: nursing ethics pedagogy and praxis. Sage, Oxford
Johnstone M (ed) 2015c Nursing ethics, volume III: politics and future directions of nursing ethics. Sage, Oxford
Johnstone M 2023a Bioethics: a nursing perspective, 8th edn. Elsevier, Sydney
Johnstone M-J 2023b Nurse ethicists: innovative resource or ideological aspiration? Nursing Ethics 30(5):680–7
Johnstone M-J 2023c Bombing hospitals, destroying ambulances and the ethics of (un)just war. Australian Nursing and Midwifery Journal (ANMJ). Online. Available: https://anmj.org.au/bombing-hospitals-destroying-ambulances-and-the-ethics-of-unjust-war/
Johnstone M-J 2024 Taking a stand against attacks on healthcare: a call to support ICN's #nursesforpeace campaign. International Nursing Review
Lehoux P, Roncarolo F, Silva H P et al 2019 What health system challenges should responsible innovation in health address? Insights from an international scoping review. International Journal of Health Policy Management 8(2):63-75. doi: 10.15171/ijhpm.2018.110. PMID: 30980619; PMCID: PMC6462209.

Lucero-Prisno III D E, Shomuyiwa D O, Kouwenhoven M B et al 2023 Top 10 public health challenges to track in 2023: shifting focus beyond a global pandemic. Public Health Challenges 2(2):e86
Mansted K, Smith H 2020 Deep fakes will exacerbate challenges Australia already faces in the digital age. Online. Available: https://www.aspistrategist.org.au/deep-fakes-will-exacerbate-challenges-australia-already-faces-in-the-digital-age/
New Zealand Nurses Organisation (NZNO) 2019 Guideline—Code of ethics. NZNO, Wellington
Nursing and Midwifery Board of Australia (NMBA) 2008 Code of ethics for nurses in Australia. NMBA, Canberra
Nursing and Midwifery Board of Australia (NMBA) 2016 Registered nurse standards for practice. NMBA, Canberra
Nursing Council of New Zealand (NCNZ) 2012 Code of conduct for nurses. NCNZ, Wellington
Nursing Council of New Zealand (NCNZ) 2016 Competencies for registered nurses. NCNZ, Wellington
Qiu M, Jessani N, Bennett S 2018 Identifying health policy and systems research priorities for the sustainable development goals: social protection for health. International Journal for Equity in Health 17(1):1–4
Sazgarnejad S, Takian A 2022 The universal triangle to ensure health security. International Journal of Public Health 67:1605443
The Free Legal Dictionary nd Moral turpitude. Online. Available: https://legal-dictionary.thefreedictionary.com/Moral+Turpitude 30 November 2023
Wikipedia contributors 2023 Moral turpitude. In: Wikipedia, The Free Encyclopedia. Online. Available: https://en.wikipedia.org/w/index.php?title=Moral_turpitude&oldid=1183110525
World Health Organization (WHO) 2023a Climate change and health. WHO. Online. Available: https://www.who.int/news-room/fact-sheets/detail/climate-change-and-health
World Health Organization (WHO) 2023b Regulatory considerations on artificial intelligence for health. WHO. License: CC BY-NC-SA 3.0 IGO. Online. Available: https://iris.who.int/handle/10665/373421
World Health Organization (WHO) 2023c People-centred approach to addressing antimicrobial resistance in human health: WHO core package of interventions to support national action plans. Geneva: World Health Organization; Licence: CC BY-NC-SA 3.0 IGO. Online. Available: https://www.who.int/publications/i/item/9789240082496
World Health Organization (WHO) 2023d World Health Day 2023: Health for all. Online. Available: https://www.who.int/campaigns/75-years-of-improving-public-health

CHAPTER 4

AN INTRODUCTION TO LEGAL ASPECTS OF NURSING PRACTICE

Jayne Hewitt

KEY WORDS

assault
code of conduct
common law
complaints
conduct
consent
ethics
health law
health practitioner regulation
legislation
negligence

LEARNING OBJECTIVES

After reading this chapter, readers should be able to:

- understand the basics of the Australian legal system
- understand basic principles of law and regulation applicable to nursing practice
- understand the legal rights of patients, women and their infants
- understand the role of the civil and criminal law in nursing practice
- understand the registration and standards for the nursing profession.

INTRODUCTION

Nursing takes place within an environment regulated by law. It is important, therefore, that nurses are aware of the legislation, regulations and decisions from the tribunals and courts that both prescribe and impact their practice to ensure safe and competent patient care.

This chapter serves as an introduction to the legal system, laws and regulations relevant to nursing practice. It is necessarily brief and cannot cover all aspects of the law that affect nursing practice. The law evolves, and changes are made as required, particularly to legislation. Nurses should keep up to date and develop a sound understanding of the legal system in which they work, and of the laws that govern their clinical practice, through active participation in continuing professional development (CPD), clinical research and education.

Australia's common law system

Common law refers to judge-made law and is based upon the doctrine of precedent. That is, by looking at how cases have been decided in the past and applying the principles developed in those cases to the present. Legal systems based on common law are referred to as common law systems. Australia inherited a common law system when it was colonised by England.

Although founded on judge-made law, common law countries include a combination of common law, equity and legislation.

The second type of law is *legislation*, or statutory law. This is a law developed by parliamentarians through the parliamentary processes at federal, state and territory levels. A piece of legislation is referred to as a statute or an Act of Parliament. Valid legislative provisions prevail where there is inconsistency with the common law. Thus, parliamentary law can be used to change the law where it is considered that the common law is deficient or to govern new circumstances.

Law is divided into civil and criminal. *Civil law* involves legal actions taken by a complainant (plaintiff) against another or others seeking a civil remedy for a legally recognised wrong—for example, a plaintiff seeking compensation for injury sustained if a nurse gives an incorrect medication. The alleged negligent practitioner is normally referred to as the defendant. The task (onus) of proving the case rests with the plaintiff 'on the balance of probabilities'.

Most *criminal law* consists of prosecutions brought on behalf of a state or territory to punish breaches of criminal offences, and a guilty verdict results in a fine and/or custodial sentence. The onus of proving a criminal offence lies with the prosecution, which must prove its case 'beyond a reasonable doubt'. The criminal offences of manslaughter, grievous bodily harm and criminal negligence are some of the major criminal offences that can apply to nursing practice.

Civil law and healthcare

Nurses need to work within the context of civil law, as it relates to patient safety; negligent advice; patient consent; and patient freedom of movement.

PATIENT SAFETY AND NEGLIGENCE

Negligence is a *tort*, which means a civil wrong resulting in an injury. The tort of negligence arises from the common law. To succeed in an action of negligence against a nurse, the plaintiff (patient) must prove, on the balance of probabilities, that:

1. the nurse owed the person a legal duty of care
2. the nurse breached this duty of care
3. the person suffered harm because of that breach.

A duty of care exists when a person can reasonably foresee that their acts or omissions are likely to place another at risk. In a healthcare context, a nurse–patient therapeutic relationship, in all but the most unusual circumstances, will evidence the existence of a duty of care. 'That duty is a single comprehensive duty covering all the ways in which a doctor [and all other health professionals] is called upon to exercise his skill and judgement ...' (*Rogers v Whitaker* (1992) 175 CLR 479 at 483 per Mason CJ, Brennan, Dawson, Toohey and McHugh JJ).

Once a duty of care is established, the plaintiff must prove that the defendant did something, or failed to do something, which amounted to a breach of that duty. Whether or not a breach has occurred requires consideration of the standard of care required in the circumstances. When considering the standard of care required from skilled professionals such as nurses, case law (see *Bolam v Friern Hospital Management Committee* [1975] 1 WLR 582 and *Rogers v Whitaker* (1992) 175 CLR 479) and civil liability legislation provides the benchmark against which the conduct will be considered. The standard of care is not perfect care, but reasonable care. It is an objective test and therefore is not dependent upon the particular skills and knowledge of the healthcare professional. The standard expected is that which is attributed to the class of healthcare professionals to which the defendant belongs. Thus, the conduct of a nurse will be measured against that of the hypothetical, reasonably competent nurse. It is when the defendant's standard of care falls below that of the reasonably competent nurse that a breach of care is found.

Damage is the gist of an action of negligence; a plaintiff must prove that foreseeable damage resulted from a breach of duty by the nurse. Damage may be physical harm, psychological harm, economic harm or a combination of these. Once the plaintiff has proved that the nurse's breach of duty caused damage that was reasonably foreseeable, the defendant will be liable to compensate for that damage and any further loss that flows reasonably to and naturally from the initial injury. Pain and suffering, loss of enjoyment of life, loss of expectation of life, loss of opportunity in life and financial consequences are examples of accepted heads of damage (categories of damage recognised by the courts) for which compensation can be sought in a negligence action.

Finally, the plaintiff must prove that the breach of duty caused the harm now claimed. To prove a causal connection, the plaintiff must demonstrate that 'but for' the act or omission of the defendant, they would not have suffered the harm. The civil liability legislation in each of the states and territories, except the Northern Territory, requires a two-stage approach to finding a causal link between the act/omission and the harm. A determination that the negligence caused the harm requires that the 'negligence was a necessary condition of the occurrence of the harm ("factual causation"), and … that it is appropriate for the scope of the negligent person's liability to extend to the harm so caused ("scope of liability")' (see, e.g., *Civil Liability Act 2002* (NSW) s 5D).

STORY

Reina Choy works for a nursing agency and has been allocated a shift in the high-dependency unit at the local general hospital. She is caring for Zyg Oagie who has returned from the operating theatre following abdominal surgery. Although Zyg has a narcotic infusion in situ he is complaining of severe pain. Reina has not used the infusion pump before but is keen to do what she can to alleviate Zyg's pain, so she administers a bolus of medication. In her haste, she inadvertently administers 10 times the prescribed dose of medication. Shortly after, Zyg suffers a respiratory arrest, and although he is successfully resuscitated, he now has a hypoxic brain injury.

Reflective questions

Reflect on the scenario and answer the following questions:
1. What factors may have contributed to Reina's error?
2. What could have been done to avoid this error?
3. Who could be liable to pay Zyg's compensation if his negligence action is successful?

The principles of negligence also apply to giving professional advice. Nurses must exercise reasonable care to avoid the person suffering harm as a result of following the advice. Patients should be informed of all 'material risks' inherent in a procedure or treatment, together with any risks that are of particular importance to the person. A risk is material if a reasonable person in the patient's position would be likely to attach significance to the risk, and thus require a warning. It would be reasonable for a person with one good eye to be concerned about the possibility of injury to it from an elective procedure. In *Rogers v Whitaker* (1992) a patient agreed to eye surgery on one eye without being advised that there was a remote risk she could become blind, which was what happened. She was awarded compensation for the ophthalmologist's failure to warn her of the remote risk.

DEFENCES TO AN ALLEGATION OF NEGLIGENCE

The main defences to an allegation of negligence are:
- *No duty of care*—the defendant may show there was no duty of care owed to the plaintiff
- *No breach of the duty*—the defendant may successfully argue that their act or omission was consistent with competent professional practice and did not amount to a breach of the duty of care
- *No causation*—the defendant may show on the evidence that their act or omission was not causally linked to the damage claimed
- *Contributory negligence*—a defendant can argue that the plaintiff was partially or totally responsible for the harm that eventuated (under the provisions of the civil liability legislation by reason of contributory negligence a court may consider a reduction of 100% with the result that the action for damages is defeated). The court will award damages in proportion to the extent it accepts that the plaintiff was negligent. A woman who successfully sued a doctor for his failure to refer her to an alternative specialist when she advised him she was unable to use the referral he had given her had the amount of her damages reduced by 20% because of her subsequent failure to seek medical attention for 4 months despite suffering continued and severe vaginal bleeding (*Kalokerinos v Burnett* [1996] NSWSC 288).

Trespass to person and consent

All competent adults have the right to determine what care, treatment or diagnostic tests they will undergo, unless there is some overriding law that allows treatment without consent. When an adult with decision-making capacity is treated without valid consent, they have a right to sue under the tort of trespass to the person. This tort includes assault (words or actions that give rise to an apprehension of imminent harmful or offensive contact), battery (when actual contact occurs) and false imprisonment (where there is a total deprivation of liberty). The torts of battery and assault are frequently referred to as 'assault' (Luntz et al 2021:733).

A battery is complete once touching has occurred without lawful justification; there is no need for a person to prove that damage occurred. It is not a defence to battery that treatment was carried out in good faith for the benefit of the patient when the patient could consent but has not done so. It is a defence that the person consented to the touching.

The requirements for valid consent are:
1. Consent must be freely and voluntarily given
2. The person must have decision-making capacity
   - They must be able to take in and retain the information

- Believe the treatment information
- Use that information to balance the risks posed by the treatment with their health needs

3. The person must be informed in broad terms about the procedure
4. The consent must cover the procedure that is being performed (Richards 2024).

Voluntary consent is given freely by the patient in the absence of fraud, coercion or duress. Advising a patient of the risks and benefits of nursing treatment is part of a nurse's role but if the nurse becomes overbearing and the patient feels they have no choice, then the person's consent is not voluntary. A patient who wanted general anaesthesia for surgery gave up and agreed to spinal anaesthesia at the insistence of a doctor and suffered injuries. It was held that her consent had been overborne by the insistence of the anaesthetist and others (see *Beausoleil v Sisters of Charity* (1964) 53 DLR 2d 65). The person must be advised in 'broad terms' of the nature of the procedure to be performed and agree to it being performed (see *Chatterton v Gerson* [1980] WLR 1003). Concerns relating to the degree of information given regarding risks involved is a matter for the law of negligence, as discussed previously. The consent must cover the treatment to be carried out and any related treatment. Any procedures carried out beyond that for which the patient consented (except in an emergency where the patient is incapable of giving or withholding consent) can result in a complaint of battery (*Murray v McMurchy* [1949] 2 DLR 442).

The tort of false imprisonment compensates a person who has been subjected to an intentional and total restraint of movement without lawful justification. False imprisonment is defined as: 'Unlawfully restraining the liberty of another person' (*R v Banner* [1970] VR 240). The restraint must be total, not merely a partial obstruction of a person's free movement (*Bird v Jones* (1845) 7 QB 742; 115 ER 668). Restraint is either by total confinement or by preventing the person from lawfully leaving the place where they are. The tort can be committed when a patient is too ill to move or is unaware of the fact that they were imprisoned by reason that they were in a state of drunkenness or while asleep (see *Meering v Grahame-White Aviation Co Ltd* (1920) 122 LT 44. See also *Hart v Herron and Anor* [1996] NSWSC 176). In the latter case, Mr Hart was detained and treated with electroconvulsive therapy (ECT) and deep sleep therapy at a private psychiatric hospital without proof of his consent. He successfully sued the psychiatrist for assault and false imprisonment.

The plaintiff must prove the confinement was total. If the person can leave by some reasonable alternative exit, there is no false imprisonment. Locking a patient in a room with no reasonable avenue of escape or barring a patient from lawfully leaving a healthcare institution by the use of bed rails, manacles and chemical restraints could amount to false imprisonment in the absence of lawful justification.

It can also amount to false imprisonment if a patient reasonably believes that any attempt to leave a healthcare institution will be prevented by a nurse, even if there are no physical restraints (psychological restraint). This could occur if a nurse gave the patient the impression that they would be prevented from leaving if they tried to do so; for example, telling the patient they could not leave until they saw a doctor and signed a release form. However, the patient would have to prove the submission to the nurse was complete and that it was a reasonable response.

Hospitals develop policies requesting that patients see a doctor and must sign a release form if they wish to leave the hospital against medical advice. There is no problem if a patient voluntarily agrees to the request. Some doubt exists as to whether hospital staff could detain a patient without consent to fulfil the hospital requirements. If a patient leaves without advising staff or refuses to stay to sign a release form and see a doctor, the patient should not be prevented from leaving and the events should be clearly and contemporaneously documented in the hospital notes.

The fact that a patient wishes to leave the hospital against medical advice does not relieve the staff from advising the patient of any deleterious effects that could arise if they leave. Wherever possible, staff should ensure that the patient fully appreciates the risks involved in leaving against medical advice.

Obtaining consent

Consent may be obtained by asking a person's permission before commencing treatment. Consent may also be implied by the person's overt physical response to suggested treatments; for example, if the patient lifts their arm to have a blood pressure cuff put on when the nurse approaches with a sphygmomanometer or other blood pressure measuring device. Consent in writing, and witnessed, is usually sought for major intrusions of the body, such as surgery. It is best practice for the person undertaking the procedure to obtain consent. In an emergency where a person is unable to give consent, a nurse may institute measures aimed at saving life or avoiding severe injury while the emergency exists.

Consent can be withdrawn at any time; however, the person withdrawing consent must inform the person undertaking the procedure.

Defences to an allegation of trespass

The first, and most obvious defence to an allegation of trespass is that the nurse obtained legally valid consent from the person or the person's substitute decision maker. The defence of necessity operates in those circumstances when patients are unable to give consent and the treatment is necessary to preserve them from imminent danger to their life. An example would be a patient who has suffered head injuries in a car accident and is unconscious. It would be lawful to perform whatever surgery is necessary to save the patient from death or a serious risk to their health.

Defences that can be raised against an allegation of false imprisonment include the defence of necessity, which permits the restraint of persons who are a danger to themselves or others. The restraint of a patient attempting to jump off the roof of a hospital, or threatening staff and other patients with violence, would be justified on this basis. A second defence exists where legislation authorises the detention of persons (e.g. mental health and public health legislation). A third lawful means of detaining patients is where a court authorises the detention of a person for treatment. Such orders are usually reserved for the detention of children when parents wish to remove a child in need of care from a healthcare institution.

Obtaining consent when a person lacks decision-making capacity

The law presumes that all adults have decision-making capacity. However, a person's decision-making capacity may be affected by an intellectual disability, conditions such as dementia, acquired brain injury or other injury. When a person lacks decision making capacity, alternate arrangements for providing consent are required. This primarily occurs through state and territory-based guardianship legislation that identifies and authorises a substitute decision maker for the period in which the adult is incapable of consenting to treatment (see Queensland University of Technology [QUT] 2020). It is the substitute decision maker who takes responsibility for deciding to consent, or refusing to consent, to the treatment or procedure.

Australia, like other countries worldwide, has an ageing population. With ageing comes the increased likelihood of developing conditions that can impact a person's decision-making capacity. However, people can make known their future wishes (and consent) for care or treatment should they lose decision-making capacity. Different jurisdictions use different terminology for the mechanisms and documentation produced by their legislation to do this, such as advance health directives. New South Wales (NSW) does not have statutory provisions in place, but the health department has policies that create the possibility for patients to make advance care directives and provide forms and advice on how to do so.

People with mental health issues

There are occasions when mental illness affects a person's decision-making capacity. Most adults within the mental health system are voluntary patients with the same legal rights to consent or refuse to consent to treatment as any other patient within a healthcare facility. Some patients, however, have mental illnesses that periodically render them a danger to themselves and/or others and, for a time, are incapable of seeking appropriate assessment and treatment. For those patients, mental health legislation in each state may authorise non-voluntary examination, admission and treatment.

Children

A combination of common law principles and legislation applies when obtaining consent to provide treatment for children. Where a child is an infant or very young, the child's parent or guardian may consent to treatment, provided the treatment is in the child's best interest. Parental authority is subject to some limitations where the proposed treatment involves major, irreversible and invasive surgery (Smith & Mathews 2024). At common law a child may consent to treatment that is therapeutic, provided they understand the nature and consequences of the proposed treatment. The application of this principle requires a balance between the intellectual and emotional maturity of the minor and the complexity and seriousness of the proposed treatment (see *Gillick v West Norfolk and Wisbech Area Health Authority* [1985] 3 All ER 402, approved by the High Court in the case of *Department of Health and Community Services v JWB and SMB* [1992] HCA 15 'Marion's Case').

Legislation can change or modify the common law. In NSW, legislation provides that consent to medical and dental treatment is given by a parent or guardian of a minor aged less than 16 years, or by a minor aged 14 years or upwards. Between the ages of 14 and 16, consent can be given by a parent or the child, provided the child has sufficient maturity to understand the nature of the treatment. Below the age of 14 years, the consent of the parent or guardian is required (except in an emergency to save the life of the child) (*Minors (Property and Contracts) Act 1970* (NSW) s 49). In South Australia, children over the age of 16 can make decisions about their healthcare treatment (*Consent to Treatment and Palliative Care Act 1995* (SA) s 6).

Where a child, their parents or guardians refuse to consent to healthcare treatment that a doctor believes is in the child's best interest, consent may be obtained by a state or territory Supreme Court exercising its *parens patriae* jurisdiction.

Vicarious liability

When a nurse's act or omission has caused harm to a patient and the patient has successfully sued to recover compensation for that harm, the question arises as to who is responsible for providing the compensation. Under the doctrine of vicarious liability, an employer can be held responsible for the acts of its employees carried out in the course of their employment. The employer is liable without any blame or fault. In some states, the employer cannot chase the employee for damages paid.

An employer's responsibility is limited to those acts an employee performs during the 'course of employment'. However, this term is broad and encompasses all acts, authorised or not, which are reasonably within the scope of the employee's duties. Therefore, an employer can be legally responsible for compensating an injured patient whose injuries resulted from an employee's negligence. It is only when a nurse's actions are so far removed from anything that can reasonably be held to be part of a nurse's role that an employer will escape responsibility. A nurse's failure to follow guidelines in a procedure manual would generally not be enough to excuse the employer unless there was a gross departure from standards.

Vicarious liability means that the healthcare employer will generally be held responsible for compensating a successful plaintiff but this may not negate the nurse's personal liability. The nurse may be joined as a co-defendant. Also, responsibility under vicarious liability applies to civil wrongs but normally does not apply to criminal acts. Therefore, a health service may be found vicariously liable for a nurse who commits a civil assault by giving an injection without consent, but not if the nurse angrily punched a patient (a criminal offence).

Even when an employer is not vicariously liable because a person committing a wrong is not an employee, the courts have been prepared to find that an organisation such as a hospital has a duty of care towards patients and others that is non-delegable. Consequently, a hospital can be found negligent for harm caused to a patient by an act or omission of a visiting medical officer responsible for causing the alleged harm. When a hospital's policies and procedures could expose a patient to an unreasonable risk of harm, a duty arises to avoid that harm.

Criminal law

There may be occasions when a nurse causes serious bodily harm or death to patients. As well as providing facts that may be the subject of a civil action, such events may result in charges of criminal assault, criminal negligence, manslaughter or, rarely, murder. The prosecutor must prove both *mens rea* (guilty mind) as well as *actus reus* (an unlawful act). The *mens rea* element can be satisfied by proving that the accused committed an unlawful act, either with intent or could have foreseen that someone could suffer harm but proceeded to commit the act.

CRIMINAL ASSAULT

Assault can be the subject of a criminal charge as well as a tort. In addition to the elements required to prove civil assault, there must be proof of an intentional forcible or hostile act of the accused or recklessness as to the outcome of the conduct. If a patient is criminally assaulted (e.g. threatened, punched, grabbed or kicked), the matter must be reported to the appropriate health service managers, and, most importantly, to the police, who can charge the responsible party with criminal assault. The same legal redress is available to nurses who are assaulted by others. Conduct that is driven with malice and intended to cause harm, or a reckless indifference to the harm, amounts to criminal assault. Touching a person in the course of diagnosis or treatment without consent may give rise to an action to recover compensation at civil law but is unlikely to be regarded as a criminal assault where the intent is to benefit the patient.

Criminal negligence, manslaughter

Although exceedingly rare, nurses can be charged with criminal negligence where an act causing serious bodily harm or death shows such a high disregard for the life and safety of another and is so reckless that it goes beyond a mere matter of compensation at civil law and amounts to a crime. Where the death of a patient results from conduct that would give rise to a charge of criminal negligence it is generally referred to as involuntary manslaughter. This could occur where the nurse's practice, though not intended to bring about the death of the patient, was so grossly negligent it amounted to something no reasonably skilled person would have done. This was the case where a nurse was charged with manslaughter by criminal negligence after crushing an elderly patient's oral medication and injecting it intravenously. Although the patient subsequently died, the jury in the trial could not reach a verdict, and she was not re-tried (Bibby 2015).

RECORDING PATIENT INFORMATION

The recording of patient and client information is continuing in a process of transition from hard copy to electronic version. Nonetheless, the documentation of patient care is fundamental to good patient care. This proposition is supported in the guidelines and codes published by the respective professional regulatory authorities (e.g. International Council of Nurses 2021, Nursing and Midwifery Board of Australia 2016); and government policies and directives (e.g. NSW Department of Health 2012). Patient records are legal documents and, therefore, it is important to keep accurate and complete records of all treatment and care provided to patients. The documents record the progress of patients admitted to healthcare services for the time that they are receiving care. Accurate and complete documentation can provide a good defence for a nurse who is faced with legal action if the medical record discloses that appropriate, timely and reasonable nursing care was delivered.

Even when appropriate treatment may have been administered, failure to keep accurate, concise, objective and contemporaneous patient records can lead to a finding of liability on the part of a nurse. Failure to record treatment may be accepted as evidence that such treatment was not in fact given (see, e.g., *Albrighton v Royal Prince Alfred Hospital* [1980] 2 NSWLR 542). Overall failure to keep complete and adequate records can be regarded as a negligent omission because a reasonable nurse would be expected to keep all patient record notes in order and up to date. It is reasonably foreseeable that a patient may suffer harm from failure to record a treatment given (e.g. a patient may be given two doses of a drug because a first dose was not recorded).

Patient records should be objectively written, and those responsible for writing records should avoid making value judgments. 'Patient has a headache' is a subjective statement and should be recorded as 'patient complaining of headache'. A description of the nature of the headache, the nursing action taken and the outcome of that action should follow this statement.

Records should be as near as possible contemporaneous with the event for both quality ongoing care and if they are to be accepted as reliable evidence in a court action. Delays in recording make the record less reliable as a true description of an event. A record made days after an event can be made to look as though it was an afterthought. Interlineations and notes made in margins should also be avoided, as they can suggest that information has been added to a record at a later date. It is for this reason that nurses who are still recording patient information in hard copy are advised not to leave lines between individual reports.

Nurses should be aware that personal information given by patients in the course of providing care is to be kept confidential. The legal obligations of confidentiality and privacy arise when creating, managing or using healthcare records. However, these two areas deal with matters that are broader than healthcare records, as they also apply to relationships, trust and having adequate information to provide safe, competent care for patients while ensuring their dignity and integrity are maintained. Although confidentiality and privacy are often used interchangeably, they have distinct meanings and should be differentiated. Confidentiality is a vital element of the nurse–patient relationship, and protects information given in confidence (Prictor & Taylor 2024). Privacy encompasses many concepts, including bodily privacy and privacy of information kept about a person (Prictor & Taylor 2024).

Patients are entitled to expect that nurses will maintain a high degree of confidentiality and protect their privacy. Should a nurse breach a patient's confidentiality, the patient may be able to sue in defamation for unlawful disclosure if their reputation has been harmed; in negligence if they suffer foreseeable loss or damage; or in breach of contract.

Regulation of nursing practice

In Australia, since 2010, specified disciplines of health professionals are registered to practise under the National Registration and Accreditation Scheme (the 'National Scheme' or 'NRAS') facilitated by the *Health Practitioner Regulation National Law Act 2009* (the 'National Law'). The National Law was enacted in each of the states and territories with New South Wales (*Health Practitioner National Law (NSW) No 86a*) and Queensland (*Health Ombudsman Act 2013*) retaining a co-regulatory system.

The object of national registration is to protect the public by ensuring that only suitably trained and qualified health practitioners are registered to practise. However, it also facilitates workforce mobility across Australia; the provision of high-quality education and training of health practitioners; rigorous and responsive assessment of overseas-trained practitioners; access to services provided by health practitioners in accordance with the public interest; and the continuous development of a flexible, responsive and sustainable Australian health workforce and innovation in the education of, and service delivery by, health practitioners (*Health Practitioner Regulation National Law*, s 3).

The Australian Health Practitioner Regulation Agency (Ahpra) is the national body responsible for the regulation, national registration and accreditation of health practitioners and the registration of students. Ahpra supports 15 national health practitioner boards that are responsible for regulating each profession. The primary role of the National Boards is to ensure the protection of the public and to set standards and policies for the professions. The Nursing and Midwifery Board of Australia (NMBA) is the National Board for nurses.

National Boards must develop registration standards for their health profession. These include standards for professional indemnity insurance, criminal history checks, CPD, English language skills and recency of practice (*Health Practitioner Regulation National Law Act 2009*, s 38). In all states and territories other than NSW and Queensland, Ahpra, on behalf of the boards, manages investigations into the health, performance or professional conduct of registered health practitioners in conjunction with relevant health complaints entities in the states and territories.

To be eligible for general registration in a health profession, the applicant must hold an approved qualification for the health profession or one that is substantially equivalent, or gained under a corresponding prior Act (*Health Practitioner Regulation National Law Act 2009*, s 53). The National Board has the power to check an applicant's proof of identity and criminal history (*Health Practitioner Regulation National Law Act 2009*, ss 78–79). The National Board is authorised to decide if a person is unsuitable to hold registration as a health professional. Issues the Board may consider include: an impairment that would 'detrimentally affect the individual's capacity to practise the profession'; the particulars of the criminal history; competency to speak or otherwise communicate in English; current suspension or cancellation of registration in another jurisdiction; or a failure to meet other requirements about suitability to be registered or to competently and safely practise the profession.

Nurses must apply annually for renewal of registration or endorsement if they wish to continue to practise. In addition to reapplying for registration annually and paying a fee, all practising registered practitioners must undertake CPD for each profession they wish to remain registered for (*Health Practitioner Regulation National Law Act 2009*, s 128) and be able to demonstrate recency of practice. Nurses must annually declare that they do not have an impairment and that they have not practised the health profession during the preceding year without appropriate indemnity insurance (*Health Practitioner Regulation National Law Act 2009*, s 109). Other requirements include the disclosure of criminal charges and convictions, or disciplinary actions taken with respect to their profession in another jurisdiction (*Health Practitioner Regulation National Law Act 2009*, s 130).

The above discussion provides an overview of some of the provisions of the National Law. It is not definitive, and nurses should obtain a copy of the Act in the jurisdiction in which they practise and be aware of how it applies. Nurses should also acquaint themselves with the various nationally agreed codes of conduct and ethics, practice standards, frameworks and guidelines for professional practice governing their practice.

Complaints and notifications

During their practice, nurses may observe behaviour, conduct or situations they believe to be inappropriate or wrong and feel obliged to report another health practitioner for their actions. Reporting issues of unsatisfactory professional conduct or unethical behaviour through the proper channels is important in maintaining public confidence in the profession and maintenance of standards.

Notifications or complaints about nurses generally fall into three categories:

1 PERFORMANCE

Performance can be defined as the knowledge, skill or judgment possessed, or care exercised by, a registered health practitioner in the practice of the health profession in which the practitioner is registered. The NMBA may require a nurse to undergo a performance assessment if it reasonably believes that the nurse practises in a way that is unsatisfactory (*Health Practitioner Regulation National Law 2009*, s 170). Examples of unsatisfactory professional performance may include carrying out procedures to a poor standard or making and acting on decisions that are not clinically justified or evidence-based.

2 PROFESSIONAL CONDUCT

Unprofessional conduct of a nurse means professional conduct that is of a lesser standard than that which might reasonably be expected of the health practitioner by the public or the practitioner's professional peers (*Health Practitioner Regulation National Law 2009*, s 5). Professional misconduct is more serious and relates to unprofessional conduct that is substantially below the standard reasonably expected of a registered health practitioner of an equivalent level of training or experience. Complaints that are substantiated can result in the suspension or cancellation of the practitioner's registration (*Health Practitioner Regulation National Law 2009*, s 5).

Conduct issues are generally related to behavioural acts or omissions. Following the investigation of a complaint, disciplinary action may be taken by a professional standards committee or tribunal, depending on the seriousness of the complaint (AHPRA & National Boards 2023b).

3 HEALTH

Health (impairment) is defined under section 5 of the National Law as 'physical or mental impairment, disability, condition or disorder (including substance abuse or dependence), that detrimentally affects or is likely to detrimentally affect' a registered health practitioner's capacity to safely practise the profession. The NMBA may establish a panel to assess if a nurse has an impairment and determine a course of action. This may result in assisting impaired nurses to manage their condition while they remain employed or there may be a recommendation to make their registration conditional; for example, suspension of practice (Ahpra & National Boards 2023b).

Mandatory notifications

The National Law requires mandatory notification of notifiable conduct by registered health practitioners and employers. Notifiable conduct includes:
- intoxication by alcohol or drugs while practising the profession
- sexual misconduct in connection with their profession
- having an impairment that places the public at substantial risk of harm, or
- a significant departure from accepted professional standards that places the public at risk of harm (*Health Practitioner Regulation National Law 2009*, s 140).

Registered health practitioners, in the course of practising their profession, must report other health practitioners whom they reasonably believe have behaved in a way that constitutes notifiable conduct, or students who have an impairment that may place the public at substantial risk of harm while undertaking clinical training (*Health Practitioner Regulation National Law 2009*, s 141). Obligations regarding mandatory notifications extend to employers of a registered health practitioner (*Health Practitioner Regulation National Law 2009*, s 142). Education providers must notify Ahpra if a student has an impairment that may place the public at risk while undertaking clinical training (*Health Practitioner Regulation National Law 2009*, s 143).

Grounds for a voluntary notification or complaint against a registered health practitioner include a criminal conviction or criminal finding, unsatisfactory professional performance, unprofessional conduct or professional misconduct, lack of competence, impairment and/or that the practitioner is not a suitable person (*Health Practitioner Regulation National Law 2009*, s 144). The fact that a matter complained of has occurred in the personal life of the nurse does not exclude it from giving rise to disciplinary proceedings to determine whether the behaviour is such that the nurse is not a fit and proper person to practise nursing. For example, information that a registered nurse has been convicted of downloading child pornography will be referred and can lead to a disciplinary hearing with the prospect that disciplinary action will be taken and that the nurse's name may be removed from the register.

If a nurse enters into a financial, personal and/or sexual relationship with a patient or former patient, this can give rise to a complaint. The fact that the nurse–patient relationship has ceased does not legitimise the relationship if the circumstances were such that the profession regards the relationship as unethical. Such matters are regarded as 'boundary crossings' or 'boundary violations', depending on the extent of the conduct. Whether or not such a relationship falls within prohibited behaviour will be decided on its facts. Nurses are advised to seek advice regarding such actual or potential relationships, as it could lead to disciplinary action.

> **STORY**
>
> **Professional boundaries**
>
> A patient you have been caring for in the medical ward is preparing for discharge after a long admission. He knows you will be having days off when he is discharged, so as a token of his appreciation for the excellent care you have provided, he presents you with a box of chocolates. Because it is a relatively low-value gift, you accept it with thanks. When you arrive home and open the gift you find $100 inside the box, and a thank you note with his mobile phone number.
>
> **Reflective questions**
>
> Reflect on the scenario and answer the following questions:
>
> 1. What is the most appropriate action or response in these circumstances?
> 2. What could you do in future to avoid being placed in this situation?
> 3. When would this situation become a potential boundary violation?

Decisions of the courts and tribunals in each state and territory dealing with nursing matters are excellent sources of real-life case studies about complaints such as these. The Ahpra and the NMBA publish case studies that provide guidance about the application of the Code of Conduct for nurses, summaries of court and tribunal decisions, and links to the full decision (Ahpra & National Boards 2023a).

CONCLUSION

Knowledge of the law and its application to nursing practice has become a necessary component of a nurse's knowledge base. Nurses must be aware of and respect the legal rights of patients and the corresponding obligations of nurses providing nursing care. Failure to appreciate the legal rights of patients can lead to a nurse being open to legal action initiated by a patient or disciplinary action taken by a professional regulatory authority. Acknowledgment of, and adherence to, the legal rights of patients also underpins quality nursing care and the respect to be accorded to the profession. It is a professional obligation of all nurses to acquaint themselves with current legal issues touching upon the profession, and to do so by remaining up to date with their legal knowledge.

The discussion of the law and legal issues in this chapter is necessarily brief. This basic introduction does not purport to give legal advice. Should a nurse require legal assistance they should seek advice from their professional indemnity provider or a legal practitioner at the time that an adverse event that could give rise to legal action occurs.

REFLECTIVE QUESTIONS

1. Identify the legislation in your state or territory that impacts on nursing practice. How do you ensure the legislative obligations are incorporated into your practice?
2. Consider the codes of conduct and ethics and the standards of practice that apply to nurses in Australia. To what extent do you consider these documents adequately provide for the complexities of nursing practice?
3. Consider how you would ensure you had a valid consent for treatment from: a child; an adult with a significant acquired brain injury; and a person regulated as a non-voluntary patient under the mental health legislation.
4. Identify the basis upon which a complaint about a health practitioner may be lodged with the relevant authority and the possible outcomes that may result from the conduct.
5. Consider attending a Coroner's Inquest in your state.

Recommended readings

Johnstone M J 2022 Bioethics: a nursing perspective, 8th edn. Elsevier, Sydney
Staunton P, Chiarella M 2020 Law for nurses and midwives, 9th edn. Elsevier, Australia – new edition pending
White B, McDonald F, Willmott L 2023 Health law in Australia, 4th edn. Lawbook Company, Sydney

Cited legislation

Civil Liability Act 2002 (NSW)
Consent to Treatment and Palliative Care Act 1995 (SA)
Health Ombudsman Act 2013 (Qld)
Health Practitioner National Law (NSW) No 86a
Health Practitioner Regulation National Law Act 2009
Minors (Property and Contracts) Act 1970 (NSW).

Case law

Albrighton v Royal Prince Alfred Hospital [1980] 2 NSWLR 542
Beausoleil v Sisters of Charity (1964) 53 DLR 2d 65
Bird v Jones (1845) 7 QB 742; 115 ER 668
Bolam v Friern Hospital Management Committee [1975] 1 WLR 582
Chatterton v Gerson [1980] WLR 1003
Department of Health and Community Services v JWB and SMB [1992] HCA 15 'Marion's Case'
Gillick v West Norfolk and Wisbech Area Health Authority [1985] 3 All ER 402
Hart v Herron and Anor [1996] NSWSC 176.
Kalokerinos v Burnett [1996] NSWCA 288
Meering v Grahame-White Aviation Co Ltd (1920) 122 LT 44
Murray v McMurchy [1949] 2 DLR 442
R v Banner [1970] VR 240
Rogers v Whitaker [1992] 175 CLR 479

References

AHPRA & National Boards 2023a Court and tribunal decisions. Online. Available: https://www.ahpra.gov.au/Resources/Tribunal-decisions.aspx 18 March 2024

AHPRA & National Boards 2023b How we manage concerns. Online. Available: https://www.ahpra.gov.au/Notifications/How-we-manage-concerns.aspx 18 March 2024

Bibby P 2015 Prosecution of nurse Mavis Lopez over death of Nymphea Anderson permanently stayed. Sydney Morning Herald June 21 Online. Available: https://www.smh.com.au/national/nsw/prosecution-of-nurse-mavis-lopez-over-death-of-nymphea-anderson-permanently-stayed-20150621-ghtlez.html.

International Council of Nurses 2021 The ICN code of ethics for nurses, revised edn. Online. Available: https://www.icn.ch/resources/publications-and-reports/icn-code-ethics-nurses

Luntz H, Hambly D, Burns K et al 2021 Luntz and Hambly's torts: cases, legislation and commentary, 9th edn. LexisNexis Butterworths, Chatswood

New South Wales (NSW) Department of Health 2012 Policy directive: health care records – documentation and management. Document number: PD 2012-069, 21 Dec 2012. Online. Available: https://www1.health.nsw.gov.au/pds/ActivePDSDocuments/PD2012_069.pdf

Nursing and Midwifery Board of Australia (NMBA) 2016 Registered nurse standards for practice. Online. Available: https://www.nursingmidwiferyboard.gov.au/Codes-Guidelines-Statements/Professional-standards/registered-nurse-standards-for-practice.aspx 25 March 2024

Prictor M, Taylor M 2024 Privacy and confidentiality in healthcare. In: White B P, McDonald F, Willmott L (eds) Health law in Australia, 4th edn. Thomson Reuters, Australia, pp 411–464

Queensland University of Technology 2020 End of life law for clinicians: treatment decisions. Online. Available: https://end-of-life.qut.edu.au/treatment-decisions 8 Jan 2024

Richards B 2024 General principles of consent to medical treatment. In: White B P, McDonald F, Willmott L (eds) Health law in Australia, 4th edn. Thomson Reuters, Australia, pp 137–163

Smith M, Mathews B 2024 Children and consent to medical treatment. In: White B P, McDonald F, Willmott L (eds) Health law in Australia, 4th edn. Thomson Reuters, Australia, pp 165–220

CHAPTER 5

CULTURAL SAFETY IN NURSING AND MIDWIFERY

Rakime Elmir and Zoe Tipa

KEY WORDS

Australia
Aboriginal
colonisation
cultural capability
cultural safety
culturally safe nursing care
culture
First Nations peoples
Māori
multiculturalism
New Zealand (Aotearoa)
social determinants of health
Torres Strait Islander

LEARNING OBJECTIVES

After reading this chapter, readers should be able to:

- explain the concept of culture
- define the terms cultural safety and cultural capability and how these concepts inform nursing care
- discuss culture in the context of nursing and the healthcare system
- examine the role of cultural safety in improving access to healthcare services
- reflect and think critically about own values and beliefs when caring for First Nations and people from cultural and ethnic backgrounds that differ from your own
- identify specific considerations for the delivery of culturally safe nursing care for First Nations peoples and people from cultural and ethnic backgrounds that differ from your own
- understand how the social determinants of health can impact First Nations peoples and people from cultural and ethnic backgrounds that differ from your own.

INTRODUCTION

The populations of Australia and New Zealand (Aotearoa) have increased in cultural and social diversity. One of the most obvious contributors to this diversity is immigration. Migration impacts the host country's economic and health system.

Nurses are frontline workers in contact with patients, individuals, families and communities. To provide person-centred care for all people, it is important that nurses are aware of their own biases, are able to accommodate cultural considerations and understand differing constructs of health in their work. In recognition of Indigenous peoples as the original inhabitants, and their unique healthcare needs that stem from a history of colonisation, marginalisation and racism in both Australia and New Zealand (Aotearoa), in this chapter we will differentiate the healthcare needs of Indigenous peoples from the needs of people from other culturally and linguistically diverse (CALD) backgrounds.

Reflections

Think about what culture means to you. Think about your understanding of the word culture. What factors have contributed to your understanding of culture? How do you think culture influences nursing and healthcare practices? List any cultures you believe you belong to. Try and think more broadly than just your ethnicity.

Culture

Culture is a multi-faceted phenomenon that encompasses the common beliefs, values, behaviours, traditions and symbols of a group of people. Within a culture, particular behaviours are constructed and form part of an individual's identity (Drevdahl 2018, Ting-Toomey & Dorjee 2019). Although frequently associated with ethnicity, the concept of culture is broader and the word is generally used to describe subcultures, or groups of people with shared values who live similar lives. Belonging to a culture, cultural practices, beliefs and values influence social and emotional wellbeing (Taylor & Thompson Guerin 2019, Ting-Toomey & Dorjee 2019, Wilson et al 2019).

The concept of culture and its relationship to nursing
CULTURE IS DYNAMIC

The Nursing Council of New Zealand (NCNZ 2016) defines the concept of culture as 'the beliefs and practices common to any particular group of people' under the broad categories of: 'age or generation, gender, sexual orientation, occupation and socio-economic status, ethnic origin or migrant experience, religious or spiritual belief and disability' (32). A number of authors argue that assigning a set of differences to each of the categories that people other than the dominant cultural group can use as a method of identification or signification is an essentialist view of culture (Blanchet Garneau & Pepin 2015, Cormack et al 2019, Drevdahl 2018), which can marginalise individuals in the context of mainstream healthcare services. Using an essentialist definition of culture implies that cultures are static, that there are a set of characteristics and issues that members of each cultural group face regardless of context and that these cultural norms are handed down from generation to generation (Blanchet Garneau & Pepin 2015, Taylor & Thompson Guerin 2019). This concept of culture is problematic.

It is important to understand that just because people come from the same culture, it does not mean they will all believe the same things and act in the same ways. For example, consider Aboriginal people in Australia; there are hundreds of different groups who speak many different languages. Like all people, Aboriginal people vary in ethnicity, gender, spiritual beliefs and adherence to cultural practices (Červený et al 2022). Assuming all Aboriginal people can be considered a homogeneous group with a singular set of beliefs or qualities is misleading. Unfortunately, an essentialist view of culture can result in clinicians developing stereotypes and using a blueprint approach to try and explain the actions of peoples from specific cultural groups (Cox & Taua 2016). Having a stereotypical view of certain groups of people, such as First Nations, migrant and refugee peoples, can affect how we as health providers engage with communities, and could cause people to disengage or not access treatment or care when required. This disengagement can occur because healthcare professionals holding stereotypes can lead to biased treatment, discrimination and a lack of culturally sensitive care, making individuals feel misunderstood, unwelcome and mistrustful of healthcare providers.

Reformulating the concept of culture as a dynamic process, as opposed to a static entity, informs the concept of cultural constructivism (Blanchet Garneau & Pepin 2015, Cox & Taua 2016) whereby nurses and midwives begin with the individuals with whom they practise, and seek to understand their worldviews and their ways of being and knowing. In using this approach, people of a different culture are seen as individuals rather than as a member of a group with similar beliefs and qualities. This approach allows clinicians to work with people from different cultures by seeking to understand each individual as a unique person with qualities, beliefs and unique circumstances while taking their social context into account (Cox & Taua 2016).

REFLECTION

Before moving on to the next section, take a moment to reflect on your own definition of culture and decide if your initial ideas have most in common with either an essentialist or constructivist view of culture and think about what has influenced your understanding of 'culture'.

CULTURAL SAFETY

Dr Irihapeti Ramsden (2002) has had significant influence in New Zealand (Aotearoa) and internationally through her contribution to the concept of *cultural safety*. Originally proposed as a political response to the long-term effects of colonisation on the Māori people, cultural safety is situated within a framework of biculturalism between the Māori and non-Māori New Zealanders with the goal of better healthcare for all (Kurtz et al 2018, Ramsden 2002). Importantly, the notion rests on the principle that culturally safe healthcare is determined by end-users themselves, rather than by healthcare providers (NMBA 2018, Taylor & Thompson Guerin 2019). Cultural safety recognises the importance of individuals, families and communities being able to judge the quality and appropriateness of care provided to them (Taylor & Thompson Guerin 2019). The National Aboriginal and Torres Strait Islander Health Plan 2021–2031 states:

> Cultural safety is about how care is provided, rather than what care is provided. It requires practitioners to deliver safe, accessible and responsive care that is free of racism by recognizing and responding to the power imbalance between practitioner and patient and reflecting on their knowledge, skills, attitudes, practicing behaviours, and conscious and unconscious biases.

Much has been written about the importance of cultural safety in nursing and midwifery practice, particularly in colonised countries such as New Zealand (Aotearoa) and Australia, which are becoming increasingly multicultural and diverse. To guide the provision of healthcare, cultural safety is now a pivotal component of nursing and midwifery curricula (Australian Nursing and Midwifery Council 2016, NCNZ 2019) and nursing and midwifery registration (Nursing and

Midwifery Board of Australia [NMBA] 2016, 2018, NCNZ 2011). Cultural safety is not about developing in-depth knowledge about diverse cultures. It is about addressing structural inequities and power imbalances in health, education and research (Curtis et al. 2019). Grounded in critical social theory, cultural safety calls upon health professionals to continually reflect on their own sociopolitical contexts and how these influence their values, beliefs, assumptions and professional practice (Cox & Taua 2016, NMBA 2018). Health professionals have the right to differing cultural and religious views; however, they must ensure their views do not impede the provision of appropriate and culturally safe healthcare practice.

Cultural safety is about recognising barriers to clinical practice as a result of power imbalance between the healthcare professional and patient. The concept of cultural safety supports the idea that effective healthcare is possible and is better achieved through being aware of difference, decolonising health settings and practices, considering power difference, practising self-reflection and allowing a space for patients to assess whether a clinical encounter is safe (Curtis et al 2019). We will return to the concept of cultural safety and how you embed it in your practice later in this chapter.

Aboriginal and Torres Strait Islander peoples in Australia

In 2016 there were nearly 800,000 self-identified Aboriginal or Torres Strait Islander people in Australia, equalling 3.3% of the total Australian population (Australian Institute of Health and Welfare [AIHW] 2019). Despite their right to equal health status, Aboriginal and Torres Strait Islander peoples experience health disparities when compared with non-Indigenous populations (Davey 2022). For example, while the life expectancy of Australians is high when compared with that of the rest of the world, the life expectancy of Australia's First Peoples is among the lowest worldwide (less 10.2–10.8 years for men and 9.6–10.6 years for women) and they continue to experience poorer health and higher death rates than non-Indigenous Australians (AIHW 2017). Aboriginal and Torres Strait Islander peoples in Australia are hospitalised for intentional self-harm at 2.7 times the rate of the general population (AIHW 2024). The suicide rate is also double (Australian Indigenous HealthInfoNet 2019). Aboriginal and Torres Strait Islander peoples have a 50% chance of surviving 5 years after a cancer diagnosis, compared with a 65% survival rate for non-Indigenous people (Australian Indigenous Health*InfoNet* 2019).

The marked disparity in health between First Nations peoples and others has been directly attributed to colonisation and resulting marginalisation and discrimination (Wilson et al 2019). Prior to colonisation, Australia's First Peoples had a healthy, active lifestyle that included governance of the land and natural resources. Their lives and societies were complex, and rich with tradition and spiritual practices (Sherwood 2018). The arrival of British settlers in 1788 marked the beginning of systematic cultural destruction resulting in the loss of language, ceremony and customs; separation from country and natural resources; the introduction of devastating diseases; and racist policies and practices that disintegrated families and kinship networks (Cox & Taua 2016, Sherwood 2018, Wilson et al 2019).

Despite their poorer health, many Aboriginal and Torres Strait Islander peoples are reluctant to access health services because of the reliance on Westernised biomedical models of service delivery that fail to accommodate alternative constructions of health (Sherwood 2018). A lack of culturally capable practitioners providing care in settings that support cultural safety practices results in reduced access to health services. Discrimination and systematic racism in mainstream health services is well documented (Aitken & Seaton 2019). One important strategy to reduce the health disparity is the education and recruitment of Indigenous health professionals. Indigenous health professionals bring an understanding of shared lived experience, history, cultural skills and knowledge and contribute to culturally safe healthcare (Wilson et al 2019).

Māori people in New Zealand (Aotearoa)

In New Zealand (Aotearoa), Māori people represent 16.5% of the population (Stats NZ 2019). Like other colonised peoples, Māori have poorer health and social outcomes than other New Zealanders. While non-Māori life expectancy has continued to improve, there has been little change in the life expectancy of Māori. Similarly to Australian Aboriginal and Torres Strait Islander peoples, the disparity in health can be attributed to colonisation, historical trauma, damage to culture and family networks and racist policies and practices (Reid et al 2019, Wilson et al 2019). Māori have longer and slower pathways through the healthcare system and also experience difficulty accessing cultural and affordable healthcare (Reid et al 2019).

The Treaty of Waitangi (Te Tiriti o Waitangi), signed in 1840, is the founding document of New Zealand (Aotearoa). The Treaty is the basis for all legislation, and its principles are incorporated into all health service initiatives in New Zealand (Aotearoa) (Came et al 2018). The Treaty contains three Articles: Article 1 (Kāwanatanga) refers to self-governance, Article 2 (Tino Rangatiratanga) to Māori self-determination and Article 3 to the rights and protection of Māori (Orange 1989). The Treaty is simplified into three guiding principles: partnership, participation and protection. Together, these form the basis of cultural safety within the New Zealand (Aotearoa) health services and are intended to guide health service delivery (Came et al 2018, Cox & Taua 2016). However, there is a current debate that reference to these principles in health policies is sparse and largely rhetorical (Came et al 2018). The continuing disparities in Māori health has led to a tribunal to investigate the enactment of the Treaty of Waitangi in primary healthcare (Waitangi Tribunal 2019).

See Box 5.1 for other key dates in New Zealand's (Aotearoa's) history.

Box 5.2 identifies some suggestions to consider when working with First Nations peoples. It is important to remember not to expect individuals from a particular culture to be uniform; hence, these are offered as suggestions only.

Multicultural Australia

Australia has one of the largest proportions of immigrant populations in the world, with an estimated 29.7% of the total population born overseas (Australian Bureau of Statistics 2020). A further 21% of second-generation Australians (born in Australia) had at least one parent born overseas (Australian Bureau of Statistics 2017).

The Australian Government (2017:4) describes multiculturalism as being: '… one of our greatest strengths; … that equips us to build a future where everyone belongs and has the chance to live a great life.'

From a historical perspective, Australia's policies on immigration have evolved in response to social changes and a commitment to the development of society as a whole (Table 5.1). Since 1947, Australia's immigration policies have shifted between phases of assimilation, integration, multiculturalism and mainstreaming, to inclusiveness and being united in diversity.

Australia's multicultural strategic plan 2023–2025 states inclusivity and belonging are achieved through service delivery, community development, advocacy, building cultural capability and community

BOX 5.1
Key dates in New Zealand's (Aotearoa's) history

1300	East Polynesian people arrive—now known as Māori
1642	Abel Tasman visits
1769	James Cook arrives and claims New Zealand (Aotearoa) for Great Britain
1835	Declaration of Independence signed by 34 Māori chiefs
1840	Treaty of Waitangi
1865	Wellington declared capital in place of Auckland
1893	New Zealand (Aotearoa) becomes the first country to give all women the right to vote
1907	New Zealand (Aotearoa) becomes a dominion
1908	Population reaches 1 million
1933	Adopts own currency
1947	Adopts the Statute of Westminster (1931) and becomes independent of Great Britain
1952	Population reaches 2 million
1967	Decimalisation of currency
1973	Population reaches 3 million
1983	Closer Economic Relations (CER) agreement signed with Australia
1985	Waitangi Tribunal given power to hear Māori land grievances going back to 1840
2003	Population reaches 4 million
2020	Population reaches 5 million

BOX 5.2
Working with Indigenous people

Things to be aware of when working with Indigenous people include:
- Indigenous people perceive health and illness differently from the Western biomedical model. Be sensitive to alternative worldviews
- It may not be appropriate for a nurse to care for an Indigenous consumer of a different gender. Where possible ask that a nurse of the same gender is assigned to care for that person or ask if a family member is able to assist in any way. If this is not possible, explore solutions with the consumer; for example, delaying personal care till the next shift
- Indigenous consumers must be consulted and included in all decisions about their care. Sometimes this may also mean involving family members. Be guided by the consumer in this matter. Indigenous consumers often have an extended family and group of carers who all should be consulted
- Avoid asking questions about ceremonial business, bereavement, sexuality, fertility, domestic habits and other similar sensitive issues. If you are unsure regarding what is appropriate to ask, meet with an Aboriginal Liaison Officer for guidance. Engage in ongoing professional development regarding Indigenous culture

Adapted from Haswell et al 2009, Westerman 2004

TABLE 5.1
Periods in Australian immigration policy development

YEARS	POLICY	FEATURES	HEALTH POLICY IMPLICATION
1945–70	Assimilation	Predominantly White Australian Anglo-Saxon policies	Absence of government assistance
1970–80	Integration	White Australia policy relaxed and gradually abandoned	Relevant services provided
		Some cultural characteristics tolerated	Welfare needs of migrants being addressed
1980–89	Multiculturalism	Pluralistic approach to immigration Policies to limit discrimination on racial and ethnic grounds Cultural and ethnic diversity becoming more accepted in Australian society Cultural identity, social justice and economic efficiency were adopted	Provision of various health services Equality of access to culturally appropriate services
1983	Mainstreaming	Redirecting service delivery from marginal to a central base	Promotion of culturally sensitive health services
		Concern of government institutions based on social equity and access; economic efficiency and cultural identity	Equality of access to health services by immigrants
1999	Inclusiveness	Diversity Multicultural policies built upon civic duty, cultural respect, social equity and productive diversity The term *multiculturalism* to remain Inclusiveness	Promotion of culturally sensitive health services Equality of access to health services by immigrants
2000–08	United in diversity	National agenda for a multicultural Australia Policy framework including: all Australians are expected to have a 'loyalty to Australia and its people, and to respect the basic structures and principles underpinning our democratic society. These are: Constitution, Parliamentary democracy, freedom of speech and religion, English as the National language, the rule of law, acceptance and equality' (Commonwealth of Australia 2008:1–2)	Main components of 'Multicultural Australia: united in diversity policy 2003–06': responsibility, respect, fairness and benefits for all
2008–12	Benefits of cultural diversity	Celebrate and value the benefits of cultural diversity Emphasis on justice, inclusivity, trade, racism and discrimination	The People of Australia: Australia's multicultural policy launched in 2011
2013–17	Strength in diversity	Recognise the strength inherent in a multicultural society	Multicultural Australia—united, strong, successful: multicultural statement released 2017

Source: Commonwealth of Australia 1999, 2003, 2008, Department of Home Affairs 2020, Spinks 2009

events, working with people, and community, business and government working together (Federation of Ethnic Communities' Councils of Australia [FECC] 2021). Australia's multicultural society has benefits to social, economic and political advancement of the nation, and in the global exchange of skills and knowledge (FECC 2021). As migration to Australia increases, there is a need for health professionals to provide care that is culturally appropriate and sensitive to their unique healthcare needs (Tremblay et al 2023). People who experience healthcare as discriminative when they enter the health system tend to disengage with healthcare services and are less likely to seek healthcare advice when being faced with symptoms that warrant investigation or follow up (Tremblay et al 2023).

Refugees and asylum seekers

The United Nations estimated that in 2023, 2.9 million people globally sought refugee status or resettled and that approximately 1.4 million people sought refugee status in 2019 (Department of Home Affairs 2019, Refugee Council of Australia 2024). The Australian Government's Humanitarian Program aims to protect refugees who have been forced to leave their country due to a dereliction of human rights and warfare. In 2022–2023, 19,641 visas were granted under the Humanitarian Program (Refugee Council of Australia 2024). Over the past 10 years 8727 women who were considered 'at risk' were granted a visa (Refugee Council of Australia 2024).

People arriving as refugees and asylum seekers have complex health needs—they may have experienced severe deprivation, trauma and torture that can lead to post-traumatic stress disorder (PTSD), a condition that can profoundly affect a person's health and capacity to resettle (Patel et al 2022, Ziersch et al 2020). Despite the provision of comprehensive and cost-effective primary healthcare, people arriving as refugees face barriers to access such as lack of familiarity with the health system, differing health beliefs and/or cultural and language barriers, and lack of cultural awareness among health professionals (Lloyd et al 2023). In addition, many newly arrived immigrants and refugees transfer to regional and rural locations for employment and affordable housing (Lloyd et al 2023). However, social support networks and access to culturally appropriate services are reduced in regional areas, in comparison with urban and metropolitan regions in Australia, which can add to the barriers to access healthcare and contribute to poor mental health (Lloyd et al 2023).

Multicultural New Zealand (Aotearoa)

New Zealand (Aotearoa) has a diverse multicultural population of approximately 4.7 million people (Stats NZ 2019). While British migrants predominated during the first half of the twentieth century, the 1950s saw an increasing number of migrants come from the Pacific Island countries. However, since the 1990s there has been a rapid diversification of migrants arriving in New Zealand (Aotearoa) with increasing numbers coming from Asia. In the 2018 census, over a quarter of the total New Zealand (Aotearoa) population had been born overseas (Stats NZ 2020). In the 2018 census, 70.2% of New Zealanders claimed European ancestry, Māori represented 16.5%, Asian people accounted for 15.1% and Pacific Islanders 8.1% (Stats NZ 2019).

Correlations between disadvantage and the social determinants of health

The World Health Organization (WHO) defines health as a state of complete physical, mental and social wellbeing, not merely the absence of disease or infirmity (WHO 2024). The degree to which a society experiences health and wellbeing is largely dependent upon the social and cultural structures in place to support the nation's most vulnerable populations (AIHW 2018). Compared with those who have social and economic advantages, disadvantaged Australians, for example First Nations peoples, are more likely to have shorter lives, higher levels of disease risk factors and lower use of preventive health services (AIHW 2024). Australia and New Zealand's (Aotearoa's) Indigenous populations have some of the worst health indicators globally.

In contrast to the poor health status of Australian and New Zealand (Aotearoa) Indigenous peoples, most immigrants to these countries enjoy health that is at least as good as, if not better than, that of the Australian-born population. Immigrants often have lower death and hospitalisation rates, as well as lower rates of disability and lifestyle-related risk factors (AIHW 2018). The 'healthy migrant effect' is believed to result from two main factors. First, a self-selection process includes those who are willing and economically able to migrate and excludes those who are sick or disabled. Second, the government selection process involves certain eligibility criteria based on health, education, language and job skills (AIHW 2018). However, as migrants acculturate to their host country and make changes to lifestyle factors such as diet, the healthy migrant effect tends to deteriorate with increased length of stay. This is particularly evident in people who speak a language other than English at home (AIHW 2018).

Providing culturally safe nursing care

In New Zealand (Aotearoa), cultural safety education is underpinned by five principles. These principles address 'communication, recognition of the diversity in worldviews (both within and between cultural groups), and the impact of colonisation processes on minority groups' (NCNZ 2011:4, Wilson et al 2022). As it is beyond the scope of this chapter to explore the five principles in depth, we will instead discuss the overarching elements involved in achieving cultural safety in practice (Fig. 5.1).

CULTURAL AWARENESS

Cultural awareness is defined as 'understanding that differences exist' (Australian Human Rights Commission 2018:4). Developing cultural awareness is considered the first step towards cultural safety. In the context of working towards providing culturally safe care, it is important to understand that culturally safe practice is considerate of difference. It is also important to be aware of how cultures might be similar. Although this sounds like an easy thing to do, cultural awareness does not come naturally and must be cultivated (Taylor & Thompson Guerin 2019).

The objective is to care for a person in a way that respects their individual values and beliefs, culture and history (Cox & Taua 2016, Ramsden 2002). Attempting to treat every person the same fails to take into account inequitable access to privilege and opportunity (Cox & Taua 2016, Taylor & Thompson Guerin 2019). Once differences are acknowledged, their legitimacy can be accepted (Australian Human Rights Commission 2018).

CULTURAL SENSITIVITY

Accepting that all people are different is the beginning of developing cultural sensitivity. Cultural sensitivity is further developed through nurses and midwives reflecting on how their own cultures and life experiences influence their attitudes, values and beliefs about people from other cultures (Australian Human Rights Commission 2018), and ability to care for others. Cultural sensitivity is described as '… the ability to recognise, understand, and react appropriately to behaviours of persons who belong to a

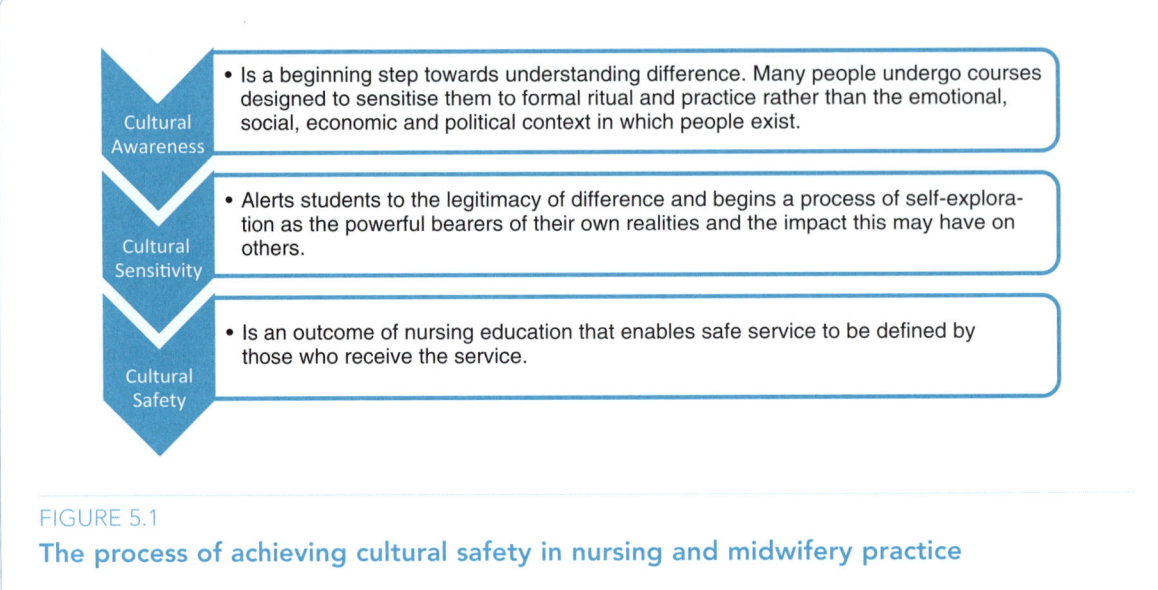

FIGURE 5.1

The process of achieving cultural safety in nursing and midwifery practice

- Cultural Awareness: Is a beginning step towards understanding difference. Many people undergo courses designed to sensitise them to formal ritual and practice rather than the emotional, social, economic and political context in which people exist.
- Cultural Sensitivity: Alerts students to the legitimacy of difference and begins a process of self-exploration as the powerful bearers of their own realities and the impact this may have on others.
- Cultural Safety: Is an outcome of nursing education that enables safe service to be defined by those who receive the service.

cultural or ethnic group that differs substantially from one's own' (Brooks et al 2019:385). In other words, cultural sensitivity is about applying knowledge gained from developing cultural awareness (Yu et al 2021). To be culturally sensitive, Best (2018:58), citing Cox and Taua (2013), stated the need for nurses to consider:

- their own cultural identity
- their assumptions about health, illness and people
- their personal definitions of health
- their patients' definition of health
- whose definitions of health are legitimised (by law and society)
- the implications of these definitions for nursing practice
- the consequences of these definitions for clients' healthcare.

It is also important that nurses reflect on how the colonial histories of both Australia and New Zealand (Aotearoa) have influenced issues of power and control in healthcare. Both healthcare systems are based on a 'white' biomedical model. This has resulted in an uneven power differential, inequity in health outcomes and structural racism (Best 2018, Cox & Taua 2016).

REFLECTIONS

Reflecting on the beginning activity, where you were asked to list the cultures you belong to, how do you think these cultures impact on your values and beliefs about other people?

CULTURAL SAFETY

Cultural awareness and cultural sensitivity precede cultural safety. Aspiring to be a culturally safe health professional means nurses and midwives have engaged in significant self-reflection on their own culture. They have thought deeply about the historical and social influences that govern healthcare in their countries and how this has manifested in biomedical dominance and power imbalances (Best 2018). Culturally safe nurses seek to mitigate imbalances between themselves and those they care for, through engaging authentically and respectfully with individuals to ensure that they understand their needs, preferences and beliefs about health and healthcare.

Culturally safe health professionals actively try to avoid cultural harm and are patient-centred (Červený et al 2022). They build rapport with their patients through respectful communication that involves active listening and responding appropriately to verbal and non-verbal cues through a process of cultural humility (Stubbe 2020). Where appropriate, patients' families are included in care planning and decision making. Above all, they understand that cultural safety is achieved when the recipient of care feels that their cultural needs have been satisfied (Yu et al 2021). Appropriate education and training can increase the cultural competence of nurses and midwives (Červený et al 2022). Cultural competence training and a 'person-centred' approach can increase a nurse's ability to acknowledge the differing cultural backgrounds and needs that people may have. Training can provide insight into customs of certain cultures that differ from one's own ideology (Kaihlanen et al 2019).

CONCLUSION

Meeting the healthcare needs of individuals living in multicultural countries such as Australia and New Zealand (Aotearoa) requires nurses to careful reflect and consider the impact of their interactions with individuals and their families. This chapter has provided an overview of each country's Indigenous and CALD populations and the ways this composition impacts on the role and function of nurses. A number of strategies to promote critical thinking and reflective practice around particular issues that impact nursing care are provided.

REFLECTIVE QUESTIONS

1. What are some of the factors influencing healthcare for culturally diverse populations and minority or vulnerable groups in Australia and New Zealand (Aotearoa)? Reflect upon those discussed in this chapter.
2. How are social context and cultural beliefs linked to health and wellbeing outcomes?
3. Take some time to think about your own cultural beliefs in relation to health and healthcare. How might your own beliefs be similar or different from those of someone from another culture? Consider how you will navigate similarities and differences in a sensitive and culturally respectful manner.
4. Consider the importance of changing the existing view of culture from a static to a dynamic process. What does this mean and how can a person achieve this?

Recommended readings

Best O, Fredericks B 2021 Yatdjuligin: Aboriginal and Torres Strait Islander nursing and midwifery care. University Printing House, Cambridge
Mkandawire-Valhmu L 2018 Cultural safety, healthcare and vulnerable populations: a critical theoretical perspective. Routledge, London
Willaims R, Dune T, McLeod, K 2021 Culture, diversity and health in Australia. Principles of cultural safety, 1st edn. Routledge, London

References

Aitken R, Seaton L 2019 Health inequities and cultural care. In: Brown D, Edwards H, Buckley T et al (eds) Lewis's medical-surgical nursing: assessment and management of clinical problems, 5th edn. Elsevier, Sydney
Australian Bureau of Statistics 2017 2071.0—Census of population and housing: reflecting Australia—stories from the census, 2016. Online. Available: https://www.abs.gov.au/ausstats/abs@.nsf/Latestproducts/2071.0Main%20Features602016?opendocument&tabname=Summary&prodno=2071.0&issue=2016&num=&view=
Australian Bureau of Statistics 2020 3412.0—Migration, Australia, 2018–2019. Online. Available: https://www.abs.gov.au/ausstats/abs@.nsf/mf/3412.0
Australian Government 2017 Multicultural Australia: united, strong, successful—Australia's multicultural statement. Online. Available: https://www.homeaffairs.gov.au/mca/Statements/english-multicultural-statement.pdf
Australian Human Rights Commission 2018 Cultural safety for Aboriginal and Torres Strait Islander children and young people: a background paper to inform work on child safe organisations. AHRC, Sydney
Australian Indigenous Health*InfoNet* 2019 Overview of Aboriginal and Torres Strait Islander health status, 2018. Australian Indigenous Health*InfoNet*, Perth
Australian Institute of Health and Welfare (AIHW) 2017 Trends in Indigenous mortality and life expectancy, 2001–2015: evidence from the Enhanced Mortality Database. Cat no. IHW 174. AIHW, Canberra
Australian Institute of Health and Welfare (AIHW) 2024 Aboriginal and Torres Strait Islander health performance framework (HPF) report 2017. Online. Available: https://www.aihw.gov.au/reports/indigenous-health-welfare/health-performance-framework/contents/tier-3-effective-appropriate-efficient/3-10-access-to-mental-health-services
Australian Institute Health and Welfare (AIHW) 2018 Australia's health 2018: Australia's health series no. 16 AUS 221. Online. Available: https://www.aihw.gov.au/getmedia/7c42913d-295f-4bc9-9c24-4e44eff4a04a/aihw-aus-221.pdf
Australian Institute of Health and Welfare (AIHW) 2019 Australia's welfare 2019 in brief. Cat. no. AUS 227. AIHW, Canberra
Australian Institute of Health and Welfare (AIHW) 2024 Health and wellbeing of First Nations people. AIHW, Canberra.
Best O 2018 The cultural safety journey: an Aboriginal Australian nursing and midwifery context. In: Best O, Fredericks B (eds) Yatdjuligin: Aboriginal and Torres Strait Islander nursing and midwifery care. Cambridge University Press, Cambridge, pp 46–66
Blanchet Garneau A, Pepin J 2015 Cultural competence: a constructivist definition. Journal of Transcultural Nursing 26(1):9–15 doi:10.1177/1043659614541294
Brooks L A, Manias E, Bloomer M J 2019 Culturally sensitive communication in healthcare: a concept analysis. Collegian 26(3):383–391 doi:10.1016/j.colegn.2018.09.007
Came H, Cornes R, McCreanor T 2018 Treaty of Waitangi in New Zealand public health strategies and plans 2006–2016. New Zealand Medical Journal 131(1469):32–37
Červený M, Kratochvílová I, Hellerová V et al 2022 Methods of increasing cultural competence in nurses working in clinical practice: a scoping review of literature 2011–2021. Frontiers in Psychology 13:936181 doi: 10.3389/fpsyg.2022.936181. PMID: 36092120; PMCID: PMC9449514.
Commonwealth of Australia 1999 Australian multiculturalism for a new century: towards inclusiveness. Online. Available: http://www.multiculturalaustralia.edu.au/doc/mcc_1.pdf

Commonwealth of Australia 2003 Multicultural Australia: united in diversity. Updating the 1999 new agenda for multicultural Australia: strategic directions for 2003–06. Online. Available: http://www.multiculturalaustralia.edu.au/doc/ma_1.pdf

Commonwealth of Australia 2008 National agenda for a multicultural Australia. Online. Available: http://www.multiculturalaustralia.edu.au/doc/multoff_1.pdf

Cormack D, Reid P, Kukutai T 2019 Indigenous data and health: critical approaches to 'race'/ethnicity and Indigenous data governance. Public Health 172:116–118 doi:10.1016/j.puhe.2019.03.026

Cox L, Taua C 2013 Sociocultural considerations and nursing practice. In: Crisp J, Taylor C, Douglas C, Rebeiro G (eds) Potter and Perry's fundamentals of nursing, 4th edn. Elsevier, Sydney

Cox L, Taua C 2016 Understanding and applying cultural safety: philosophy and practice of a social determinants approach. In: Crisp J, Douglas C, Rebeiro G, Waters D (eds) Potter & Perry's fundamentals of nursing—Australian version. Elsevier, Sydney, pp 260–287

Curtis E, Jones R, Tipene-Leach D et al 2019 Why cultural safety rather than cultural competency is required to achieve health equity: a literature review and recommended definition. International Journal of Equity in Health 18:174 https://doi.org/10.1186/s12939-019-1082-3

Davey R X 2022 Decoding the gap: Australia's ongoing struggle to address Indigenous health outcomes. Centre for Independent Studies Limited. Sydney. Online. Available: cis.org.au, ap37-web1.pdf

Department of Health 2021 National Aboriginal and Torres Strait Islander Health Plan 2021–2031. Department of Health. Online. Available: https://www.health.gov.au/resources/publications/national-aboriginal-and-torres-strait-islander-health-plan-2021-2031

Department of Home Affairs 2019 Discussion paper: Australia's Humanitarian Program 2019–2020. Australian Government. Online. Available: https://www.homeaffairs.gov.au/reports-and-pubs/files/2019-20-discussion-paper.pdf

Department of Home Affairs 2020 Australia's multicultural policy history. Online. Available: https://www.homeaffairs.gov.au/about-us/our-portfolios/multicultural-affairs/about-multicultural-affairs/our-policy-history

Drevdahl D J 2018 Culture shifts: from cultural to structural theorizing in nursing. Nursing Research 67(2):146–160 doi:10.1097/NNR.0000000000000262

Federation of Ethnic Communities' Councils of Australia (FECCA) 2021 Strategic Framework 2023-2028. FECCA, Canberra

Haswell M, Hunter E, Wargent R et al 2009 Protocols for the delivery of social and emotional wellbeing and mental health services in Indigenous communities: guidelines for health workers, clinicians, consumers and carers. University of Queensland and Queensland Health, Cairns

Kaihlanen AM, Hietapakka L, Heponiemi T 2019 Increasing cultural awareness: qualitative study of nurses' perceptions about cultural competence training. BMC Nursing 18:38 https://doi.org/10.1186/s12912-019-0363-x

Kurtz D L M, Janke R, Vinek J et al 2018 Health Sciences cultural safety education in Australia, Canada, New Zealand, and the United States: a literature review. International Journal of Medical Education 9:271–285 doi:10.5116/ijme.5bc7.21e2

Lloyd A, Wattis L, Devanney C et al 2022 Refugee and asylum seeker communities and access to mental health support: a local case study. Journal of Immigrant and Minority Health 25(1):176–180 doi: 10.1007/s10903-022-01367-z. Epub 2022 May 4. PMID: 35507214; PMCID: PMC9065235

Nursing and Midwifery Board of Australia (NMBA) 2016 Registered nurse standards for practice. NMBA, Melbourne

Nursing and Midwifery Board of Australia (NMBA) 2018 Midwife standards for practice. NMBA, Melbourne

Nursing Council of New Zealand (NCNZ) 2011 Guidelines for cultural safety, the Treaty of Waitangi and Maori health in nursing education and practice. NCNZ, Wellington

Nursing Council of New Zealand (NCNZ) 2016 Competencies for registered nurses: regulating nursing practice to protect public safety. NCNZ, Wellington

Nursing Council of New Zealand (NCNZ) 2019 Handbook for pre-registration nursing programmes. NCNZ, Wellington

Patel P, Muscat D M, Bernays S et al 2022 Approaches to delivering appropriate care to engage and meet the complex needs of refugee and asylum seekers in Australian primary healthcare: a qualitative study. Health & Social Care in the Community 30: e6276–e6285 https://doi.org/10.1111/hsc.14065

Ramsden I 2002 Cultural safety and nurse education in Aotearoa and Te Waipounamu. PhD thesis, Victoria University of Wellington, Wellington

Refugee Council of Australia 2024 Who are they? Where do they come from? Refugee Council of Australia, Surry Hills

Reid P, Cormack D, Paine S J 2019 Colonial histories, racism and health—the experience of Māori and Indigenous peoples. Public Health 172:119–124 doi:10.1016/j.puhe.2019.03.027

Sherwood J 2018 Historical and current perspectives on the health of Aboriginal and Torres Strait Islander people. In: Best O, Fredericks B (eds) Yatdjuligin: Aboriginal and Torres Strait Islander nursing and midwifery care. Cambridge University Press, Cambridge

Spinks H 2009 Research paper no. 29 2008–09: Australia's settlement services for migrants and refugees. Online. Available: https://www.aph.gov.au/About_Parliament/Parliamentary_Departments/Parliamentary_Library/pubs/rp/rp0809/09rp29#:~:text=The%20Integrated%20Humanitarian%20Settlement%20Strategy,assistance%20to%20humanitarian%20entrants%20today

Stats NZ 2019 2018 Census population and dwelling counts. Online. Available: https://www.stats.govt.nz/information-releases/2018-census-population-and-dwelling-counts

Stats NZ 2020 2018 Census totals by topic—national highlights. Online. Available: https://www.stats.govt.nz/information-releases/2018-census-totals-by-topic-national-highlights-updated

Stubbe D E 2020 Practicing cultural competence and cultural humility in the care of diverse patients. The Journal of Lifelong Learning in Psychiatry 18:49–51

Taylor K, Thompson Guerin P 2019 Health care and Indigenous Australians: cultural safety in practice, 3rd edn. Red Globe Press, London

Ting-Toomey S, Dorjee T 2019 Communicating across cultures. The Guilford Press, New York

Tremblay M-C, Olivier-D'Avignon G, Garceau L et al 2023 Cultural safety involves new professional roles: a rapid review of interventions in Australia, the United States, Canada and New Zealand. AlterNative: An International Journal of Indigenous Peoples 19(1):166–175 https://doi.org/10.1177/11771801221146787

Yu Y, Xioa L, Chamberlain D J 2021 Perceptions of care in patients from culturally and linguistically diverse background during acute and critical illness: an integrative literature review. Australian Critical Care 34:486–495

Waitangi Tribunal 2019 Hauora: report on stage one of the health services and outcomes Kaupapa inquiry. Waitangi Tribunal, Lower Hutt

Westerman T 2004 Engagement of Indigenous clients in mental health services: what role do cultural differences play? Australian e-Journal for the Advancement of Mental Health (AeJAMH) 3(3)

Wilson D, Aitken R L, West R F 2019 Working with Indigenous peoples of Australia and New Zealand. In: Brown D, Edwards H, Buckley T et al (eds) Lewis's medical-surgical nursing: assessment and management of clinical problems, 5th edn. Elsevier, Sydney, pp 68–83

Wilson D, Heaslip V, Jackson D 2022 Improving equity and cultural responsiveness with marginalised communities: understanding competing worldviews. Journal of Clinical Nursing 27:19–20, 3810–3819 doi.org/10.1111/jocn.14546

World Health Organization (WHO) 2024 WHO remains firmly committed to the principles set out in the preamble to the constitution. Constitution of the World Health Organization. Online. Available: who.int

Ziersch A, Due C, Walsh M 2020 Discrimination: a health hazard for people from refugee and asylum-seeking backgrounds resettled in Australia. BMC Public Health 20, 108 https://doi.org/10.1186/s12889-019-8068-3

CHAPTER 6
KEY CONCEPTS INFORMING NURSING: CARING, COMPASSION AND EMOTIONAL COMPETENCE

Jacqueline Bloomfield

KEY WORDS

care
compassion
compassion fatigue
emotional competence
empathy
kindness

LEARNING OBJECTIVES

After reading this chapter, readers should be able to:

- define compassion in the context of professional nursing
- explain the impact of compassion on patient health outcomes and the experience of healthcare
- describe the attributes of empathy and kindness and their relationship to compassion
- identify enablers and barriers to compassion and discuss ways in which these can be overcome
- explain what is meant by compassion fatigue and how this can be prevented by developing emotional competence.

INTRODUCTION

The importance of compassion in healthcare has attracted increased attention over the past few decades with patients consistently identifying its important contribution to their overall experience and quality of care (Malenfant et al 2022). Compassion has long been shown to positively impact a variety of patient-reported outcomes, including reduced symptom burden, enhanced quality of life and improved ratings of care quality (Watts et al 2023). Despite being recognised as a fundamental aspect of patients' healthcare experiences, and an indicator of high-quality care, the provision of compassionate care has often been found lacking in some healthcare organisations and in need of considerable improvement. In this chapter we will explore the concept of compassion within the context of nursing and identify its contribution to the professional nurse interactions involving caring. We will also discuss the importance of empathy, kindness and engagement when communicating with people and their families in the healthcare setting. Some of the enablers and barriers to the provision of compassionate nursing care will also be explored. Finally, we will draw our attention to the need for nurses to develop emotional competence through strategies such as self-care and self-compassion.

Compassion in nursing: a foundation of care

Compassion in nursing is more than just a concept—it is the cornerstone of patient care, and the essence of human connection that should underpin every interaction with people in healthcare settings. Although there is no universally agreed definition of compassion, it is acknowledged that compassionate nursing care is a complex process that necessitates a distinct set of skills and that is an essential element of professionalism in nursing (Bloomfield et al 2015). At its core, compassion can be described as the ability to understand the emotional state of another person along with the desire to alleviate their suffering. A more detailed definition of compassion from the perspective of a healthcare professional is 'a virtuous and intentional response to know a person, discern their needs and ameliorate their suffering through relational understanding and action' (Sinclair et al 2018).

We can see that this definition extends beyond empathy, a concept closely related to compassion, to encompass a proactive response that seeks to comfort, support and empower patients during what are frequently their most vulnerable moments.

Often when new nursing students are asked what influenced their decision to become a nurse, they speak of an important person in their life who was a nurse and the contribution of that person to people's wellness and comfort, including theirs. They may have experienced being cared for by nurses themselves or may have seen nurses in their work with close friends and family. Many students also describe themselves as being 'people-orientated' and that they like working with others, value health and helping others and want to make a difference.

REFLECTION

What or who influenced your decision to become a nurse? What personal attributes do you have that you think align with compassionate nursing? Nurses are the largest health workforce and are often described as the 'heart' of healthcare. Compassion can, therefore, be considered an essential element in the delivery of effective, quality nursing care (Ghafourifard et al 2022, Waird 2023). Compassionate care can be demonstrated through actions such as therapeutic touch, attentively listening to a patient's concerns, and the willingness to go that 'extra step' to promote comfort and ensure holistic care (Aagard et al 2018). Compassion is particularly crucial in the context of healthcare where patients may be experiencing anxiety, fear, pain or uncertainty about their condition or health outcomes. In such situations, a compassionate nurse will provide holistic care, and not only attend to a person's physical or clinical needs but will also provide emotional reassurance and psychological support.

One of the fundamental outcomes of compassion in nursing is its role in building trust between patients and healthcare providers. When patients feel understood and cared for on a deeper, individual level, they are more likely to openly communicate their symptoms, concerns and preferences. This, in turn, enables nurses to deliver more person-centred and effective care that respects the dignity and autonomy of each individual (Vujanic et al 2022).

Importantly, compassion in nursing extends not only to patients but also to their families and loved ones. During times of illness or crisis, family members often experience their own emotional turmoil and uncertainty. A compassionate nurse acknowledges and addresses these concerns with sensitivity and empathy, fostering an environment where everyone feels supported and valued (Ghafourifard et al 2022). Research has also consistently shown that compassionate care correlates with improved patient outcomes, increased patient satisfaction, and enhanced job satisfaction among healthcare providers. Nurses who embody compassion report a greater sense of fulfilment in their roles, knowing that they have made a meaningful difference in the lives of those they have cared for (Younas & Maddigan 2019).

> ## REFLECTION
> Have you or any of your family members ever been admitted to hospital? Can you remember how you felt at this time? It is likely that you may have felt a mix of anxiety, fear and uncertainty. How did the nurses caring for you help to alleviate these feelings?

Developing compassion in caring

In practice, compassionate nursing involves a combination of skills, attitudes and behaviours that can be developed through education, experience and personal reflection. It begins with the development of emotional intelligence, which allows nurses to recognise and manage their own emotions while empathising with others. We will discuss this later in the chapter.

Caring as a human encounter involves many aspects of human experiences. Caring occurs at the interface of interaction between the cared-for and the carer and has become in nursing a moral imperative focused on protection, participation and partnership (Donley 2014). Nurses can develop awareness of the needs of those receiving care and develop compassionate caring through physical, intellectual and emotional presence.

Empathic communication is a key component of compassionate caring that includes active listening, touch, eye contact and facial expressions. Effective communication enables nurses to fully understand a patient's perspective and to 'tune into' the values and needs of people and their families with whom they work alongside (Den Hertog & Niessen 2019). Active listening skills are also essential for compassionate care, as they enable nurses to respond accordingly and in an authentic manner.

Empathy and compassion

Empathy and compassionate nursing share a symbiotic relationship that is essential to providing holistic patient care. As you read the literature related to these concepts, you will see that the terms empathy and compassion are often used interchangeably. However, it is important to understand that there is a difference. Empathy, put simply, is the ability to understand and share another person's feelings. It is the ability to connect with the life of another person and to accurately perceive their current feelings and their meaning. Empathy begins with putting your own concerns and needs aside and being open to the other person's perspective and experience. You may have heard empathy colloquially described as 'the ability to walk in someone else's shoes'.

Empathy is fundamental in nursing and forms the basis on which compassionate nursing is developed. It involves nurses actively listening to patients, perceiving their emotions and comprehending their perspectives without judgment. Respecting patients' opinions, values and beliefs is also imperative (Babaei & Taleghani 2019). This empathetic understanding lays the groundwork for compassionate actions that aim to facilitate trust, alleviate distress and promote wellbeing.

In practice, empathy enables nurses to connect with patients on a deeper level. By tuning into patients' emotional states and experiences, nurses can provide care that is not only clinically effective but also emotionally supportive. This connection fosters trust and builds rapport, creating an environment where patients feel valued and understood (Vujanic et al 2022).

Compassionate nursing, on the other hand, takes empathy a step further by translating understanding into action. It involves responding to patients' emotional and physical needs with kindness, sensitivity and a genuine desire to improve their quality of life. For example, compassionate nurses not only empathise with patients' pain and discomfort but also proactively seek ways to alleviate suffering and promote healing (Nijboer & Van der Cingel 2019).

You may now be beginning to understand that empathy is the antecedent, or prerequisite, to compassionate care. When nurses empathise with patients, they are more likely to advocate for their needs, communicate effectively, and tailor care plans to individual preferences and circumstances. This compassionate and person-centred approach not only enhances patient outcomes (Byrne et al 2024) but also reinforces the therapeutic relationship between nurses and patients.

Ultimately, the relationship between empathy and compassionate nursing is reciprocal and mutually reinforcing. Empathy forms the foundation of understanding, while compassion transforms understanding into meaningful action. Together, they enable nurses to provide patient-centred care that respects dignity, promotes healing and cultivates trust in healthcare relationships.

STORY

Read the scenario below, reading through the perspectives of Bill and Chen.

Bill is an 82-year-old man who recently lost his wife to cancer. They had been married for 60 years. Bill now lives alone. Bill was admitted to hospital following a fall in the local shopping centre. He has a fractured wrist and lacerated shoulder that requires daily dressing. It is evening shift on the ward and Chen, a registered nurse, has been assigned to care for Bill.

Bill's story

I don't like being in hospital. I just want to go home. The nurses seem so busy, and no-one ever talks to me, especially as I am in a room on my own. I try to stay quiet and not ask for anything. I am frightened that if I ask for help, the doctors and nurses will think I am not able to look after myself at home and I will have to stay here for longer. I feel so sad that my wife has died, and I really miss her. Sometimes I feel so alone. The young nurse looking after me tonight seems so busy. I asked her for another pillow to put under my arm, but I don't think she heard me as she was looking at a computer, so I asked again very loudly.

Chen's story

It's another busy shift today and there have been some new admissions and some discharges. I haven't had time for my break yet. I have been assigned the six-bedded ward, as well as the single room with the old man. Once I have done his dressing, I hope that I won't have to go in there too often. He seems grumpy all the time and never talks, except for just now when he yelled at me … it was something about a pillow. I hope I don't have to care for him again tomorrow.

Reflective question

1. How may this situation have come about?
2. How could it have been avoided?

Enablers to compassion in nursing: cultivating a culture of care

Compassion in nursing thrives under the influence of various enablers, encompassing personal attributes, role models, leadership and organisational culture. These elements collectively foster an environment where nurses can consistently deliver empathetic, patient-centred care that goes far beyond simply following checklists or clinical protocols.

Personal attributes: at the heart of compassionate nursing are personal attributes such as kindness, empathy and emotional intelligence. Kindness, often expressed through simple gestures of comfort and understanding, forms the basis of compassionate interactions between nurses and patients. Kindness involves acts of sensitivity and consideration that go beyond the technical aspects of healthcare, demonstrating genuine concern for the wellbeing of patients. Using positive body language, communicating with warmth and genuine interest, engaging in short conversations to establish rapport and the use of humour are some strategies that can be used to demonstrate compassion (Ferraz et al 2020).

Empathy, closely linked to kindness, allows nurses to connect emotionally with patients by understanding their feelings, concerns and perspectives. As previously discussed, it enables nurses to provide care that is not only effective but also responsive to the unique needs of each individual. Emotional intelligence further enhances these attributes by helping nurses manage their own emotions while navigating the emotional landscapes of patients and their families.

Role models and leadership: effective role models within nursing play a crucial role in shaping compassionate care practices. Experienced nurses who exemplify empathy, professionalism and patient advocacy serve as inspiration and guides for newer generations of nurses. By observing and learning compassion from these role models, nurses can develop the skills and attitudes necessary to provide compassionate care consistently (Gharourifard et al 2022).

Leadership and a supportive team environment within healthcare organisations also play a pivotal role in facilitating a culture of compassion (Robinson et al 2023). Strong leadership emphasises the importance of and commitment to empathy and kindness in patient care, setting clear expectations and providing support for nurses to prioritise compassionate practices. Leaders who prioritise staff wellbeing, promote teamwork and advocate for patient-centred care create an environment where compassion is valued and encouraged at all levels (de Zulucta 2021).

Organisational culture: the organisational culture within healthcare settings significantly influences the practice of compassionate nursing (Robinson et al 2023). A culture that values empathy, respect and patient-centred care allows nurses to prioritise compassion in their daily interactions with patients and others. Policies and practices that support work–life balance, education and professional development, and recognition of compassionate efforts can be used to reinforce these values and encourage nurses to consistently demonstrate empathy and kindness (Tehranineshat et al 2019). Organisational structures that facilitate interdisciplinary collaboration and communication enhance the ability of nurses to deliver person-centred care and improve patient outcomes (McLaney et al 2022). Team-based approaches to care allow nurses to draw on the expertise of colleagues from different disciplines, promoting a comprehensive approach to patient wellbeing that is grounded in compassion.

Barriers to compassion in nursing: challenges and impact on patient care

Compassion lies at the core of nursing practice, yet several barriers can hinder its integration into nursing care, impacting both nurses and patients. These obstacles range from systemic issues within healthcare organisations to personal challenges faced by nurses in their daily roles.

Workplace stress: high levels of workplace stress, often exacerbated by heavy workloads, long hours, high workplace expectations and emotionally demanding situations, can diminish nurses' capacity for compassion (Maddigan et al 2023). When nurses feel overwhelmed or burned out, they may struggle to maintain empathy and respond compassionately to patient needs. Chronic stress can also lead to emotional and spiritual exhaustion and compassion fatigue, where nurses experience a reduced ability to empathise with patients' suffering and willingness to help the patient (Gustafsson et al 2021).

Personal stress: nurses also face personal stressors outside of work, such as family responsibilities, relationship issues, financial concerns or personal health worries. These stressors can impact their emotional resilience and ability to provide compassionate care consistently. When nurses bring personal stress into the workplace, it can affect their interactions with patients and their overall job satisfaction.

Time constraints: in fast-paced healthcare environments, time constraints pose a significant barrier to compassionate nursing care (Robinson et al 2023). Nurses may feel pressured to prioritise tasks and adhere to strict/rigid nursing care schedules, leaving limited time for meaningful interactions with patients or to assess their individual needs (Robinson et al 2023). This can result in rushed bedside manner and a perceived lack of attentiveness to patients' emotional needs.

Lack of human resources: a lack of human resources and understaffing is a prevalent issue in many healthcare settings, leading to increased workloads and decreased availability of nurses to provide timely and person-centred care. Vast amounts of paperwork or administrative tasks, and a lack of support and appreciation from managers have also been reported as barriers to nurses providing compassionate care (Valizadeh et al 2018). When nurses are stretched thin, they may struggle to allocate sufficient time and attention to each patient, compromising their ability to deliver compassionate care effectively (Naseri et al 2022).

Impact on patient care: the barriers to compassion in nursing not only affect nurses' wellbeing but also have profound implications for patient care outcomes. Patients who perceive a lack of empathy or rushed interactions may experience reduced satisfaction with their care. Importantly, compassionate care has been linked to improved clinical outcomes, increased patient compliance with treatment plans, greater satisfaction and an improved sense of responsibility for health (Younas & Maddigan 2019). When barriers prevent nurses from providing compassionate care, patients may feel overlooked or misunderstood, potentially impacting their trust in healthcare providers, their experiences of healthcare and their overall recovery.

Addressing these barriers requires a multi-faceted approach that includes organisational strategies to reduce workplace stress, improve staffing levels and engender a workplace culture that values empathy, supports teamwork and facilitates the promotion of compassionate care (Tierney et al 2019). Additionally, supporting nurses in managing personal stress and providing opportunities for professional development in compassionate care can enhance their resilience and ability to deliver high-quality, patient-centred care consistently. By addressing these barriers, healthcare organisations can create environments where compassion flourishes, ultimately benefiting both nurses and the patients they care for.

> ## REFLECTION
> Reflect on the recent COVID-19 pandemic and how this may have impacted the delivery of compassionate nursing care. Consider factors such as stringent infection control measures and the use of personal protective equipment (PPE), isolation policies and staffing shortages. What are some of the ways that nurses adapted to these challenges to demonstrate empathy and compassion?

Understanding compassion fatigue in nursing and its prevention through self-care and self-compassion

By now, you should recognise that compassion is one of the core elements of nursing care and have an appreciation of the role that personal attributes such as kindness, empathy and effective communication skills play. It is also important to consider the impact that practising compassionate nursing may have on the nurse themselves, especially if actions focused on self-care are not implemented. Nurses who are consistently exposed to patient distress, pain and suffering are at risk of developing what is known as compassion fatigue (Dobrina et al 2023, Oktay & Ozturk 2020). Compassion fatigue is the emotional and physical exhaustion that arises from the constant demands of caring for patients who are suffering or experiencing trauma and has been defined as: 'a state of exhaustion and dysfunction—biologically, physically and socially, as a result of prolonged exposure to compassion stress and all that it evokes' (Figley 1995). It is often exhibited as a diminished ability to empathise with patients and/or a negative response to repeated exposure to patients' suffering (Peters 2018).

Nursing students, as they transition into clinical practice, may encounter situations that challenge their emotional resilience. For instance, witnessing patients in pain, dealing with death and end-of-life care, or managing high-stress environments. These can all contribute to compassion fatigue over time. When empathy becomes overwhelming and difficult to sustain, nurses and nursing students may find themselves experiencing symptoms such as irritability, detachment and a decreased sense of personal accomplishment, which, among others, are all symptoms of burnout (Finnerty et al 2022).

PREVENTING COMPASSION FATIGUE

1. **Self-care practices:** engaging in regular self-care activities is crucial for nursing students to maintain their emotional and physical wellbeing. This includes prioritising adequate sleep and rest, diet and nutrition, exercise and leisure activities that provide enjoyment, relaxation and stress relief. For example, taking short breaks during shifts to practise mindfulness techniques or going for a walk during breaks can help recharge and maintain their emotional balance.
2. **Seeking support:** nursing students should seek out support from peers, mentors and facilitators to discuss challenging experiences and share emotions in a safe environment. Peer support groups or debriefing sessions after particularly difficult patient encounters can provide opportunities for validation, empathy and coping strategies.
3. **Setting boundaries:** learning to set boundaries is essential in preventing compassion fatigue. Nursing students should recognise their limitations and communicate effectively when feeling overwhelmed. This may involve prioritising tasks, delegating responsibilities when appropriate and learning to say no to additional commitments when necessary.
4. **Practising self-compassion:** self-compassion involves treating oneself with kindness and understanding during times of difficulty or perceived failure. Nursing students can cultivate self-compassion by acknowledging their own emotions and challenges without self-judgment. For example, they can adopt a mindset of learning and growth, recognising that all nurses and healthcare professionals encounter setbacks.
5. **Professional development:** continuous learning and professional development in areas related to stress management, resilience building and compassion satisfaction can equip nursing students with effective coping strategies. Workshops, seminars, in-services and online courses focused on mindfulness, emotional intelligence and communication skills can enhance students' ability to address challenging situations with compassion and resilience.

By integrating these preventive measures into their daily routines and professional development plans, nursing students can mitigate the risk of compassion fatigue and sustain their capacity to provide compassionate care throughout their careers. Recognising the importance of self-care and self-compassion not only benefits the wellbeing of nursing students but also enhances the quality of care they deliver to patients, fostering a supportive and empathetic healthcare environment.

REFLECTION

Consider the potential impact that compassion fatigue may have on you and your ability to deliver high-quality nursing care. Write some notes to identify the self-care strategies that you will implement in your daily life to mitigate the risk of this occurring.

Caring competence in nursing

Interpersonal nurse theorist Peplau (1997) coined the phrase 'caring neutrality'. She suggested that nurses are required to develop a level of congruence between what they say and how they act towards the person with whom they work. Compassionate care in nursing includes healthy communication and personal competence so it is useful for nurses to recognise and be careful about how they express their views, language, behaviour and feelings. Being authentic and hopeful are key ingredients for outcomes of the relationships in which we participate as nurses (Younas & Maddigan 2019). Consideration of our own unique capabilities and limitations can assist us to recognise this in others.

For nurses to effectively communicate, they need to develop confidence and the ability to recognise and understand emotions so they can use this awareness to manage their own responses and relationships with others. Emotional competence as a concept was developed within the fields of psychology and social science (Goleman et al 2013) and now features strongly in the nursing literature (Hurley et al 2019, Khademi et al 2021, Maya-Silva et al 2024). Many nursing theories emphasise that nurses should be able to develop relationships that include empathy to undertake the role of a professional. Moreover, the ability to manage our emotional life, while interpreting the emotional life of other people, is a prerequisite skill for any caring profession. As the students manage their emotions and tune into the needs of others, they become more able to recognise the patient's emotional needs and this enables students to engage patients in effective communication.

Humanistic nursing is a lived experience between human beings, so nurses need to move beyond the technical *doing* of nursing, to become able to experience the feeling and *being* of nursing (Richardson et al 2015). This emotionally competent approach to nursing supports the ability to move beyond the problems of health people may have, to the potential capabilities and relationships people may draw on to maintain their own health and independence. Emotional competence can foster reciprocity within nursing relationships by valuing relationships and supporting each other to create opportunities to gain confidence in relational being and a sense of trust in our ability to be with people, in ways that are meaningful and authentic. Feeling valued and supporting others extends in nursing to not only people we care for but also includes peers and colleagues from various other disciplines.

CONCLUSIONS

In conclusion, compassion in nursing is a profound expression of humanity that transcends the clinical aspects of healthcare. It is the foundation upon which trust is built, relationships are nurtured, and effective, person-centred care is facilitated. As the healthcare landscape continues to evolve and become increasingly complex, compassion remains a timeless virtue that defines the essence of nursing practice—a commitment to caring for the whole person with dignity, empathy and care.

REFLECTIVE QUESTIONS

1. Why have you chosen nursing as a profession? What compassionate attributes do you possess that align with the provision of compassionate care?
2. Compassionate nursing care includes a purposeful commitment to developing knowledge and skills to assess and intervene through nursing actions. These actions bring about positive experiences and change for people while preserving human dignity. How will you develop your ability to communicate caring?
3. Follow this link to learn more about emotional competence by taking a free emotional intelligence self-test: https://www.mindtools.com/pages/article/ei-quiz.htm

Recommended readings

Arnold E, Boggs K 2020 Interpersonal relationships: professional communication skills for nurses, 8th edn. Elsevier, St Louis

Dewar B, Adamson E, Smith S et al 2014 Clarifying misconceptions about compassionate care. Journal of Advanced Nursing 70(8):1738–1747. doi: 10.1111/jan.12322

Smith C M, Horne C E, Wei H 2024 Nursing practice in modern healthcare environments: a systematic review of attributes, characteristics, and demonstrations. Journal of Advanced Nursing 00:1–18 https://doi.org/10.1111/jan.16088

References

Aagard M, Papadopoulos I, Biles J 2018 Exploring compassion in U.S. nurses: results from an international research study. Online J Issues Nurs 23(1)

Babaei S, Taleghani F 2019 Compassionate care challenges and barriers in clinical nurses: a qualitative study. Iran Journal of Nursing and Midwifery Research 24(3):213–219 doi: 10.1136/bmjoq-2023-002651

Bloomfield J, Pegram A 2015 Care, compassion and communication. Nursing Standard (29):45–50

Byrne M, Campos C, Daly S et al 2024 The current state of empathy, compassion and person-centred communication training in healthcare: an umbrella review. Patient Education and Counselling 19 https://doi.org/10.1016/j.pec.2023.108063 doi: 10.1016/j.intcar.2021.100071

de Zulucta P 2021 How do we sustain compassionate healthcare? Compassionate leadership in the time of the Covid-19 pandemic. Clinics in Integrated Care 8:100071

Den Hertog R, Niessen T 2019 The role of patient preferences in nursing decision-making in evidence-based practice: excellent nurses' communication tools. Journal of Advanced Nursing 75:1987–1995 https://doi.org/10.1111/jan.14083

Dobrina R, Bicego L, Giangreco M et al 2023 A multi-method quasi-experimental study to assess compassion satisfaction/fatigue in nurses, midwives and allied health professionals receiving a narrative medicine intervention. Journal of Advanced Nursing 79:3595–3608 https://doi.org/10.1111/jan.15686

Donley R 2014 Teaching ethics to nurses. In: Hunt A (ed) Bioethics education in a global perspective. Springer, Pittsburgh

Ferraz S L, O'Connor M, Mazzucchelli T G 2020 Exploring compassion from the perspective of health care professionals working in palliative care. Journal of Palliative Medicine 23(11):1478–1484 10.1089/jpm.2019.0682 https://doi.org/10.1111/nuf.12274

Figley C R 1995 Compassion fatigue as secondary traumatic stress disorder: an overview. In: Figley CR (ed) Compassion fatigue. Brunner/Mazel, New York, pp 1–20

Finnerty R, Zhang K, Tabuchi R A et al 2022 The use of music to manage burnout in nurses – a systematic review. American Journal of Health Promotion 36(8):1386–1398 doi: 10.1177/08901171221105862

Ghafourifard M, Zamanzadeh V, Valizadeh L et al 2022 Compassionate nursing care model: results from a grounded theory study. Nursing Ethics 29(3):621–635 doi:10.1177/09697330211051005

Goleman D, Boyatzis R, McKee A 2013 Primal leadership: unleashing the power of emotional intelligence. Harvard Business Review Press, Boston

Gustafsson T, Hemberg J 2021 Compassion fatigue as bruises in the soul: a qualitative study on nurses. Nursing Ethics 29(1) https://doi.org/10.1177/09697330211003215

Hurley J, Hutchinson M, Kozlowski D et al 2019 Emotional intelligence as a mechanism to build resilience and non-technical skills in undergraduate nurses undertaking clinical placement. International Journal of Mental Health Nursing 29(1):47–55 doi:10.1111/inm.12607

Khademi E, Abdi M, Saeidi M et al 2021 Emotional intelligence and quality of nursing care: a need for continuous professional development. Iranian Journal of Nursing and Midwifery Research 26(4):361–367 doi: 10.4103/ijnmr.IJNMR_268_19. PMID: 34422618; PMCID: PMC8344623

Maddigan J, Brenna M, McNaughton K et al 2023 The prevalence and predictions of compassion a satisfaction, burnout and secondary traumatic stress in registered nurses in an eastern Canadian province: a cross-sectional study. Canadian Journal of Nursing Research 55(4):425–436 doi:10.1177/08445621221150297

Malenfant S, Jaggi P, Hayden A, Sinclair S 2022 Compassion in healthcare: an updated scoping review of the literature. BMC Palliative Care 21:80 https://doi.org/10.1186/s12904-022-00942-3

Maya-Silva L I, Del Gallego-Lastra R, Meneses-Monroy A et al 2024 A scale for assessing nursing students' emotional competence: a validation study. Nurse Education Today 133 https://doi.org/10.1016/j.nedt.2023.106046

McLaney E, Morassaei S, Hughes L et al 2022 A framework for interprofessional team collaboration in a hospital setting: advancing team competencies and behaviours. Healthcare Management Forum 35(2) https://doi.org/10.1177/08404704211063584

Naseri S, Ghafourifar M, Ghahramanian A 2022 The impact of work environment on nurses' compassion: a multicentre cross-sectional study. Sage Open Nursing 24(8):23779608221119124 doi:10.177/23779608221119124

Nijboer A, Van der Cingel MC 2019 Compassion: use it or lose it. A study into the perceptions of novice nurses on compassion: a qualitative approach. Nurse Education Today 72:84–89

Oktay D, Ozturk C 2020 Compassion fatigue in nurses and influencing factors. Perspectives in Psychiatric Care 58:1691–1700 doi: 10.1111/ppc.12977

Peplau H 1997 Peplau's theory of interpersonal relations. Nursing Science Quarterly 10(4):162–167

Peters E 2018 Compassion fatigue in nursing: a concept analysis. Nursing Forum 53:466–480 https://doi.org/10.1111/nuf.12274

Richardson C, Percy M, Hughes J 2015 Nursing therapeutics: teaching student nurses care, compassion and empathy. Nurse Education Today 35(5):1–5

Robinson J, Raphael D, Moeke-Maxwell T et al 2023 Implementing interventions to improve compassionate nursing care: a literature review. International Nursing Review 1–11 https://doi.org/10.1111/inr.12910

Sinclair S, Hack T F, Raffin-Bouchal S et al 2018 What are healthcare providers' understandings and experiences of compassion? The healthcare compassion model: a grounded theory study of healthcare providers in Canada BMJ Open e01970 doi: 10.1136/bmjopen-2017-019701

Tehranineshat B, Rakhshan M, Torabizadeh C et al 2019 Compassionate care in healthcare systems: a systematic review. Journal of the National Medical Association 11(5):546–554 https://doi.org/10.1016/j.jnma.2019.04.002

Tierney S, Bivins R, Seers K 2019 Compassion in nursing: solution or stereotype? Nursing Inquiry 26(1):e12271 10.1111/nin.12271

Valizadeh L, Zamanzadeh V, Dewar B et al 2018 Nurses' perceptions of organisational barriers to delivering compassionate care: a qualitative study. Nursing Ethics 25(5):580–590 10.1177/0969733016660881

Vujanic J, Miksic S, Barac I et al 2022 Patients' and nurses' perceptions of importance of caring nurse-patient interactions: do they differ? Healthcare (Basel) 10(3):554 doi: 10.3390/healthcare10030554

Watts E, Patel H, Kostov A et al The role of compassionate care in medicine: toward improving patients' quality of care and satisfaction. Journal of Surgical Research 2023 289:1–7 doi: 10.1016/j.jss.2023.03.024. Epub 2023 Apr 15. PMID: 37068438.

Younas A, Maddigan J 2019 Proposing a policy framework for nursing education for fostering compassion in nursing students: a critical review. Journal of Advanced Nursing 75(8):1621–36 https://www.ajan.com.au/index.php/AJAN/article/view/1073

CHAPTER 7

PATIENT PERSPECTIVES AND PERSON-CENTRED CARE IN NURSING

Horas Wong and Georgia Tobiano

KEY WORDS

accreditation standards
active listening
advocacy
agency
autonomy
biases
biomedical model
care continuum
clients
co-design
dignity
empathy
empowerment
ethical considerations
inclusivity
macro-level participation
meso-level participation
micro-level participation
patient-centred care
patient rights
patient safety
patients
person-centred care
person-centred practice
personhood
respect
self-management
service users
victim-blaming

LEARNING OBJECTIVES

After reading this chapter, you will be able to:

- understand the nuances of the meanings of terms such as 'patients', 'clients', 'consumers' and 'service users' in the healthcare context
- differentiate between 'patient-centred care' and 'person-centred care', comprehending both the similarities and differences in these approaches
- analyse the concepts of 'patient participation' and 'public participation', and apply these insights to develop collaborative, inclusive and respectful strategies for engaging with patients, families and communities
- assess and practise effective communication, emphasising active listening to understand the perspectives of patients and their families.

INTRODUCTION

Throughout your educational journey at the nursing school, you would have likely focused on acquiring essential medical skills and knowledge, such as understanding human pathophysiology, medications and treatments, and clinical techniques. These foundations are undeniably critical in nursing. However, it is essential to remember that nursing, at its core, is inherently a profession dedicated to caring for people. As the largest workforce within the healthcare system, nurses bear an immense responsibility that surpasses the mere biomedical aspect of life. We are not merely addressing conditions or diseases, instead we are caring for individuals, each with their own unique stories, fears, hopes and dreams.

The true art of nursing is realised in those moments of authentic human connections. It is evident when we sit beside a patient, take their hand and genuinely listen to their concerns. This practice extends beyond the application of clinical skills; it is about advocating for patients in every aspect of their care, understanding their needs comprehensively and respecting their distinct life experiences.

This chapter focuses on prioritising patient perspectives and embracing person-centred care in nursing. We will investigate the shift from perceiving individuals under our care simply as 'patients' to recognising them as complete individuals. We will discuss the significance of this perspective and explore methods for effectively engaging them in shaping healthcare. This paradigm shift profoundly influences both the quality of care and the overall healthcare experience.

In this chapter, we use 'person-centred care' to describe individualised care that emphasises the concept of personhood. While many may also refer to this as 'patient-centred care', we will discuss the nuances of these terms later in the chapter. Following this, we can maintain the use of 'person-centred care' throughout the chapter.

Who are we caring for? The patient vs client debate

When we consider who receives nursing care, the term 'patients' is typically the first to come to mind. However, in nursing and healthcare, terms such as 'patients', 'clients', 'consumers', and 'service users' are commonly used. As noted by Jackson et al (2016), the power of language and the choice of terminology can profoundly influence our perceptions and attitudes. Each term carries its own weight and meaning, reflecting the different facets of the relationship between individuals seeking healthcare services and the professionals providing them. Understanding the nuances of these terms is important, as they can subtly shape our conception of the subject of care, often without our conscious awareness. This understanding is key to ensure that our care aligns with the values and needs of those we care for.

The term 'patients' has been widely used by healthcare professionals in hospitals and other clinical settings to refer to individuals receiving healthcare or treatment. In recent decades, this term has attracted criticism. Originating from the Latin 'patiēns', meaning 'to suffer', some scholars argue that 'patient' implies a passive role, emphasising a person's vulnerability and dependence on healthcare professionals. They contend that the term aligns with a biomedical model that focuses on diagnoses and treatments, potentially diminishing the agency and autonomy of the individuals under care (Christmas & Sweeney 2016, Jackson et al 2016, Speed 2006). However, it is still regarded as the only term that reflects the uniqueness of the relationship between the care receiver and health professionals in the healthcare context, whereby the nurse has a crucial role in facilitating recovery and promoting health.

As healthcare models evolve towards more collaborative, autonomous and empowering frameworks, the term 'clients' has gained popularity, especially in mental health, psychology and social care. Originating from non-medical fields like law and business, some scholars believe 'client' carries a stronger connotation that the individual is an active participant in their care, indicative of a more holistic and partnership-based approach (Speed 2006). Other terms like 'service users', 'consumers' and 'customers' have also emerged in healthcare terminology (Christmas & Sweeney 2016, Jackson et al 2016). These terms are introduced to counteract the power imbalances and medical dominance associated with 'patient', promoting empowerment of those seeking healthcare.

Each term, however, has its advantages and limitations. While 'patient' has faced criticism for implying passivity, 'clients' and 'consumers' have also been critiqued for reflecting a business model of healthcare that emphasises efficiency and cost-effectiveness, potentially overlooking the altruistic aspects of healthcare (Goldstein & Bowers 2015, Gusmano et al 2019). Additionally, by emphasising the agency and choice of the care recipient, there is a risk of inadvertently encouraging victim-blaming attitudes towards those unable or unwilling to actively engage in their healthcare management (Cui et al 2019, Gusmano et al 2019).

There is still no consensus on preferred terminology. Many healthcare recipients may prefer 'patient' due to familiarity, but usage varies across settings and countries (Costa et al 2019). The Australian Commission on Safety and Quality in Health Care (ACSQHC), for example, uses both terms but they distinguish 'patient' as someone receiving services, and 'consumer' as a user or potential user, or their representative (ACSQHC 2023:149, 151). In comparing mental health policies, Cui et al (2019) observed 'patient' as preferred in policy documents in Hong Kong, while 'consumer' appears more often in Australia. Such a difference in terminological preference, as they argued, indicates underlying conceptualisations of mental health subjects and the sociopolitical, cultural influences on the healthcare models in each region. In Hong Kong, mental health *patients* are encouraged to depend on healthcare professionals for reintegration into the 'normal' community. In contrast, in Australia mental health *consumers* are expected to take responsibility in guiding the delivery of mental healthcare, and are respected as a part of the diverse Australian community (Cui et al 2019).

As healthcare models continue to evolve, the debate over the most appropriate terminology to describe those receiving care is likely to persist. More recently, with the shift towards person-centred language, terms like 'persons', 'people with lived experience' and 'survivors' have become more prevalent in certain fields of healthcare (Betriana & Locsin 2022, Costa et al 2019, Hunt et al 2022). In real-world settings, the choice of terms is influenced by individual practice, the values and culture of healthcare settings, and the broader sociocultural context. For nurses, being adaptable to different terminologies is important, but it is equally crucial to understand the nuances of terms, critically examine the assumptions they carry, and recognise how they shape our perspectives of the individuals we care for.

REFLECTION

In your clinical practice, have you noticed variations in the terminology used to refer to individuals seeking healthcare across different settings? What are the characteristics of these settings? Additionally, have you perceived any differences in the service models or in the underlying concepts of care in these environments?

From patient-centred care to person-centred care

Now that you have an understanding of the importance of being conscious of the terminology used to describe individuals receiving care, let's explore the nuances and distinction between 'patient-centred care' and 'person-centred care'.

Understanding the difference between 'patient-centred care' and 'person-centred care' is not an easy task, as the terms have overlapping meanings. Additionally, many people tend to use them interchangeably without thinking much about the philosophical meanings of what constitutes personhood, or how we perceive the body beyond merely flesh and bones (Gibson et al 2021). This has made the literature quite messy, as different authors use the same term to refer to different concepts.

Historically, the concept of patient-centred care emerged alongside the rise of the biopsychosocial model proposed by Engel in 1977, recognising the importance of psychological and social factors in health (Eklund et al 2019). Since then, it has played a central role in healthcare. Conversely, person-centred care, first proposed by Kitwood in 1997 in the context of caring for older people, is informed by the Rogerian principles in non-directive counselling and emphasises the philosophical concept of *personhood* (McCormack et al 2021, Tieu et al 2022). In the past 20 years, person-centred care has received increasing attention in the nursing literature, partly due to the negative connotation attached to the term 'patient' as we have discussed previously (Lambert et al 1997).

Several scholars have attempted to compare the core principles of patient-centred and person-centred care. In this context, Eklund et al (2019) undertook a comprehensive literature review, examining studies published between 2000 and 2017 that explored both approaches. They discovered that patient-centred and person-centred care share several key elements but diverge significantly in their primary goals. Both approaches emphasise empathy, respect and effective communication, along with tailoring care to individual needs and fostering participation, relationship-building, and a holistic perspective. However, the primary focus of patient-centred care is to improve functional outcomes. In contrast, person-centred care is dedicated to enabling a meaningful and purposeful life for the individuals receiving care (Eklund et al 2019).

Let's consider an example of an individual diagnosed with diabetes. Under patient-centred care, the primary goal for the nurse is to ensure the individual receives optimal care to maintain the highest level of functionality (Eklund et al 2019). Aligning with the biopsychosocial model, the care plan may include blood sugar monitoring and medication review. The nurse empathises with the patient's frustration or anxiety about frequent blood sugar testing and diet modifications, offering emotional support and building rapport with the patient. They may involve the patient's family members in supporting the patient through health education and clear communication of treatment plans and options. In the process of caregiving, the nurse respects the values, preferences, choices and relationships of the patient (McCormack et al 2021). This approach empowers patients to make informed decisions about their condition, encouraging them to actively involve themselves in health-related choices impacting their lives.

In the context of person-centred care, caregiving is deeply rooted in profound respect for the concept of personhood. This approach, as highlighted by McCormack et al (2021), stems from the philosophical questions regarding our identity as persons and our distinction from other entities. Key to this approach is to 'see the person', and the acknowledgment that a person is not merely an isolated, autonomous and fixed entity defined by physical and psychological characteristics. Rather, a person should be recognised as being embedded in their social environments and relationships, which are dynamic and evolve over time (McCormack et al 2021, Tieu et al 2022).

In this approach, nurses view the individual not only as a diabetic patient seeking healthcare, but also as a *person* with unique life stories, values and aspirations. The nurse also needs to recognise their own personhood and 'know their own self', by reflecting on their own history, values and beliefs, and understanding how these might influence their interactions with the care recipient (McCormack et al 2021). Empathy and therapeutic communication are utilised not just for building rapport and exchanging information, but they are also crucial in forming a comprehensive picture of what the individual values in their life and how they make sense of their experiences (McCormack 2004). For instance, the person living with diabetes may tell the nurse that they want to participate in a marathon, so the management plan would be centred around supporting the person to adjust their diet and medication around training schedules. The nurse also understands cultural dietary practices (e.g. religious fasting and food preferences) and other social constraints (e.g. limited time for meal preparation), while remaining aware of their own biases towards these practices. The healthcare team collaborates with the individual to develop a care plan that not only addresses medical needs associated with diabetes but also supports their broader aspirations for an active and fulfilling life. This approach embraces a more humanistic understanding of life. It acknowledges and integrates the patient's unique life goals into the care plan, fostering a more comprehensive and meaningful healthcare experience.

In a sense, patient-centred care revolves around an individual's role as a patient within the healthcare system, with a particular emphasis on the relationships between healthcare providers and patients. Conversely, person-centred care underscores the significance of looking beyond the patient's role, centring care around the individual's social life and relationships. In more recent years, McCormack et al (2021) have broadened the concept of person-centred care to encompass a wider application of person-centred practice. They propose a shift in focus from merely how healthcare professionals deliver care to a recipient towards fostering a healthcare ecosystem that nurtures a supportive and healthful environment. In this expanded view, the personhood of everyone involved in healthcare—not just patients but also staff, caregivers and other stakeholders—is respected. The aim is to create a setting where all individuals involved in the healthcare system can flourish, grow and transform (McCormack et al 2021).

It is crucial to emphasise that patient-centredness and person-centredness are not inherently contradictory, nor is one superior to the other. In the dynamic landscape of healthcare, these approaches often intersect in practice. The key takeaway is that both concepts, while grounded in distinct philosophies, focus on different aspects of care. Each approach offers unique contributions to the healthcare field, underscoring the importance of a comprehensive, integrated care model.

From theoretical debates to practice: keeping the individual and the public at the forefront

As we have seen, the essence of person-centred care (and patient-centred care) is placing people at the heart of healthcare services through individualised care. This approach requires actively exploring and comprehending the priorities of the patient, their family, caregivers and support network, thereby building trust and establishing mutual respect. It also highlights the practical necessity of aligning nursing practice with both the individual needs and the broader perspectives of the community.

There are several compelling reasons to adopt person-centred care. First, *consequential arguments* propose that such approaches ultimately lead to beneficial outcomes. Indeed, substantial evidence indicates that centring care on the needs of the individual improves health outcomes, as seen in reduced falls rates, and reduced agitation among people with dementia (Rossiter et al 2020), enhanced care quality and better experiences for patients and their families (Janerka et al 2023). Additionally, healthcare professionals report more fulfilling experiences of providing care and noticeable shifts in attitudes and empathy (Janerka et al 2023). At the organisational level, benefits include increased efficiency and service cost reduction (Janerka et al 2023).

On the other hand, the *ethical argument* posits that adopting person-centred care frames it as a fundamental human rights approach to health. This perspective is rooted in recognising the agency and autonomy of patients, as well as their rights to participation. Globally, the emphasis on patient rights highlights the importance of such approaches. For example, the Australian Charter of Healthcare Rights describes what Australian patients can expect when receiving healthcare. Statements such as 'be treated as an individual and with dignity and respect' and 'ask questions and be involved in open and honest communication' (ACSQHC 2020:1) affirm the expectation for healthcare practices that centre around patients' needs and voices.

Furthermore, *regulatory factors* also provide a strong basis for the practice of person-centred care (ACSQHC 2020). Worldwide, healthcare organisations are increasingly championing a person-centred approach, guided by specific organisational policies and guidelines. From a pragmatic standpoint, for many organisations, this shift is not just a matter of best practice but also a requirement for accreditation. For example, centring patients' and their families' wellbeing is a core principle embedded in the accreditation standards set by the Australian Commission on Safety and Quality in Health Care. Consequently, for Australian hospitals to be accredited, they must actively implement practices that keep patients and the public at the forefront of care (ACSQHC 2024).

> ## REFLECTION
> Think about a time when you promoted person- or patient-centred care in your practice. What made this encounter a satisfying experience for you? How could you continue to embed these practices to reap the rewards in your practice?

Encourage participation to shape healthcare practices

Beyond treating and respecting each person as an individual, person-centred care encompasses a collaborative approach in shaping healthcare. This collaborative approach encourages active participation, fostering a partnership where patients and healthcare professionals, educators or researchers or health organisations and authorities work together to involve patients in their direct care, or shape others' healthcare more broadly through activities like policy making.

Participation in healthcare can be conceptualised as a multi-level ladder, as illustrated in Table 7.1. Climbing higher on the ladder, more information flows between patients and healthcare professionals, and the patient or member of the public becomes more actively engaged in shaping their care or

TABLE 7.1
The continuum of engagement (Carman et al 2013), using the example of improving vaccination among people with disability

LEVEL OF PARTICIPATION	DESCRIPTION OF LEVEL OF PARTICIPATION	INDIVIDUAL-LEVEL ACTIONS	MESO-LEVEL ACTIONS	MACRO-LEVEL ACTIONS
High: partnership and shared leadership	**Information flow:** bidirectionally throughout the process of engagement **How patient or public input is used:** decision-making responsibility is shared; there is a promise to incorporate patient or public input	A nurse establishes mutual respect with a person with disability and their family members, and together they co-create an individualised vaccination plan and catch-up schedule that is based on the person's unique needs, accessibility requirements, and health concerns	A healthcare facility and local disability support organisations work together to design an inclusive vaccination program, involving individuals with disability in decision-making processes, from addressing accessibility barriers to implementing targeted strategies for vaccination outreach	Health authorities and disability advocacy groups collaborate to co-design a national vaccination strategy, engaging individuals with disability in decision making, from identifying vaccination accessibility challenges to developing and implementing inclusive vaccination strategies
Intermediate: involvement	**Information flow:** two-way interactions occur throughout the process, including understanding patient or public concerns and needs **How patient or public input is used:** final decision-making power lies with healthcare professionals, educators, researchers, health authorities or organisations	A nurse actively listens to a person with disability and their family to understand the vaccination history and unique considerations before providing tailored information and recommendations about vaccination	A healthcare organisation conducts a series of workshops with individuals with disability to gather insights into their vaccination experiences and needs, using this feedback to improve service	Health authorities create a committee with individuals from disability-focused organisations and conduct public consultations to assess the opinions and sentiments of the community regarding a pre-drafted vaccination policy
Low: consultation	**Information flow:** little interaction, tends to be one-way, such as obtaining patient or public feedback **How patient or public input is used:** their input may be listened to, but not always acted upon	A nurse educates a person with disability about the importance of vaccination, providing information without considering the person's concerns and social challenges	A healthcare organisation conducts a survey on attitudes towards a standardised vaccination program for all patients	A public health authority conducts one-off focus groups about a proposed mandated national vaccination program for certain conditions among people with disability However, they are not directly involved in the planning or execution of the program

Source: Based on Carman et al, 2013. Carman K L, Dardess P, Maurer M, Sofaer S, Adams K, Bechtel C, & Sweeney J 2013. Patient and family engagement: a framework for understanding the elements and developing interventions and policies. Health Affairs, 32(2):223–31 https://doi.org/10.1377/hlthaff.2012.1133

healthcare at the organisation or policy level. At the base of this ladder is a form of healthcare that is *'done to'* patients; patients are involved, but the healthcare professionals, organisations or systems have a set agenda and simply seek patient input (Carman et al 2013).

Climbing higher on the ladder, we encounter processes that more actively engage people, soliciting their views. At this intermediary level, healthcare is *'done for patients'*. Patients' concerns and voices may be considered when shaping the patient's own care, or shaping decisions made by organisations and policy makers (Carman et al 2013). Most clinical encounters and service development fall within this level. In these scenarios, while patient concerns are listened to, the care provided is still predominantly guided by a biomedical framework, with healthcare professionals, or educators, or researchers or health authorities and organisations retaining most of the power, and patients having a minimal role. This level of engagement can sometimes lead to tokenism, where superficial or symbolic efforts are made to involve patients and the public (Carman et al 2013).

In recent years, in Australia and other parts of the world, there has been a growing recognition of the importance of designing and providing healthcare services *with* patients and the public as integral team members or partners in the healthcare process. At this advanced level of the ladder, care recipients, families and their communities engage in a reciprocal partnership and share power with healthcare professionals, educators, researchers or health authorities, thus fostering a more inclusive and collaborative approach to healthcare (Carman et al 2013). It is important to note that higher levels of engagement are not appropriate for every situation, and we must work with the patient or member of the public to determine the right level of participation for them (Carman et al 2013).

As Table 7.1 indicates, participation can also be viewed through the socioecological framework, which encompasses actions at the micro-, meso- and macro-levels (Castro et al 2016), which will be elaborated on below.

MICRO-LEVEL PATIENT PARTICIPATION

At the micro-level, the focus is the individual patient and their interactions with healthcare professionals at the bedside, clinic or hospital. This level requires establishing a respectful, mutual relationship that addresses power dynamics. It is all too common for nurses to assume the role of an expert, perceiving the patient as ignorant or illiterate about their condition. This can lead to healthcare education and recommendations being made without considering the patient's lived experiences, often resulting in impractical advice and the unfair labelling of patients as non-compliant or difficult when they cannot meet the standards set by nurses. Such an approach disempowers the patient and discourages their participation in care.

Many terms are often used synonymously for participation, such as engagement and involvement in this context. Regardless of the term used, the essence remains that patient participation is about patients and nurses interacting in a mutual partnership (Jerofke-Owen et al 2023). Both parties bring different attributes to the partnership; for example, patients bring their lived experience of illness and nurses bring expertise learned from the nursing curricula, and they work together to enable the patient to have an active role in their care, at a level of participation that aligns with the patient's preferences (Jerofke-Owen et al 2023).

To foster a successful partnership, nurses must critically reflect on their own assumptions and social standings, understanding how these may impact their relationship with patients.

This becomes particularly important when working with socially marginalised and disadvantaged groups, such as First Nations peoples, refugees and asylum seekers, people with disability, and those living with HIV/AIDS. As nurses, we have to remind ourselves not to bring our implicit biases to the care.

Therapeutic communication skills are fundamental, including proper introductions, active listening, empathy, reflection on content and emotions, and effective summarising of conversations. Nurses should inform patients to prepare them for participation and explicitly invite and encourage patients to participate in their care (Thórarinsdóttir & Kristjánsson 2014, Tobiano et al 2015). When working with culturally and linguistically diverse patients, nurses need to consider factors such as involving interpreters and peer workers, to address language needs and different cultural expectation in healthcare. When caring for individuals who may not be able to fully participate, such as young children, people with impaired cognition and people with intellectual disability, nurses have a responsibility to consider who should be involved in the decision-making process. Typically, this will be guided by respective service guidelines and regulations. Decisions should be made collaboratively, involving people such as the patient's carers, family, physicians, allied health professionals and social workers, to ensure a comprehensive and inclusive approach to patient care.

There are many simple ways to encourage the patient to participate in their care, in partnership with nurses. Let us consider a patient's admission to a hospital. Participation can encompass both verbal and physical activities that are already integrated into routine nursing care (Castro et al 2016, Thórarinsdóttir & Kristjánsson 2014). For instance, bedside handovers during shift change, where outgoing and incoming nurses exchange information about the patient, can be conducted at the patient's bedside instead of at the nursing station. This practice encourages active verbal patient participation by sharing of information *with* the patient, as outlined in Table 7.2, which shows examples of how a patient can participate in, and the information they could contribute to, the handover (Tobiano et al 2018).

Physical forms of participation that can be encouraged in hospital settings include encouraging patients in activities such as washing and dressing, engaging in medication management and working on enhancing their mobility (van Belle et al 2020). These activities not only promote patient independence, but also prepare them for self-management once discharged home (Thórarinsdóttir & Kristjánsson 2014, Tobiano et al 2015). However, a challenge arises when nurses inadvertently maintain control over these activities, limiting patient participation in their own care (Tobiano et al 2015). Therefore, patient involvement in these aspects of care is essential for their successful transition back to daily life after hospitalisation.

TABLE 7.2
How patients can verbally participate in bedside handover

ACTIONS	INFORMATION CONTENT AREAS
Listening	• Nursing care (conducted on previous shift or upcoming shift and beyond) and medical treatment • Patient status (how the patient is progressing and feeling, their readiness for discharge, and symptoms)
Adding information	
Asking and answering questions	
Identifying misses or wrong information	

> **STORY**
>
> Jane Smith, 42 years old, was recently admitted to the hospital for an amputation procedure due to complications arising from prolonged injecting drug use. Jane, who has been using drugs for several years, developed a severe infection in her left leg, ultimately necessitating amputation.
>
> Jane's journey into substance use began in her late twenties as a way to cope with personal stress and psychological trauma. Despite multiple attempts at rehabilitation, Jane struggled to maintain long-term abstinence.
>
> The decision to amputate was a difficult but necessary one, given the severity of the infection and the risk it posed to her overall health. Post-amputation, Jane is experiencing a mix of emotions, including grief over the loss of her limb and anxiety about the future. She is also struggling with feelings of guilt and shame related to her drug use and its consequences.
>
> **Reflective questions**
>
> You are the nurse who is taking care of Jane after her surgery; reflect on the following questions:
>
> 1. What do you think about people who inject drugs? How might these perceptions affect your interactions with Jane?
> 2. How could you encourage verbal patient participation from Jane, and what benefit would this have for her?
> 3. How could you encourage physical patient participation to enhance Jane's self-management practices once home?
> 4. What behaviours could you display to encourage Jane to actively participate in her own care? What behaviours should you avoid?

MESO- AND MACRO-LEVEL PATIENT AND PUBLIC PARTICIPATION

We must not overlook the crucial role that nurses play beyond bedside care. At the meso-level, the primary objective is to encourage participation in interactions with various organisations, institutions, networks and agencies. Meanwhile, macro-level participation involves engaging patients and the public at a collective and societal level, with the goal of benefiting healthcare service users and the large population. Here, patients and the public collaborate with health services, authorities and researchers to make a substantial impact on the healthcare landscape. Taking a broader perspective of participation at the meso- and macro-levels, terms like 'consumer', 'citizen', 'public', 'community' and 'service user' are more commonly used than 'patient' to encompass a wider range of people with shared health experiences. This includes not only the patient themselves but also their family, carers, significant others, and the broader community (Carlini et al 2023, Hoddinott et al 2018).

Table 7.3 presents a range of examples of activities that patients and the public can undertake at the meso- and macro-level, which will be elaborated on. For example, many hospital and community health services have consumer groups to ensure those utilising their services have a meaningful and effective voice in shaping healthcare delivery (Carlini et al 2023). These groups enhance and evaluate the services by providing insider insights and knowledge based on their lived experiences, suggesting areas for improving healthcare quality and accessibility (Carlini et al 2023).

TABLE 7.3
Examples of patient and public participation at the meso- and macro-level

LEVEL OF PARTICIPATION	TYPE OF PARTICIPATION	EXAMPLES OF SOME ACTIVITIES (LIST NOT EXHAUSTIVE)	REFERENCES
Meso-level	Service development and evaluation	Participate in facilitated meetings or workshops by sharing their perspectives, concerns and ideas directly with decision makers. For example, patients and the public usually sit on hospital committees to ensure the Australian Commission on Safety and Quality in Health Care standards are met	Carlini et al 2023, Jamieson Gilmore et al 2023
		Participation in patient journey or touchpoint mapping whereby the patient's journey of care is visually represented, including all points of interaction within the journey	
		Share personal experiences in reflections or filmed narratives. Healthcare professionals and decision makers can watch these powerful accounts of patient and public perspectives	
		Provide feedback and complete surveys. For example, healthcare facilities may administer patient experience of care surveys on hospital discharge, and review these data to inform changes	
	Education and training	Volunteer in a scripted scenario in a classroom, which allows students to assess patient history or practise a clinical exam on a real-life member of the public	Towle et al 2010
		Share their lived experiences in a session planned by the faculty	
		Patients and the public can be teachers who deliver education and evaluate student performance	
		Contribute to curriculum development	
Macro-level	Policy	Participate in citizen juries, where 12–20 citizens meet over several days to discuss a specific health issue. After these discussions conclusions are summarised and reported to decision makers	Baumann et al 2022
		Participate in citizen advisory committees or citizen health councils, which can engage citizens in discussions about a specific issue or varying health issues, and are typically implemented as a continuing advisory group for the decision makers	
		Complete public opinion surveys, a broad approach where surveys are administered to large representative samples to get their view on a specific health issue	
	Research	Be a member of the research team, whereby two or more patients or members of the public shape all decisions throughout the life cycle of the research project, acting with the same level of decision-making power as research academics. These patients and members of the public may collect data (i.e. conduct interviews) and assist with analysis	Domecq et al 2014, Hawkins et al 2017, McCarron et al 2021, Yoshida 2016

Continued

TABLE 7.3
Examples of patient and public participation at the meso- and macro-level—cont'd

LEVEL OF PARTICIPATION	TYPE OF PARTICIPATION	EXAMPLES OF SOME ACTIVITIES (LIST NOT EXHAUSTIVE)	REFERENCES
		Participate in co-design meetings, whereby consumers and researchers collaborate together to design new approaches to healthcare, to test under research conditions. For example, co-designers may participate in a series of workshops to develop an intervention to prevent illicit drug use among secondary-school students; the co-designers would generate ideas for the program, help refine the program and provide ongoing feedback during implementation and evaluation of the program	
		Be part of a consumer reference group, who provide advice on the research project. They have set meetings throughout the project that are focused on getting patient and public input on issues like recruitment difficulties, and they may review research documents and advise on research plans	
		Taking part in priority setting activity to identify what needs to be researched. This could take the form of a community conversation where community members come to a facilitated workshop to identify research questions that are significant. Or more formal approaches can be used such as the process developed by the James Lind Alliance	

Another example is patient participation in teaching and education, an approach that has been around since the 1960s and is increasingly recognised (Towle et al 2010). Patients can take on the role of teacher in learning environments like university classrooms, directly shaping budding healthcare professionals' practice by creating more real-world learning environments. As the educator, patients may participate in scripted scenarios, give presentations, evaluate student performance or develop curriculum (see Table 7.3).

Another common form of patient participation is engaging the public in health research, which has increasingly been recognised as a highly effective method for making a significant impact on improving people's lives. This approach contrasts with more traditional medical research where patients and the public are typically passive participants, merely providing data for researchers. Table 7.3 outlines various ways to engage patients and the public in the research process, ensuring they are actively included and inform decisions throughout the life cycle of a research project, from the design and planning stage, to conducting the research, developing and trialling the interventions, and disseminating the results (Manafo et al 2018). As previously mentioned in Table 7.1, patients and the public can engage at various levels. Success at the 'partnership' level in health research requires establishment and maintenance of an equal, reciprocal, ongoing relationship among patients and the public and researchers. An increasingly popular approach to achieving this level of engagement is co-design; nurses have led and participated in co-design research on various topics, such as co-developing communication tools to facilitate better interactions between practitioners and older patients in transitional care (Allen et al 2022), co-creating nurse-led models of care to increase access to medical abortion and contraception in rural and regional areas (Mazza et al 2023), and enhancing the engagement of First Nations Australians in emergency departments (Davison et al 2024).

Participation also plays a significant role in policy making. Policy participation involves decision makers at state and national levels cooperating with the public on healthcare decisions (Baumann et al 2022). A case in point is in Australia, where the Queensland Ministry of Health collaborates with Health Consumers Queensland to provide a platform for senior leaders in health to listen to and learn from health consumers, as well as to gather feedback on policies during the initial stages of planning (https://www.hcq.org.au/collaborative/). Furthermore, the Australian Government facilitates public health policy consultations through initiatives like the Consultation Hub, where the public can express opinions and engage in various health policies and programs (https://consultations.health.gov.au/). The rise of social media has further revolutionised the manner in which health consumers advocate for and participate in the public health policy arena, especially in the context of the COVID pandemic (Tsao et al 2021). This digital transformation has opened new avenues for public engagement, allowing for broader and more diverse input into health policy development and reform.

> ### REFLECTION
> 1. Often when working in a clinical role, you may only think of patient participation at the micro-level, as this is what you experience daily. What activities in Table 7.3 were unknown or surprising to you?
> 2. When working clinically, how do you think the activities in Table 7.3 could ultimately influence your clinical practice?

Ethical considerations in person-centred care and patient participation

Before we wrap up this chapter, it is crucial to highlight the ethical considerations intertwined with person-centred care and participation. For instance, how do we maintain a balance between respecting patient autonomy and ensuring the safety and wellbeing of the patient themselves and the people around them, especially in cases like anti-vaccination beliefs or refusal of treatment? Additionally, how can we enable meaningful participation in decision making for individuals who might have limited cognitive capacity or maturity, such as those with dementia, intellectual disabilities or children? These questions highlight the complexities in providing person-centred care while navigating ethical and practical challenges.

These are complex issues without straightforward solutions. The bottom line for nurses is to adhere to legal guidelines and ethical principles, including informed decision making and respect for autonomy, as you have seen in another chapter of this book. Nurses should endeavour to work collaboratively with the patient or individuals who know them well, like their caregivers and family members, and with the other members of the healthcare team. This collaborative approach aims to maximise participation in the decision-making process, while upholding the patient's and their loved ones' dignity and wellbeing. This includes ongoing reflections, dialogues and considering alternative strategies that might deviate from traditional biomedical perspectives.

> **STORY**
>
> Let's reconsider the case of Jane Smith. After being discharged home, Jane is facing difficulties managing her pain post-amputation. During a follow-up visit, she reveals to the community nurse that she has resumed using drugs to cope with the physical pain.
>
> Reflective questions
>
> 1. How can a nurse effectively advocate for individuals like Jane at meso- or macro-levels, such as through hospital committees or nursing organisations, to ensure the development of better policies for those with a history of drug use?
> 2. In what ways can a nurse collaborate with interdisciplinary teams or community groups to develop and propose comprehensive care models that include mental health support, counselling for drug use and social support for individuals like Jane post-rehabilitation?
> 3. How can the community nurse navigate the ethical challenge of intervening in situations where Jane's choices might pose a risk to her health or safety, while still maintaining a respectful and supportive patient–nurse relationship?

CONCLUSION

This chapter has introduced you to the essential concepts of patient perspectives and person-centred care in nursing, providing a foundation for your journey as future healthcare professionals. We have guided you through the nuanced meanings of terms like 'patients', 'clients', 'consumers' and 'service-users', highlighting how language shapes our approach to care. We have explored the differences and overlaps between patient-centred and person-centred care, gaining insight into the importance of considering each individual's unique story, values and life context.

Throughout this chapter, we have emphasised the need for nurses to transcend traditional biomedical approaches, advocating for meaningful and multi-level participation in healthcare. Ranging from the intimate micro-level of bedside interactions to the expansive meso- and macro-levels involving healthcare systems and policies, your role as a nurse is central in holistically and ethically shaping patient experiences and outcomes. As you progress in your nursing education and embark on your career, carry with you the principles highlighted in this chapter. Commit to the transition from viewing individuals merely as patients to seeing them as complete beings with diverse stories and life aspirations.

Recommended readings

Costa D S J, Mercieca-Bebber R, Tesson S, Seidler Z, Lopez A L 2019 Patient, client, consumer, survivor or other alternatives? A scoping review of preferred terms for labelling individuals who access healthcare across settings. BMJ Open 9(3):e025166 https://doi.org/10.1136/bmjopen-2018-025166

Hoddinott P, Pollock A, O'Cathain A et al 2018 How to incorporate patient and public perspectives into the design and conduct of research. F1000Research 7:752 https://doi.org/10.12688/f1000research.15162.1

McCormack B, McCance T, Bulley C et al (eds) 2021 Fundamentals of person-centred healthcare practice. John Wiley & Sons

Thórarinsdóttir K, Kristjánsson K 2014 Patients' perspectives on person-centred participation in healthcare: a framework analysis. Nursing Ethics 21(2):129–147 https://doi.org/10.1177/0969733013490593

Tobiano G, Marshall A, Bucknall T et al 2015 Patient participation in nursing care on medical wards: an integrative review. International Journal of Nursing Studies 52(6):1107–1120 https://doi.org/10.1016/j.ijnurstu.2015.02.010

References

Allen J, Hutchinson A M, Brown R et al 2022 Improving transitional care communication for older Australians from hospital to home: co-design of the TRANSITION tool. Health & Social Care in the Community 30(6):e4223-e4238.

Australian Commission on Safety and Quality in Health Care (ACSQHC) 2020 Australian Charter of Healthcare Rights. Online. Available: https://www.safetyandquality.gov.au/our-work/partnering-consumers/australian-charter-healthcare-rights

Australian Commission on Safety and Quality in Health Care (ACSQHC) 2023 Annual Report 2022-2023. ACSQHC, Sydney

Australian Commission on Safety and Quality in Health Care (ACSQHC) 2024 Person-centred care. Online. Available: https://www.safetyandquality.gov.au/our-work/partnering-consumers/australian-charter-healthcare-rights

Baumann L A, Reinhold A K, Brütt A L 2022 Public and patient involvement in health policy decision-making on the health system level – a scoping review. Health Policy 126(10):1023–1038 https://doi.org/10.1016/j.healthpol.2022.07.007

Betriana F, Locsin R C 2022 Variations on a theme: labeling patients as persons, the nursed, or client in nursing. Belitung Nursing Journal 8(6):466–469 doi: 10.33546/bnj.2427. PMID: 37554238; PMCID: PMC10405649

Carlini J, Muir R, McLaren-Kennedy A et al 2023 Transforming health-care service through consumer co-creation: directions for service design. Journal of Services Marketing https://doi.org/10.1108/JSM-12-2022-0373

Carman K L, Dardess P, Maurer M et al 2013 Patient and family engagement: a framework for understanding the elements and developing interventions and policies. Health Affairs 32(2):223–31 https://doi.org/10.1377/hlthaff.2012.1133

Castro E M, Van Regenmortel T, Vanhaecht K et al 2016 Patient empowerment, patient participation and patient-centeredness in hospital care: a concept analysis based on a literature review. Patient Education and Counseling 99(12):1923–1939 https://doi.org/10.1016/j.pec.2016.07.026

Christmas D M B, Sweeney A 2016 Service user, patient, survivor or client ... has the time come to return to 'patient'? The British Journal of Psychiatry 209(1):9

Costa D S J, Mercieca-Bebber R, Tesson S, Seidler Z, Lopez A L 2019 Patient, client, consumer, survivor or other alternatives? A scoping review of preferred terms for labelling individuals who access healthcare across settings. BMJ Open 9(3):e025166 https://doi.org/10.1136/bmjopen-2018-025166

Cui J, Lancaster K, Newman C E 2019 Making the subjects of mental health care: a cross-cultural comparison of mental health policy in Hong Kong, China and New South Wales, Australia. Sociology of Health & Illness 41(4):740–754 https://doi.org/10.1111/1467-9566.12851

Davison M, Chan J, Clarke M et al 2024 Yarning to reduce take own leave events in First Nations patients presenting to the Emergency Department: presenting the qualitative themes and co-design of the Deadly RED project. Health Promotion Journal of Australia 35(4):1060–1066

Domecq J P, Prutsky G, Elraiyah T 2014 Patient engagement in research: a systematic review. BMC Health Services Research 14(1):1–9 https://doi.org/10.1186/1472-6963-14-89

Eklund J H, Holmström I K, Kumlin T et al 2019 'Same same or different?' A review of reviews of person-centered and patient-centered care. Patient Education and Counseling 102(1):3–11

Goldstein M M, Bowers D G 2015 The patient as consumer: empowerment or commodification? Journal of Law, Medicine & Ethics 43(1):162–165. https://doi.org/10.1111/jlme.12203

Gusmano M K, Maschke K J, Solomon M Z 2019 Patient-centered care, yes; patients as consumers, no. Health Affairs (Millwood) 38(3):368–373 doi: 10.1377/hlthaff.2018.05019. PMID: 3083081

Hawkins J, Madden K, Fletcher A et al 2017 Development of a framework for the co-production and prototyping of public health interventions. BMC Public Health 17(1):1–11 https://doi.org/10.1186/s12889-017-4695-8

Hoddinott P, Pollock A, O'Cathain A et al 2018 How to incorporate patient and public perspectives into the design and conduct of research. F1000Research 7:752 https://doi.org/10.12688/f1000research.15162.1

Hunt D, Lamb K, Elliot J et al 2022 A WHO key informant language survey of people with lived experiences of diabetes: media misconceptions, values-based messaging, stigma, framings, and communications considerations. Diabetes Research and Clinical Practice 193:110109

Jackson D, Hutchinson M, Wilson S 2016 Editorial: in defence of patients. Journal of Clinical Nursing 25(9–10): 1177–8

Jamieson Gilmore K, Corazza I, Coletta L et al 2023 The uses of patient reported experience measures in health systems: a systematic narrative review. Health Policy 128:1–10 https://doi.org/10.1016/j.healthpol.2022.07.008

Janerka C, Leslie G D, Gill F J 2023 Development of patient-centred care in acute hospital settings: a meta-narrative review. International Journal of Nursing Studies 140 https://doi.org/10.1016/j.ijnurstu.2023.104465

Jerofke-Owen T A, Tobiano G, Eldh A C 2023 Patient engagement, involvement, or participation – entrapping concepts in nurse-patient interactions: a critical discussion. Nursing Inquiry 30(1):e12513 https://doi.org/10.1111/nin.12513

Kitwood T 1997 Dementia reconsidered: the person comes first. Buckingham: Open 4University Press

Lambert B L, Street R L, Cegala D J et al 1997 Provider-patient communication, patient-centered care, and the mangle of practice. Health Communication 9(1):27–43

Manafo E, Petermann L, Mason-Lai P et al 2018 Patient engagement in Canada: a scoping review of the 'how' and 'what' of patient engagement in health research. Health Research Policy and Systems 16(1):1–11 https://doi.org/10.1186/s12961-018-0282-4

Mazza D, Shankar M, Botfield J R et al 2023 Improving rural and regional access to long-acting reversible contraception and medical abortion through nurse-led models of care, task-sharing and telehealth (ORIENT): a protocol for a stepped-wedge pragmatic cluster-randomised controlled trial in Australian general practice. BMJ Open 13(3):e065137

McCarron T L, Clement F, Rasiah J et al 2021 Patients as partners in health research: a scoping review. Health Expectations 24(4):1378–1390 https://doi.org/10.1111/hex.13272

McCormack B 2004 Person-centredness in gerontological nursing: an overview of the literature. Journal of Clinical Nursing 13:31–38

McCormack B, McCance T, Bulley C et al (eds) 2021 Fundamentals of person-centred healthcare practice. John Wiley & Sons

Rossiter C, Levett-Jones T, Pich J 2020 The impact of person-centred care on patient safety: an umbrella review of systematic reviews. International Journal of Nursing Studies 109 https://doi.org/10.1016/j.ijnurstu.2020.103658

Speed E 2006 Patients, consumers and survivors: a case study of mental health service user discourses. Social Science & Medicine 62(1):28–38

Thórarinsdóttir K, Kristjánsson K 2014 Patients' perspectives on person-centred participation in healthcare: a framework analysis. Nursing Ethics 21(2):129–147 https://doi.org/10.1177/0969733013490593

Tieu M, Mudd A, Conroy T et al 2022 The trouble with personhood and person-centred care. Nursing Philosophy 23(3):e12381

Tobiano G, Bucknall T, Sladdin I et al 2018 Patient participation in nursing bedside handover: a systematic mixed-methods review. International Journal of Nursing Studies 77:243–258 https://doi.org/10.1016/j.ijnurstu.2017.10.014

Tobiano G, Marshall A, Bucknall T et al 2015 Patient participation in nursing care on medical wards: an integrative review. International Journal of Nursing Studies 52(6):1107–1120 https://doi.org/10.1016/j.ijnurstu.2015.02.010

Towle A, Bainbridge L, Godolphin W et al 2010 Active patient involvement in the education of health professionals. Medical Education 44(1):64–74 https://doi.org/10.1111/j.1365-2923.2009.03530.x

Tsao S F, Chen H, Tisseverasinghe T et al 2021 What social media told us in the time of COVID-19: a scoping review. The Lancet Digital Health 3(3):e175–e194

Van Belle E, Giesen J, Conroy T et al 2020 Exploring person-centred fundamental nursing care in hospital wards: a multi-site ethnography. Journal of Clinical Nursing 29(11–12):1933–1944 https://doi.org/10.1111/jocn.15024

Yoshida S 2016 Approaches, tools and methods used for setting priorities in health research in the 21st century. Journal of Global Health 6(1) https://doi.org/10.7189/jogh.06.010507

CHAPTER 8

NURSING AND THE QUEST FOR CARE QUALITY AND PATIENT SAFETY

Brigid Gillespie and Debra Jackson

KEY WORDS

adverse event
communicating for safety
missed care
patient safety model
preventable harm
safety culture

LEARNING OBJECTIVES

After reading this chapter, readers should be able to:
- define patient safety and explain its significance in healthcare
- explain the key principles and elements of patient safety
- describe the nurse's role in maintaining patient safety in the clinical environment
- discuss strategies to prevent the reoccurrence of adverse events and enhance patient safety
- outline the ethical and legal aspects of patient safety in nursing practice.

INTRODUCTION

Health services are designed to meet the needs of people across the lifespan, from prenatally until (and even after) the end of life. When people are in the care of health services it is generally because they are experiencing a significant health issue, such as a disease or episode of illness, a normal life event such as childbirth, because they require intervention such as surgery, or because of an accident or injury. People also contact health services when seeking preventive healthcare, such as seeking immunisations, participating in health screening or other services.

It is important that people are safe and that they feel safe when they, their family members or friends are in the care of health services. However, people can and do experience preventable harms while in the care of health services. These harms can occur in any care setting, including the community, but when acquired in hospital, these harms are sometimes referred to as hospital-acquired complications or 'HACS' (Australian Commission on Quality and Safety in Health Care 2023). Preventable harm can encompass issues such as medication errors, pressure injuries, diagnostic errors, patient misidentification, falls, hospital-acquired infections and other problems. It has been recently estimated that up to 40% of patients in primary and ambulatory care settings experience patient harm and that up to 80% of this harm is avoidable (World Health Organization [WHO] 2023).

The WHO (2021) estimates that on average, 1 in 10 patients in high-income countries experiences some sort of harm when in hospital, while the problem is much worse in low- and middle-income countries. International data suggests that unsafe care in hospitals contributes to more than 3 million deaths a year and the social costs of patient harm have been estimated at between 1 and 2 trillion US dollars per year (WHO 2021, 2023).

Concern about preventable harms experienced by patients led to the concept of 'patient safety', which is a fundamental aspect of healthcare. Nurses, along with everyone in the healthcare environment, have a crucial role to play in promoting patient safety so students of nursing need to develop familiarity with this important concept. Patient safety has also been linked to nurse wellbeing, nurse distress and intention to leave the profession because research has shown that nurses do experience distress if they feel they are unable to deliver safe care to patients (Bagnasco et al 2023).

In this chapter, we will introduce patient safety and highlight the important role(s) of nurses in contributing to the creation of safe therapeutic environments for patients and others within the healthcare environment.

The importance of patient safety

The landmark report 'To err is human', published in 1999 by the Institute of Medicine (IoM), brought into sharper focus the significance of medical errors in the United States (US) healthcare system. The report was a call to action, highlighting the need for fundamental changes in the approach healthcare organisations take to patient safety. While this report was based on the US context, its recommendations have been adopted across many healthcare systems worldwide. Table 8.1 outlines the key messages in the report.

TABLE 8.1
Key messages in the Institute of Medicine report

FOCUS	EXPLANATION
Scope of medical errors	The widespread nature of medical errors estimated that tens of thousands of Americans die each year from preventable errors
Focus on systemic issues	Errors are often the result of systems failures rather than individual negligence. This encouraged a shift from a blame culture to one that acknowledges the importance of system design in preventing errors
Recommendations	Establishing a culture of safety
	Systems thinking
	Reporting and analysis
	Standardisation of processes
National patient safety goals	Setting out specific safety goals for healthcare organisations

UNDERSTANDING PATIENT SAFETY

Patient safety has been defined as:

> A framework of organized activities that creates cultures, processes, procedures, behaviours, technologies and environments in health care that consistently and sustainably lower risks, reduce the occurrence of avoidable harm, make errors less likely and reduce the impact of harm when it does occur.
>
> (World Health Organization 2021)

While this is a useful definition, there are broader understandings of safety and harm in healthcare, and these encompass recognition of cultural safety in healthcare. In Chapter 5 there is much more information and a broader discussion of cultural safety in healthcare, but we are mentioning it here too, because it is important to understand that the concept of patient safety is multifactorial.

Minimising the use of unnecessary interventions is an important component of maintaining patient safety. *Low-value care* refers to medical treatments, tests or procedures that provide little or no benefit to patients and may even cause harm. When low-value care is present in healthcare practices, it can contribute to preventable harm in various ways; for example, the overuse of procedures and medicines, hospital-acquired infections, diagnostic errors and radiation exposure, to name a few.

Addressing low-value care is a crucial aspect of patient safety initiatives. Healthcare organisations need to promote evidence-based practices, implement clinical guidelines, and encourage shared decision making among healthcare professionals, patients and families to reduce the occurrence of unnecessary and potentially harmful interventions.

Nurses play a critical role in preventing or minimising low-value care to enhance patient safety through enacting various responsibilities and strategies. Some of these strategies are outlined in Table 8.2.

Ensuring patient safety: addressing health disparities and identifying areas of increased vulnerability

It is important to remember that an adverse event or harm can occur to any patient at any time. However, some patients may be particularly susceptible to experiencing harm. These include any patients who may have impaired communication, such as infants, older people, patients in intensive care settings, comatose patients and people with cognitive disorders. Furthermore, there is compelling evidence of racial, ethnic and gender disparity with patients experiencing harm across all settings. A systematic review of the safety of healthcare for ethnic minority patients found substantial disparity in patient safety outcomes between ethnic minority and dominant populations (Chauhan et al 2020). For example, women and Black patients are more likely to experience harms in primary care (Piccardi et al 2018); children from racial minorities in inpatient settings have been found to experience higher rates of common patient safety incidents than white children (Lyren et al 2023), and people with darker skin tones are more likely to develop higher stage pressure injuries (Oozageer Gunowa et al 2018). The literature is replete with similar evidence.

In addition, there are points along the care trajectory that have been identified as placing patients at higher risk of harm and these include situations such as when being transferred from hospital to community care (Oksholm et al 2023). At these points, you may notice that health services have additional measures in place to protect patients from experiencing preventable harm. These measures may include checklists, enhanced handover procedures, and follow-up phone calls to patients to ascertain their wellbeing.

TABLE 8.2
Strategies and nurses' contributions to minimising low-value care

STRATEGY	ROLE	CONTRIBUTION
Clinical assessment and monitoring	Nurses are often the primary caregivers who assess and monitor patients regularly	Via thorough assessment, nurses can identify changes in patient conditions, ensuring that interventions are appropriate and timely, and unnecessary procedures are avoided
Collaboration with multidisciplinary, interdisciplinary and transdisciplinary teams	Nurses work closely with physicians, pharmacists and other healthcare professionals	Collaborative efforts enable the exchange of information, ensuring that the care provided is well coordinated, evidence-based and avoids unnecessary duplication of tests or procedures
Advocacy for evidence-based practice	Nurses promote evidence-based care and follow established clinical guidelines	By aligning their practice with evidence-based guidelines, nurses contribute to delivering care that is known to be effective, reducing the likelihood of unnecessary or low-value interventions
Patient education	Nurses educate patients about their conditions, treatment options and potential risks and benefits	By promoting patient understanding, nurses empower individuals to actively participate in shared decision making, helping to avoid unnecessary tests or treatments that may not align with the patient's preferences or needs
Medication management	Nurses are responsible for administering medications and monitoring their effects	Through careful medication management, nurses help prevent polypharmacy and adverse drug reactions, reducing the likelihood of unnecessary medications being prescribed or administered
Communication and shared decision making	Nurses facilitate communication between patients, families and the healthcare team	Encouraging shared decision making ensures that patients are actively involved in their care, helping to avoid unnecessary tests or treatments that may not be in line with their goals or values
Participating in quality improvement activities	Nurses actively participate in quality improvement initiatives within healthcare organisations	By identifying and addressing areas of unnecessary care, nurses contribute to organisational efforts enhancing the value of care and patient safety

STORY

Jing Li is a first-year nursing student on her first clinical placement on a rehabilitation ward and is part of a nursing team caring for eight frail older people. In this clinical setting, the nursing team carry out intentional rounding every 3 hours. The nurse unit manager explained to Jing Li that intentional rounding was an important patient safety measure in the ward.

Reflective questions

Reflect on the above scenario and consider the following questions and issues:

1. What is intentional rounding?
2. How could intentional rounding create a safer environment for patients?
3. What types of patient harm could potentially be reduced by adopting intentional rounding?

Missed nursing care

The phenomenon of *missed nursing care* has gained increasing attention over the last 20 years. Missed nursing care refers to instances where essential or planned patient care is either left undone or omitted (Chiappinotto et al 2022). It occurs when nurses are unable to provide certain aspects of care due to various reasons such as staffing shortages, time constraints, workload, resource limitations and competing priorities. Examples of missed nursing care include:

- Delays in medication administration as nurses may be challenged to administer medications on time due to high workloads, competing priorities, interruptions and time constraints
- Omissions or delays in providing hygiene and comfort measures such as bathing, oral care, and repositioning to prevent pressure injuries may be missed or delayed
- Regular monitoring of vital signs, patient risk assessments and screening, and responses to treatments may be missed, leading to delays in detecting a change in the patient's health status
- Delays in pain management practices such as administering pain medication on schedule or responding promptly to the patient's report of pain may be compromised
- Delays in documenting vital signs, wound care treatments, etc. may lead to delays in other treatments
- Omissions in patient education due to time pressures.

Missed nursing care is a patient safety issue: the omission or delay of essential nursing activities can have direct implications for the safety and wellbeing of patients. Patient safety is focused on the prevention of errors and adverse events that may lead to harm during the provision of healthcare services. Therefore, when nursing care is missed, it may contribute to adverse events such as dehydration, falls and pressure injuries.

STORY

On her third clinical shift, Jing Li is on an afternoon shift. She is caring for an 86-year-old lady, Mrs Singh, who has expressive dysphasia after experiencing a recent cerebrovascular accident (CVA). Mrs Singh has also recently had a urinary tract infection, and her fluid intake and urinary output are being recorded on a fluid balance chart. At 3 p.m., as Jing Li reads Mrs Singh's notes and care plan, she notices that the fluid balance chart has had no entries since 9 a.m. that morning. Jing Li knows from the previous two shifts she has worked on the ward that patients are offered a drink and taken to the bathroom every 3 hours, as part of the intentional rounding routine.

Reflective questions

Reflect on the above scenario and consider the following questions and issues:
1. What actions could Jing Li take in the first instance?
2. How does accurate recording of fluid intake and output contribute to maintaining safety for Mrs Singh?
3. What factors could put Mrs Singh at risk of experiencing a patient safety issue?

THE FAR-REACHING IMPACTS OF HEALTHCARE ERRORS

When healthcare errors do occur, there are said to be four sets of victims—*first victims* are the patient experiencing the harm and their family; *second victims* are the healthcare providers associated with the error; *third victims* are the hospital or facility in which the error occurs; and the *fourth victims* are the wider society and community (Ozeke et al 2019).

The *second victim* phenomenon refers to the emotional and psychological impact on healthcare professionals, particularly those involved in a medical error or adverse event. While the primary victim of a medical error is the patient, the healthcare professionals directly or indirectly involved in the incident can experience significant emotional distress, guilt and trauma. These healthcare providers become the 'second victims'.

Healthcare personnel can and do experience second victim syndrome, which is defined as 'HCPs who commit an error and are traumatised by the event manifesting psychological (shame, guilt, anxiety, grief, and depression), cognitive (compassion dissatisfaction, burnout, secondary traumatic stress), and/or physical reactions that have a personal negative impact' (Ozeke et al 2019). As is clear from this definition, the second victim phenomenon recognises that healthcare professionals, including doctors, nurses and other staff, may suffer from feelings of responsibility, self-doubt and emotional trauma after an adverse event. They may grapple with guilt, anxiety and fear of repercussions, affecting their wellbeing and professional confidence. It is important to remember that free counselling is available to all hospital staff including students (through the university) who experience these types of issues in clinical practice.

The role of nursing in patient safety

Nursing has a central role to play in contributing to safe environments for patients. Activities that aim to promote patient safety and eliminate preventable harm to patients are embedded in the clinical practices and the clinical skills of nurses (see, e.g., Redley et al 2022). There are many examples of how these practices are embedded, but just one example are the checks that are done with medication administration. In double- and sometimes triple-checking the right patient, the right drug, the right dose, the right route, the right time and the right recording of the administration of the drug, nurses are acting to reduce the chances of a medication error. While it may seem that these steps are repetitive and take time, it is important to remember that patients and their families depend on health staff to 'get it right' and, when a mistake does occur it takes much more time to mitigate the situation than it does to carry out the checks to prevent it.

Nursing's responsibility in ensuring patient safety

One of the most important responsibilities that nurses have concerning patient safety is advocacy for patient safety. That advocacy can take various forms but always includes speaking up and raising concerns where there is a potential or actual threat to patient safety. The healthcare environment is a very dynamic environment with a range of complexities, such as new technologies, that can mean new and different (potential) threats to patient safety. Speaking up for patient safety is crucial to the provision of safe environments and is vital to ensure continuous improvements. However, speaking out can also be complex, and research suggests that in some situations, nurses may be reluctant to speak up, even for patient safety (Lee et al 2022). Later in this chapter we will discuss the importance of speaking out, effective communication and the reporting of and learning from errors.

Patient safety competencies for nurses

Patient safety competencies for nurses encompass the knowledge, skills and attitudes that nurses need to promote a safety culture and deliver high-quality care while minimising the risk of harm to patients. These competencies are crucial to ensuring the safety and wellbeing of patients across all kinds of healthcare settings. Examples of key patient safety competencies include medication management, infection control, clinical assessment and monitoring, effective communications, falls and pressure injury prevention, patient education, performing regular checks on patients (e.g. intentional rounding), and cultural competence (see Chapter 5 for information on cultural safety in nursing).

Patient safety frameworks and models

There are many useful patient safety frameworks and conceptual models that have been developed to help healthcare organisations implement programs and strategies to enhance patient safety. These frameworks provide a structured approach to identifying, analysing and mitigating risks to patient safety. These frameworks and models provide healthcare organisations with the tools and methodologies to assess, prioritise and continuously improve patient safety. Healthcare organisations often include several approaches that contribute to more comprehensive and effective patient safety programs. Table 8.3 provides a summary of the most widely used frameworks and models.

TABLE 8.3
Widely used patient safety models and their descriptions

FRAMEWORK/MODEL	DESCRIPTION AND COMPONENTS
Donabedian's model of quality: structure, process, outcome (Donabedian 1988)	Assesses the quality of healthcare services through three key components: *Structure* refers to the organisational and environmental factors that influence healthcare delivery, e.g. facilities, equipment and personnel *Process* evaluates the actual delivery of care, focusing on the methods and interactions involved in providing healthcare services *Outcome* assesses the results of healthcare interventions, including the impact on patients' health and wellbeing. This model helps analyse and improve the overall quality of healthcare by addressing these interconnected elements
Systems Engineering Initiative for Patient Safety (SEIPS) model 3.0 (Carayon 2020)	Provides a comprehensive framework to analyse and improve patient safety in healthcare by focusing on the interactions between people, technology, tasks and the environment. The framework includes five key elements: person, organisation, technology, tasks and environment
Swiss cheese model (Reason 2000)	The Swiss cheese model metaphor likens the layers of defence in a healthcare system to slices of Swiss cheese, each with holes. Errors occur when the holes align. This model emphasises the need to implement multiple layers of defence that address systemic vulnerabilities to prevent accidents or failures in complex systems
The conceptual framework for International Classification for Patient Safety (ICPS) (WHO 2009)	Developed by the World Health Organization (WHO), this classification system provides a standardised language for reporting and analysing patient safety incidents. The ICPS framework categorises incidents based on contributing factors, harm caused and the healthcare process involved, allowing a systematic approach to understanding and addressing patient safety issues

Creating a culture of safety

Safety culture refers to the shared values, beliefs, attitudes and behaviours within a healthcare organisation that prioritise and promote the safety of patients (Kilcullen et al 2022). It is about creating an environment where members of the healthcare team, including nurses, actively contribute to ensuring the wellbeing of patients and minimising the risk of harm. In a strong patient safety culture, there is open communication, a focus on continuous learning and improvement, and a commitment to addressing and learning from mistakes.

Nurses play a crucial role in fostering this culture by advocating for patient safety, reporting incidents, participating in training and education and collaborating with other healthcare team members to implement best practices. A safety culture encourages reporting of near misses or adverse events without fear of blame (Kilcullen et al 2022). Effective communication is essential for creating an open reporting culture, where team members feel comfortable sharing information about incidents or potential risks (Mortensen et al 2022). Ultimately, patient safety culture in nursing is about creating a supportive and proactive atmosphere where everyone provides the highest quality of care while minimising the potential for errors and adverse events.

Teamwork and communication are fundamental pillars of a safety culture in any healthcare setting and contribute to fostering a culture of continuous improvement (Mortensen et al 2022). Regular team discussions, debriefings and reflective practices contribute to learning from experiences and implementing changes to enhance safety. Effective communication is also essential for creating an open reporting culture, where team members feel comfortable sharing information about incidents or potential risks. Teamwork promotes collective decision making, drawing on the expertise of various healthcare professionals, including nurses. This collaborative approach ensures that decisions consider multiple perspectives, enhancing the overall safety of patient care. Through effective communication, team members can maintain a heightened awareness of their environment, patient status and potential risks. This awareness is crucial for proactive decision making and preventing errors.

Learning from and reporting errors are crucial components of building and sustaining a safety culture in nursing (Mortensen et al 2022). Reporting errors allows healthcare organisations to identify systemic issues that contribute to errors and encourages open communication among healthcare team members. It fosters an environment where individuals feel comfortable sharing information about mistakes, near misses and potential risks, leading to increased awareness and collaboration in addressing safety concerns. When nurses are encouraged to report errors and near misses it empowers them to actively participate in improving patient safety. This empowerment contributes to a sense of collective responsibility for the wellbeing of patients and a shared commitment to providing high-quality care.

The information gained from the reporting process is invaluable because it may be used to implement targeted improvements in processes, protocols and systems to prevent similar errors in the future. Learning from errors promotes a culture of continuous improvement. By analysing the root causes of errors, healthcare professionals and organisations can implement changes and interventions to enhance the overall safety and quality of care provided. In the next section, we discuss the pivotal role nurses play as leaders and advocates in fostering a culture of patient safety.

Leadership for patient safety

Leadership for patient safety involves fostering a culture that prioritises and promotes the wellbeing of patients, with an emphasis on open communication and continuous improvement (Mortensen et al 2022). In the context of healthcare, key features of leadership in creating safe cultures are outlined in Table 8.4.

Continuous quality improvement (CQI) and patient safety

Continuous quality improvement (CQI) is the term to describe the ongoing systematic process of planning, implementing and evaluating clinical and organisational processes to ensure they consistently meet or exceed quality standards. CQI is critical to maintaining patient safety by providing a systematic and continuous approach to enhancing the overall quality of healthcare delivery. Because of nurses' frontline roles, close patient and family interactions, and comprehensive

TABLE 8.4
Key features of leadership in creating a patient safety culture

FEATURE OF LEADERSHIP	DESCRIPTION
Setting a clear vision	Leaders play a pivotal role in establishing a clear vision for patient safety within the healthcare organisation. This involves articulating the importance of safety, outlining specific goals and aligning the organisation's values with a commitment to providing safe and high-quality care
Cultivating a safety culture	Leaders influence the organisational culture by creating an environment where safety is a top priority. This includes encouraging open communication, learning from mistakes and fostering a sense of accountability for patient outcomes
Communication and transparency	Leaders should actively promote transparent communication regarding patient safety issues. This involves sharing information about incidents, near misses and lessons learned. Transparent communication helps build trust among team members and encourages a culture of shared responsibility for patient safety
Supporting speaking up	Leaders must actively encourage and support a culture where healthcare professionals feel empowered to speak up about concerns related to patient safety. This involves removing barriers to communication, ensuring non-punitive reporting systems and acknowledging the value of frontline input
Providing resources and training	Leaders should allocate resources for ongoing training and education related to patient safety. This ensures that healthcare professionals are equipped with the knowledge and skills necessary to identify and address safety issues effectively
Leading by example	Effective leaders model the behaviour they expect from their team. By consistently demonstrating a commitment to patient safety, leaders set a standard for others to follow. This includes prioritising safety in decision making and acknowledging and learning from mistakes
Creating a learning environment	Leaders should promote a learning culture where mistakes are seen as opportunities for improvement rather than occasions for blame. This involves conducting thorough analyses of adverse events, implementing changes based on lessons learned and sharing these insights across the organisation
Implementing patient safety initiatives	Leaders are responsible for driving the implementation of evidence-based patient safety initiatives. This may involve adopting best practices, using technology to enhance safety measures, and continuously monitoring and improving processes

TABLE 8.5
Key characteristics and principles of continuous quality improvement (CQI)

CHARACTERISTIC/PRINCIPLE	EXPLANATION
Focus on processes	CQI acknowledges the importance of analysing and improving organisational processes rather than blaming individuals. Takes a systems approach to identifying system factors and seeks to address root causes
Iterative approach	CQI is cyclical, often depicted as a continuous feedback loop in planning, implementing, monitoring, and then tailoring the approach based on the results. One example is the PDSA cycle (plan, do, study, act)
Data-driven decision making	CQI relies on the systematic collection and analysis of performance metrics and indicators (e.g. pressure injuries, falls) to measure current processes, identify areas for improvement, implement any changes and evaluate the impact of those changes
Collaborative and team-based	CQI encourages stakeholder engagement and collaboration of clinicians, patients and senior managers
Consumer focused	CQI emphasises meeting the needs of consumers, including patients, internal stakeholders and clients. Addressing consumer feedback is central to improving processes
Standardisation and innovation	CQI aims to standardise and improve existing processes; it also encourages innovation. This involves implementing new ideas and technologies to enhance healthcare quality and efficiency
Leadership support	Successful CQI initiatives require leadership commitment and involvement. Leaders set the tone for a culture of continuous improvement, allocate resources, and support staff in their efforts to enhance processes
Congruence with organisational goals	CQI needs to align with the broader needs of the organisation to ensure improvement efforts are strategically focused so they will have maximum impact on overall performance

understanding of care processes, they are key contributors to improving the quality and safety of patient care. Table 8.5 details the key characteristics and principles of CQI.

Root cause analysis (RCA)

Root cause analysis (RCA) is a structured method used to identify the underlying or systemic causes of an issue or problem (Martin-Delgado et al 2020). The process involves investigating and analysing an event, error, near miss or undesired outcome with the intent of preventing its recurrence.

Nurses play a critical role in RCA following an adverse event or incident. The insights that nurses provide into the sequence of events, system issues and human factors involved contribute to the identification of underlying causes, which may not be immediately apparent. Nurses' contributions to the RCA process include the following strategies:

- Providing timely, detailed and accurate *documentation of patient care* that can piece together a timeline of events leading up to an incident, identifying potential root causes
- Encouraging and participating in the *reporting of adverse events or near misses*. The prevailing safety culture should enable nurses to feel empowered to report incidents, without fear of retribution or reprisal
- During the RCA process, nurses can provide a *comprehensive account of the event*, including any observations, actions taken and factors that may have contributed to the incident. This may

help to identify systems failures. For instance, nurses are well positioned to identify issues such as inadequate staffing, lack of resources or equipment issues
- Nurses are often called on to *participate in RCA meetings* and discussions.

Legal and ethical aspects of patient safety

In Chapter 9, the legal and ethical aspects of patient safety are comprehensively covered. From a legal perspective, nursing practice is governed by various laws, regulations and practice standards that are enacted by the Nursing and Midwifery Board of Australia (NMBA, Australian Health Practitioner Regulation Agency). Practising nurses are legally obliged to adhere to the professional codes of conduct and standards of practice as set out by the NMBA. Some of the legal aspects of nursing practice include reporting of near misses and adverse events, informed consent, confidentiality and documentation accuracy, all of which are integral to maintaining patient safety and ensuring compliance with the law. Ethical considerations of patient safety in nursing practice are underpinned by the fundamental need to prioritise and protect the wellbeing of patients. Nursing is one of the most trusted professions; as such, nurses are entrusted with upholding the ethical principles of autonomy, beneficence, non-maleficence and justice, ensuring their actions promote the best interests of patients while avoiding harm and treating individuals fairly. In sum, the legal and ethical considerations are intrinsically interconnected in nursing practice, highlighting the importance of delivering safe and ethically sound care to patients.

STORY

During a recent clinical placement in a general surgical unit, you are assigned to shadow RN Hara, a seasoned nurse with extensive clinical experience. As you are rounding with RN Hara, you witness an incident that potentially compromises patient safety.

As you follow RN Hara, you both enter a two-bed bay where Mr Rodriguez, a postoperative patient, is recovering. RN Hara began updating Mr Rodriguez's chart, while you observed his vital signs monitor. You notice an abnormal reading on Mr Rodriguez's oxygen saturation level.

In a respectful but concerned manner, you alert RN Hara to Mr Rodriguez's low oxygen saturation level. RN Hara dismisses your concern stating that 'it's probably only a glitch and this often happens'.

After completing the documentation in Mr Rodriguez's chart, RN Hara walks out of the room to attend to something else.

Reflective questions

With a group of peers, discuss the above scenario and consider the following questions and issues:
1. How would you approach RN Hara again to express your concerns about Mr Rodriguez's low oxygen saturation level, considering her initial dismissal?
2. What immediate actions would you take to ensure the safety of Mr Rodriguez while RN Hara is attending to other tasks outside the room?
3. Reflecting on this situation, how might you communicate your observations and concerns to the nursing supervisor or another member of the healthcare team to address the potential compromise in patient safety?

CONCLUSION

Individuals are at their most vulnerable when they come into the hospital. Nurses provide patient care 24/7, and so they bear the profound responsibility of safeguarding the patients in their care. The complex nature of modern-day healthcare delivery, coupled with patients who are generally sicker, older and have shorter hospital stays, only amplifies the vulnerability and heightened likelihood of adverse events for patients. The implementation of every action and precaution by nurses, aimed at ensuring patient safety, fosters a culture of safety.

REFLECTIVE QUESTIONS

1. What changes can you make in your daily nursing practice to enhance patient safety?
2. How do you contribute to a culture of effective communication and collaboration within your healthcare team to improve patient safety?
3. Describe a situation where effective communication helped to prevent a patient safety issue.
4. In what ways does the role of the nurse as a patient advocate ensure patient safety?
5. Can you recall a personal experience where you either observed or addressed a patient safety concern? What did you learn from that experience?

Recommended readings

Australian Commission on Quality and Safety in Health Care 2023 Hospital-acquired complications (HACs). Australian Commission on Safety and Quality in Health Care. Online. Available: https://www.safetyandquality.gov.au/our-work/indicators-measurement-and-reporting/hospital-acquired-complications-hacs 1 November 2023

Lee S E, Dahinten V S, Ji H et al 2022 Motivators and inhibitors of nurses' speaking up behaviours: a descriptive qualitative study. Journal of Advanced Nursing 78:3398–408. https://doi.org/10.1111/jan.15343

Lyren A, Haines E, Fanta M et al 2023 Racial and ethnic disparities in common inpatient safety outcomes in a children's hospital cohort. BMJ Quality & Safety 33(2):86–97 doi: 10.1136/bmjqs-2022-015786

World Health Organization 2021 Global patient safety action plan 2021–2030: towards eliminating avoidable harm in health care. Online. Available: https://apps.who.int/iris/bitstream/handle/10665/343477/9789240032705-eng.pdf 1 November 2023

References

Australian Commission on Quality and Safety in Health Care 2023 Hospital acquired complications (HACs). Australian Commission on Safety and Quality in Health Care. Online. Available: https://www.safetyandquality.gov.au/our-work/indicators-measurement-and-reporting/hospital-acquired-complications-hacs 1 November 2023

Bagnasco A, Timmins F, Moro A et al 2023 The organization of nursing work in Italian hospitals—implications for job satisfaction, nurse well-being and patient safety. Journal of Advanced Nursing https://doi.org/10.1111/jan.15778

Carayon P, Wooldridge A, Hoonakker P et al 2020 SEIPS 3.0: Human-centered design of the patient journey for patient safety [Article]. Applied Ergonomics 84 https://doi.org/10.1016/j.apergo.2019.103033

Chauhan A, Walto M, Manias E et al 2020 The safety of health care for ethnic minority patients: a systematic review. International Journal for Equity in Health 19:118 https://doi.org/10.1186/s12939-020-01223-2

Chiappinotto S, Papastavrou E, Efstathiou G et al 2022 Antecedents of unfinished nursing care: a systematic review of the literature. BMC Nursing 21(1):137 doi: 10.1186/s12912-022-00890-6

Donabedian A 1988 The quality of care. How can it be assessed? JAMA 260(12):1743–48 https://doi.org/10.1001/jama.260.12.1743

Kilcullen M P, Bisbey T M, Ottosen M J 2022 The safer culture framework: an application to healthcare based on a multi-industry review of safety culture literature. Human Factors 64(1):207–27 doi: 10.1177/00187208211060891

Lee S E, Dahinten V S, Ji H et al 2022 Motivators and inhibitors of nurses' speaking up behaviours: a descriptive qualitative study. Journal of Advanced Nursing 78:3398–3408 https://doi.org/10.1111/jan.15343

Lyren A, Haines E, Fanta M et al 2023 Racial and ethnic disparities in common inpatient safety outcomes in a children's hospital cohort. BMJ Quality & Safety doi: 10.1136/bmjqs-2022-015786

Martin-Delgado J, Martínez-García A, Aranaz J M et al 2020 How much of root cause analysis translates into improved patient safety: a systematic review. Medical Principles and Practice: International Journal of the Kuwait University, Health Science Centre 29(6):524–31 https://doi.org/10.1159/000508677

Mortensen M, Naustdal K I, Uibu E et al 2022 Instruments for measuring patient safety competencies in nursing: a scoping review. BMJ Open Quality 11(2):e001751 https://doi.org/10.1136/bmjoq-2021-001751

Oksholm T, Gissum K R, Hunskår I et al 2023 The effect of transitions intervention to ensure patient safety and satisfaction when transferred from hospital to home health care—a systematic review. Journal of Advanced Nursing 79:2098–2118 https://doi.org/10.1111/jan.15579

Oozageer Gunowa N, Hutchinson M, Brooke J et al 2018 Pressure injuries in people with darker skin tones: a literature review. Journal of Clinical Nursing 27(17–18):3266–75 doi: 10.1111/jocn.14062

Ozeke O, Ozeke V, Coskun O, Budakoglu II 2019 Second victims in health care: current perspectives. Advances in Medical Education and Practice 10:593–603 doi: 10.2147/AMEP.S185912. PMID: 31496861; PMCID: PMC6697646

Piccardi C, Detollenaere J, Vanden Bussche P et al 2018 Social disparities in patient safety in primary care: a systematic review. International Journal for Equity in Health 17:114 (2018) https://doi.org/10.1186/s12939-018-0828-7

Reason J 2000 Human error: models and management. BMJ 320(7237):768–70 https://doi.org/10.1136/bmj.320.7237.768

Redley B, Douglas T, Hoon L et al 2022 Nurses' harm prevention practices during admission of an older person to the hospital: a multi-method qualitative study. Journal of Advanced Nursing 78(11):3745–59 https://doi.org/10.1111/jan.15351

World Health Organization 2021 Global patient safety action plan 2021–2030: towards eliminating avoidable harm in health care. Online. Available: https://apps.who.int/iris/bitstream/handle/10665/343477/9789240032705-eng.pdf 1 November 2023

World Health Organization 2023 Patient Safety Factsheet. Online. Available: https://www.who.int/news-room/fact-sheets/detail/patient-safety 7 January 2024

CHAPTER 9

BECOMING A CRITICAL THINKER

Marion Tower

KEY WORDS

argument
clinical reasoning
critical thinking
decision making
evaluation
evidence-based practice
habits of mind
reasoning

LEARNING OBJECTIVES

After reading this chapter, readers should be able to:

- describe the essential nature and significance of critical thinking in nursing practice
- explain the basic structure of an argument and apply it to various areas of nursing practice, including clinical reasoning
- identify resources for further reading and the study of critical thinking.

INTRODUCTION

The focus of this chapter, critical thinking, is an essential skill for nursing practice. The Nursing and Midwifery Board of Australia's *Registered Nurse Standards of Practice* (2016) recognise the importance of critical thinking for nurses. Standard 1 describes a registered nurse (RN) as one who 'thinks critically and analyses nursing practice'. This means that:

> RNs use a variety of thinking strategies and the best available evidence in making decisions and providing safe, quality nursing practice within person-centred and evidence-based frameworks.

(2016:3)

Whether we are aware of it or not, all behaviour is based on certain values, assumptions and beliefs. These form the basis for our decisions to act in certain ways. In a professional context such as nursing practice, everything that we think, say or do is the result of a complex web of beliefs, values and assumptions that have formed as a result of our life experiences. As we grow up in our family, attend school, participate in religious communities, associate with friends, watch television, read newspapers and work for various employers we develop a 'pair of spectacles' through which we understand and interpret the world and all that happens in it. Just as a person who wears glasses eventually becomes unaware that they are even wearing them, so too each of us adjusts to our worldview 'spectacles' until, often, we are completely unaware what values, beliefs and assumptions are influencing us in a specific situation.

If all behaviour is derived from our values, assumptions and beliefs, then our behaviours and decisions in professional practice are also informed by these. It follows that poor practice and decision making will occur if our values, assumptions and beliefs are incorrect or unacceptable. The consequences of this are highly significant and potentially improve or undermine patient or client health outcomes—even to the point of sometimes determining whether someone lives or dies. It is because of this link between our beliefs, values and assumptions and practice that critical thinking is essential for high-quality nursing practice.

> ## REFLECTION
> What are the three most important reasons you can think of that demonstrate the importance of critical thinking in nursing practice? Recall any work situations in which critical thinking would have improved the outcomes.

What is critical thinking?

There are a variety of definitions of critical thinking and no general consensus on any one of them (Perez et al 2015). However, it is generally accepted that critical thinking is a complex and dynamic cognitive process used to systematically analyse information to facilitate reasoning, judgment and decision making to promote positive patient or client outcomes (or minimise risk or harm) (Falcó-Pegueroles et al 2021, Karaca et al, Perez et al 2015, Urhan et al 2022). A concept analysis of critical thinking by Von Colln-Appling and Giuliano (2017) identified attributes or characteristics associated with critical thinking that are considered crucial to critical thinking. These are discussed in more detail below.

Robert H Ennis (2015:32) provides a helpful general definition when he suggests that '[c]ritical thinking is reasonable reflective thinking focused on deciding what to believe or do'.

At the heart of reasonable reflective thinking is the activity of *questioning what is usually taken for granted*. This questioning occurs best when certain *habits of mind* have been developed and *thinking skills* are used to conduct the questioning.

Critical thinking means stopping and reflecting on the reasons for doing things the way they are done or for experiencing things the way they are—focusing on what is frequently taken for granted and evaluating the values, beliefs and assumptions that are held, and asking whether what is done and thought is justifiable or not. These characteristics of critical thinking imply a self-consciousness of what, how and why we are thinking, with the intention of improving thinking. Improving thinking is essential, especially in nursing practice, which continues to become more complex, and which occurs in diverse contexts and under more challenging conditions.

An important aspect of critical thinking is healthy scepticism. This scepticism is necessary because there are many attempts to persuade us to accept various claims. These attempts to persuade also occur in professional contexts. For example, research reports suggest changes to practice; peers argue that their way of acting is the right one; therapists promote various interventions; administrators argue that certain changes need to be made to the workplace; and so on. Often these claims are contradictory, so they cannot all be acceptable.

Practitioners need to sort through these, often competing, claims. To accept them all without question will, at best, be highly confusing and, at worst, may endanger the lives of others if actions are based on wrong information or conclusions. To adopt an attitude of healthy scepticism means to cautiously listen to or read the claims that others make, carefully evaluate their legitimacy and not rush to accept a conclusion without careful thought.

The same rigorous thinking needs to be applied to our own nursing practice. We constantly make decisions that we assume are of benefit to our patients. Asking questions about the practices we engage in, including what evidence is available to support their efficacy, is essential if our nursing practice is to produce positive outcomes.

It is possible, however, to become too pedantic, which may result in inaction, especially if we are not prepared to accept anything unless it is 100% proven. This is why scepticism needs to be healthy. We need to appreciate that there is a limit to what can be known. Importantly, part of critical thinking is acknowledging these limits and making the best decisions, given the context of the situation and based on what is known.

The characteristics of critical thinking

You may now be wondering what characteristics a critical thinker will be required to demonstrate. The registered nurse standards of practice provide us with some useful suggestions. Firstly, they require the ability to access, use and analyse the best available evidence so that it can be applied to practice and, secondly, the ability to reflect on one's experience, knowledge, actions, feelings and beliefs so that one can understand how all these things influence and shape one's practice. Von Colln-Appling and Giuliano (2017) highlight the importance of nurses having a strong theoretical and practical knowledge base, the ability to analyse information and make informed decisions and, perhaps most importantly, the ability to reflect on the thinking process. They also highlighted critical thinking ability, open-mindedness and the capacity for independent thinking as antecedents for critical thinking.

There are more examples of the various ways in which the characteristics of critical thinking can be described. One way of summarising these is to focus on critical thinking as reasoning. The heart of reasoning is the argument. In what follows, the nature of argument will be described, followed by a description of the ways in which arguments 'appear' in nursing. Suggestions will then be made regarding the way in which the principles of critical thinking can be applied in these areas. In doing so, the way in which this approach synthesises the skills of critical thinking will become obvious. Before discussing all of this, though, we need to briefly focus on another dimension of critical thinking—habits of mind.

CRITICAL THINKING AND HABITS OF MIND

Like the cognitive skills of critical thinking, the habits of mind associated with critical thinking have been discussed at great length in the literature. Zmuda et al (2023) discuss 16 habits of mind based on the earlier work of Costa and Kallick (2008). These are: thinking about thinking (metacognition), which is the ability to understand what we do and do not know and being able to strategise in problem solving; persisting, which means staying focused; managing impulsivity to think before acting and consider alternatives; listening with understanding and empathy to perceive others' points of view; thinking flexibly to consider options; striving for accuracy by checking facts; questioning and posing problems by questioning data; applying past knowledge to new situations; thinking and communicating with clarity and precision in written and oral form; gathering data through all senses by paying attention to the surrounding world; creating, imagining, innovating using new ideas; responding with wonderment and awe by being intrigued with the world; taking responsible risks by enhancing competence; finding humour; remaining open to continuous learning avoiding complacency and admitting when you don't know; and thinking interdependently by working with and learning from others.

In essence, habits of mind are the *dispositions* or inclinations of a thinker that influence the way in which a person uses or applies the cognitive skills of critical thinking. For example, the habit of *inquisitiveness*, or curiosity, is fundamental to critical thinking. If a person does not have a disposition towards asking questions and constantly inquiring about what they do not know, they are very unlikely to engage in critical thinking. If a person does not demonstrate a disposition towards *open-mindedness*, they are not likely to examine other points of view that challenge their own. Because these predispositions are habits, they require ongoing practice to improve them. This takes time and *perseverance* (another one of the habits of mind) to practise them and a commitment on the part of any nurse who wants to improve their critical thinking abilities.

> ## REFLECTION
> Undertake a Google search for *critical thinking* and see if you can find some other definitions. What definition of critical thinking resonates with you?

A HOLISTIC DEFINITION OF CRITICAL THINKING

Elder and Paul (2020) provide a brief definition of critical thinking that synthesises everything we have discussed so far. For them,

> Critical thinking is the art of thinking about thinking to make thinking better. It involves three interwoven phases: It analyzes thinking. It evaluates thinking. It improves thinking.
>
> (2020:xiii)

This definition is useful because it reduces critical thinking down to the idea that an individual will become a critical thinker by applying standards of thinking to elements of thought to develop intellectual characteristics that counter negative tendencies; we all have tendencies towards poor thinking—in other words, an improvement in our thinking. Figure 9.1 presents a way this could be illustrated.

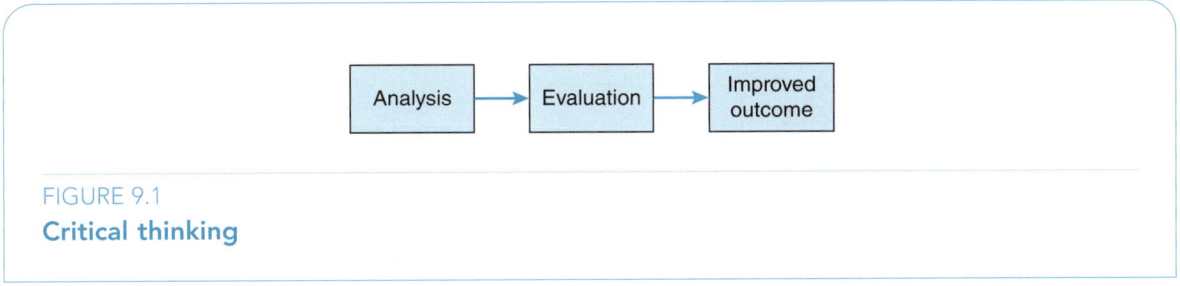

FIGURE 9.1
Critical thinking

For Elder and Paul (2020), a critical thinker is someone who asks questions and identifies problems in a clear and concise way, collects and analyses a range of information, formulates well-reasoned solutions and tests them, thinks openly and tests assumptions and consequences, and communicates effectively with others (2020:xx).

We could go into a lot more detail regarding defining critical thinking. However, rather than do that, let's now focus on one aspect of critical thinking that exemplifies what we have covered so far. That aspect is what is called *argument*. We will explore this concept in some depth and explain how it can be applied to nursing practice.

> ### REFLECTION
> Think about the characteristics of a critical thinker that have been described here. Which characteristics do you see in yourself? Reflect on the characteristics you think you need to further develop.

What is an argument?

In colloquial language the word 'argument' is often used for a shouting match between two people who are having a disagreement and may be very angry, abusive or even physically aggressive. There may be shouting, pointing of fingers, threats, crying, name-calling and so on.

In the context of critical thinking, however, the term 'argument' is very different. In fact, these situations are the very opposite of critical thinking. In critical thinking, an argument consists of a conclusion and the identification of one or more reasons that are intended to support the conclusion. Figure 9.2 shows the relationship between these parts of an argument. Each reason may or may not have evidence that is intended to support the conclusion.

Let's now look at an example of an argument:

> Every person has the right to choose how they live their lives. Therefore, a person has the right to choose to practise life-threatening behaviours if they wish.

This is an argument because it has a conclusion ('A person has the right to choose to practise life-threatening behaviours if they wish') and a reason intended to support that conclusion ('Every person has the right to choose how they live their lives'). At this stage, we are not concerned whether this is a good argument or not, but only with what makes something an argument. If it was a strong

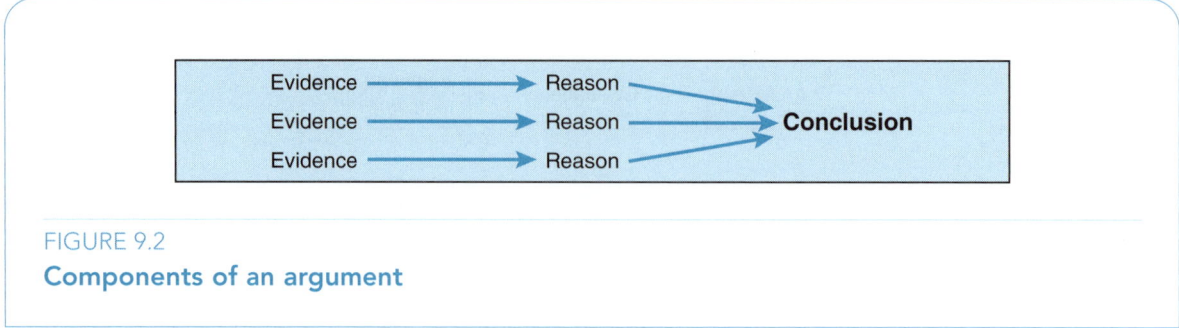

FIGURE 9.2

Components of an argument

argument, the person presenting it could provide some evidence by drawing attention, for example, to various statements of human rights, the constitutions of countries or discussions about ethics. Therefore, an argument needs the following:

- a conclusion, and
- one or more reasons intended to support the conclusion.

WHAT MAKES A SOUND ARGUMENT?

For an argument to be *sound*, three criteria need to be met. Firstly, the reasons need to be acceptable to the person evaluating the argument. Secondly, the reasons need to be relevant. Thirdly, the reasons need to provide adequate grounds for accepting the conclusion. Let us now look at each in a little more depth.

When we say the reasons need to be *acceptable*, this means that those who are on the receiving end of the argument must be able to believe the reasons offered to support it. Sometimes reasons can be evaluated as true or false. However, this is not always possible, so it is often better to think about whether a particular reason is acceptable given what is known.

Of course, if you are offering a reason in support of a conclusion, then it needs to be *relevant*. When something is relevant, it means that it contributes to answering a question, resolving an issue, or solving a problem—or, in the case of an argument, helps us to arrive at a conclusion.

When we talk about *grounds*, we are talking about the weightiness of the reasons leading us towards the conclusion. In other words, we are asking whether the reasons we are offering justify us in accepting the conclusion. Sometimes you can have lots of reasons, but they may not always directly support the conclusion.

The following example illustrates these criteria:

1 Nurses must have a practising certificate to be employed as a nurse

2 Sue does not have a practising certificate

3 Therefore, Sue is not permitted to be employed as a nurse.

Statements 1 and 2 are both reasons that are intended to support the conclusion in Statement 3. If this is a sound argument, then the reasons must be relevant and acceptable, and they must provide adequate grounds for accepting the conclusion.

Statement 1 is certainly acceptable. Most countries have a requirement that nurses need to be licensed to practise. Statement 2 is hypothetical, so we will assume that it is true for the sake of the discussion. All the reasons, then, are acceptable. The two reasons are also relevant to the issue under consideration.

The next question is whether these reasons provide adequate grounds for accepting the conclusion. We can test this by asking:

> Is it possible to reject the conclusion and still believe the reasons to be true? In other words, even though the reasons are true, is there a legitimate way that we can escape accepting the conclusion?

So, could one believe that Sue could practise and still believe that the two reasons offered are true? In this case, the answer is no. If it is true that a nurse must have a practising certificate to practise, and Sue does not have one, we are 'compelled' to accept the conclusion that Sue cannot practise. This argument, then, is a sound one.

Another example will illustrate a poor argument:

1 Everyone's hair falls out when undergoing chemotherapy

2 Jo is undergoing chemotherapy

3 Therefore, Jo's hair will fall out.

First, are the reasons acceptable? Does a person's hair fall out when they are undergoing chemotherapy? Sometimes it does, but not necessarily everyone's. Therefore, this reason is not acceptable because, although some people's hair falls out, not everyone's does. For the sake of this argument, the second reason can be accepted (that Jo is undergoing chemotherapy).

Both reasons are relevant, and so the final question is whether the reasons offered provide adequate grounds for accepting that Jo's hair will fall out. The answer is no because the first reason was false. Although it might be true that Jo's hair will fall out, it is not possible to predict it because not everyone's hair falls out when they are undergoing chemotherapy.

To summarise:
- An argument consists of a conclusion, with one or more relevant reasons that are intended to support the conclusion
- Evidence may or may not be offered to support each reason
- A sound argument is one in which the reason(s) are acceptable and provide adequate grounds for accepting the conclusion
- There are a few technical terms that need to be remembered regarding what has been covered so far
- A *reason* can also be called a premise
- The question of whether reasons provide grounds for the conclusion is a question of *validity*. In everyday conversation, the word validity often has a broader meaning. In critical thinking, it is used to refer to the logical relationship between the reasons and the conclusion
- When an argument has reasons that are acceptable and is valid (i.e. the reasons provide adequate grounds for accepting the conclusion), then the argument is said to be *sound*.

It is important to note that an argument can be valid but unsound. For example, the following argument is valid but unsound:

1 All nurses are female

2 Jo is a nurse

3 Therefore, Jo is female.

Statement 1 is not true, of course. Some nurses are male. Statement 2 can be assumed to be true. Because statement 1 is false, we already know that this argument is unsound. But is it valid? Yes, it is. If statement 1 were true, the acceptance of statement 3 would be unavoidable. This means that the argument is logically valid, but it is not sound—that is, it is not a sound argument.

REFLECTION

Arguments appear everywhere—but they are not always easy to spot. See if you can find at least three arguments in different media; for example, social media, news media or a peer-reviewed journal article. Can you identify the elements of each of these?

Critical thinking in nursing

Critical thinking, in the context of our discussion, means being able to identify the presence of an argument in any form and evaluate it. Once what makes a sound argument, and the questions needed to be asked to evaluate it, are known, it is possible to assess any argument that is encountered. Critical thinking means applying the type of thinking that has the characteristics discussed above.

This basic approach can be applied to many areas within nursing. In the following sections, some examples of these areas are provided, how the basic framework introduced above applies to that area will be discussed and some guidelines for thinking critically about issues in the respective area will be explained. The overlaying of the structure of argument onto the various areas in nursing builds on the work of Johnson-Laird et al (2017) in their discussion of reasoning and argumentation in critical thinking in psychology.

CLINICAL PRACTICE

In clinical practice, decisions are constantly being made to inform actions associated with the care of patients/clients. These actions can be beneficial or may have serious consequences for the health and wellbeing of the people a nurse is caring for. It is essential that these interventions be considered critically. Figure 9.3 illustrates the application of the basic argument framework to clinical practice.

As can be seen, very little alteration is necessary. The equivalent of the conclusion is the particular action that has been, or will be, undertaken. Each of a nurse's actions should be able to be justified by appealing to an appropriate set of reasons. These reasons, in turn, must be based on high-quality evidence.

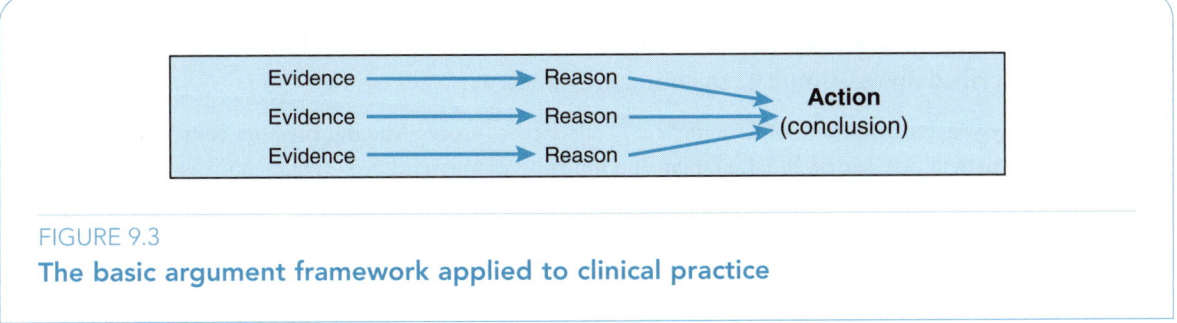

FIGURE 9.3
The basic argument framework applied to clinical practice

In the past, many of the actions and interventions of nurses have been based on tradition, folklore or no evidence at all. In recent decades, however, the professional status of nursing has resulted in more concern about the basis for nursing action. Evidence-based practice, which promotes an attitude of thinking critically about what is done by nurses and questioning the basis on which actions can be justified, is now a fundamental element of nursing.

The increasing interest of consumers in their own healthcare has also had an effect. People are no longer willing to allow health professionals to make all the decisions for them and are demanding higher-quality care. The increasing incidence of litigation has also motivated the focus on nursing care being centred on high-quality evidence.

On an individual level, a nurse should be able to justify any action performed on behalf of a person being cared for. These reasons should be based on sound evidence. The source of this evidence may take many forms, including personal experience, traditions handed down between 'generations' of nurses and what is taught during nurse education. However, on their own, these sources of knowledge are not adequate. A formal process for exploring nursing knowledge is needed, which allows the testing of ideas and the validation of actions and interventions.

The activity of formal research provides this opportunity. Nursing research will be examined below from a critical thinking perspective. Before doing so several questions that can be asked about practice, which will help nurses think critically about it, need to be considered. When reflecting on an action or intervention, ask the following questions:

- What are the reasons for acting or intervening in the way that is planned?
- What evidence is available that supports the reasons for acting in this way?
- Are the reasons relevant to the issue that is being considered?
- Are there other reasons that need to be considered?
- Is there any evidence that raises questions about the manner of acting or intervening?
- Do the reasons provide adequate grounds for acting in the planned way?
- Are there alternative actions or interventions that could be chosen, and the reasons still be acceptable in these situations?

CLINICAL REASONING

Clinical reasoning is an essential aspect of the work of nurses and should form the basis of clinical practice as described above. Clinical reasoning is defined as:

> the process by which nurses (and other clinicians) collect cues, process the information, come to an understanding of a patient problem or situation, plan and implement interventions, evaluate outcomes, and reflect on and learn from the process.
>
> (Levett-Jones 2022)

Levett-Jones identifies the following stages of clinical reasoning:
1. Consider the patient situation
2. Collect cues/information
3. Process information
4. Identify problems/issues
5. Establish goals
6. Take action
7. Evaluate outcomes
8. Reflect on process and new learning.

We do not have the space to explore these steps in depth. However, it is important to recognise that the clinical reasoning process is the predominant way of understanding what nurses do in providing high-quality care for patients and/or clients. Let us now explore how understanding the clinical reasoning process as an argument can be helpful in thinking critically about nursing practice.

The phases of clinical reasoning represented as an argument

The first three phases of the clinical reasoning process can be understood as an argument (remember the technical meaning of the term 'argument'). Figure 9.4 illustrates this.

Identifying problems and issues is the equivalent of the conclusion in an argument. The data that are collected come from observations of the patient, as well as information provided by the client, relatives, friends, history and so on. These raw data need to be processed by the nurse interpreting them and they take on meaning in the context of identifying the problems and issues. Finally, based

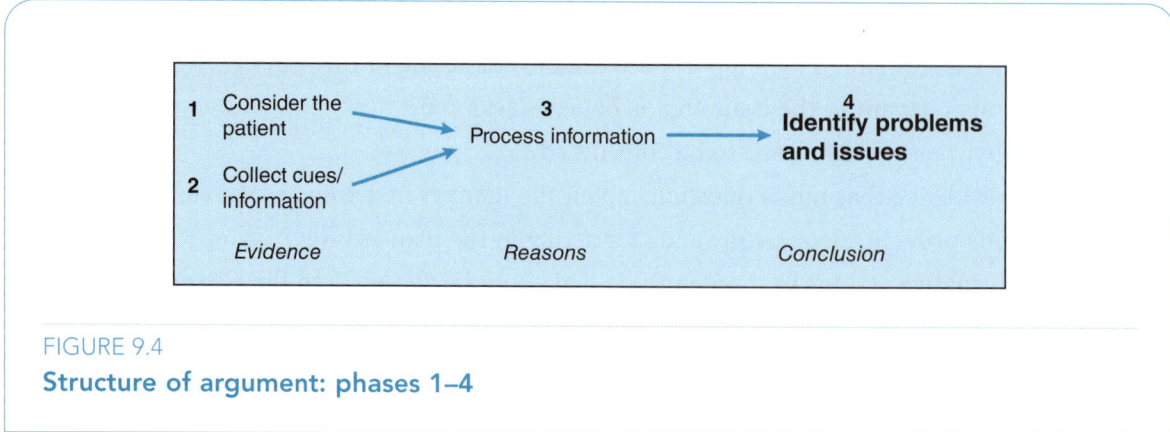

FIGURE 9.4
Structure of argument: phases 1–4

on the meaning of the data, a conclusion is arrived at in the form of a clear understanding of the problems and issues associated with a particular client.

Of course, the description here is somewhat simplistic. The actual process is much richer and more complex. However, understanding the process of arriving at the problems and issues as an argument leads us to ask the following questions:

1. Are the data collected accurate? If not, how reliable are they?
2. Have the data been understood and interpreted correctly?
3. Are the data and their interpretation relevant to the problems and issues that have been identified?
4. Does the interpretation of the data provide adequate grounds for arriving at the identified problems and issues?
5. Are there any other problems and issues that could possibly fit the data that have been collected? Are any of these more consistent with the data?

A similar process applies to the other phases of the clinical reasoning process. Establishing goals, taking action, evaluating outcomes and reflecting on the overall process all must be justified to support claims of changes such as improvement or deterioration, or preservation of the status quo. For example, does a particular intervention have adequate evidence to justify using it for a particular condition? Or is a particular evaluation criterion actually relevant to measuring real change in a condition? Figures 9.5 and 9.6 illustrate the structure of argument related to these two phases.

THINKING CRITICALLY ABOUT RESEARCH

The need for nursing research and the current focus on evidence-based practice has been described above. Nursing research provides the evidence nurses need to evaluate the appropriateness of nursing practice, helps to raise new questions for nurses to explore and provokes new ways of looking at what nurses do.

Nurses may relate to research in three ways. A nurse may be a 'consumer' of research, a researcher, or both. In this discussion, we will be focusing on the role of research consumer.

It has already been argued that nurses must base their practice on high-quality evidence. The outcomes of nursing research form the most significant source of this evidence for nurses. Nurses

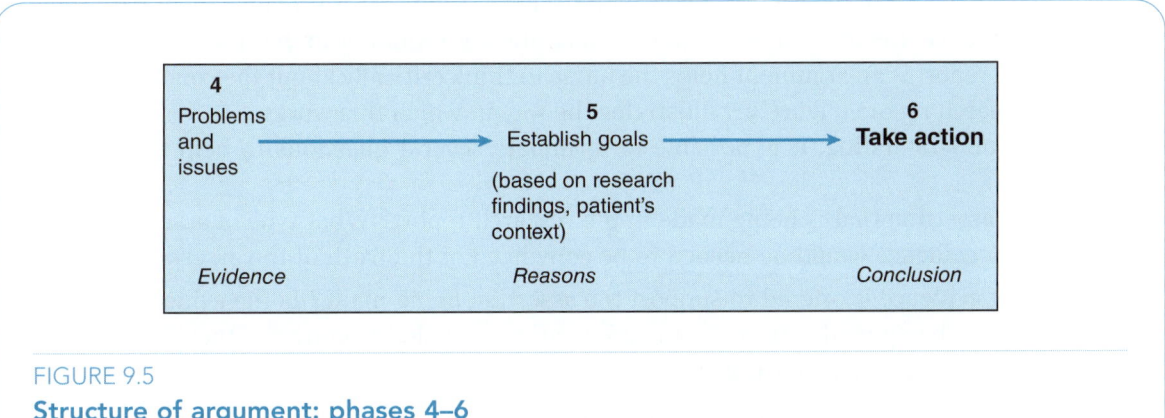

FIGURE 9.5
Structure of argument: phases 4–6

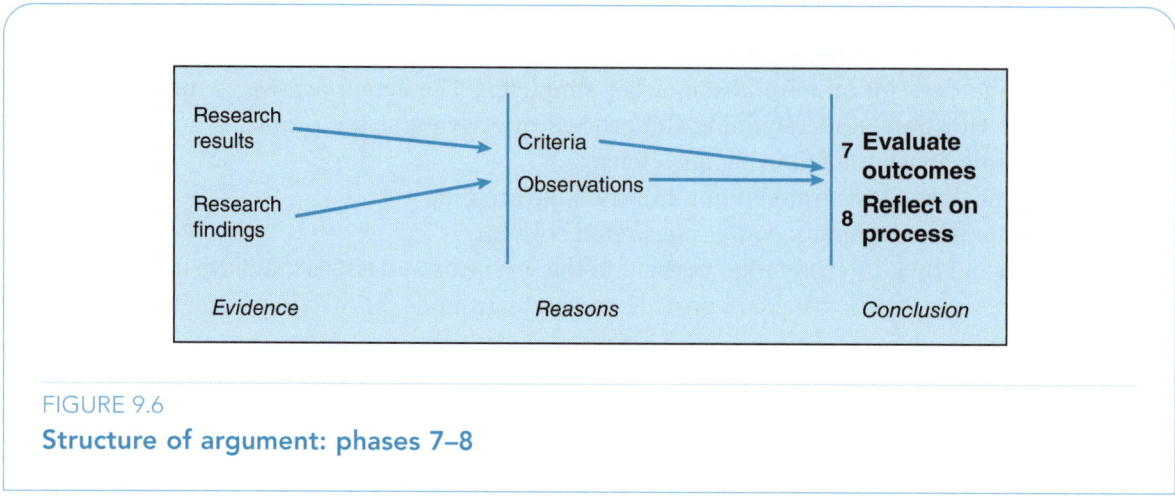

FIGURE 9.6
Structure of argument: phases 7–8

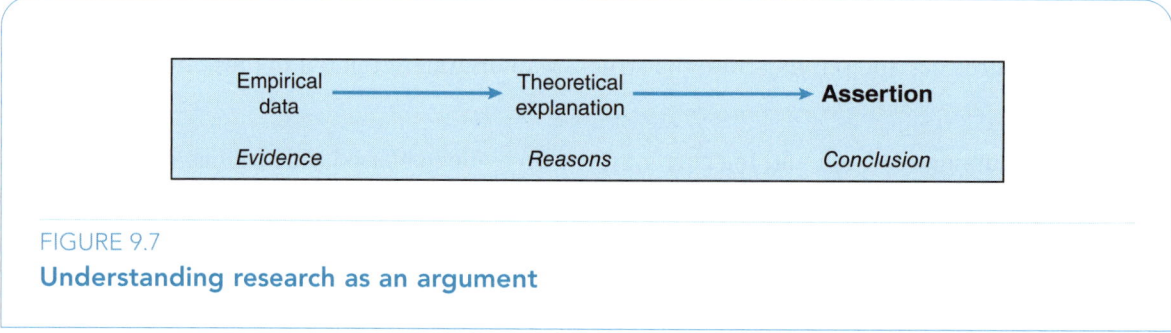

FIGURE 9.7
Understanding research as an argument

must avail themselves of the latest research in their area of practice, and this means that some understanding of the process is important.

Every research project suffers from limitations and flaws of some sort or another. Therefore, nurses cannot read a research report and automatically assume that it provides them with the best guidance for practice. Instead, nurses need to think critically about research reports. Understanding that a research report is an argument helps the nurse to think critically about the conclusions identified by the research report. Figure 9.7 illustrates the way in which this works.

Given this understanding, it is possible to formulate several questions to help think critically about research:

- What is the assertion that is being made in the research report? What type of assertion is it? What type of evidence would be needed to be convinced of the truth of the assertion?
- What sort of evidence is offered to support the assertion being made? Is the evidence relevant to the assertion being made? Is adequate information provided to convince the reader that the evidence has been collected rigorously?
- Does the evidence offered provide adequate grounds for accepting the assertion that is being made? Is it possible to think of any other conclusions that could be drawn from the evidence offered? Are these alternative solutions more reasonable than the assertion made in the report?

▸ Does the theoretical explanation make sense? Are there alternative explanations that make more sense? Does the application of Occam's razor (roughly, this is the principle that the simplest explanation is most likely to be the right one) make any difference to the likelihood of the explanation being correct?

Asking these questions in relation to any research report heightens one's awareness that the conclusions of research are not always correct, nor is the process in arriving at that conclusion automatically sound. This promotes a careful assessment of new nursing practice proposals and consequent higher levels of safety in practice.

Thinking about ethics

Another essential area that nurses need to be aware of is ethics. Thinking ethically means to be able to justify what is done in terms of ethical principles. All behaviour needs to be ethical. Although there are high-profile issues such as euthanasia, abortion and organ transplantation that demand a great deal of attention, they are, perhaps, not the most important issues for nurses.

Issues such as the style of communicating with a patient, the facilitation of the signing of a consent form, communication with other professional colleagues and patients, the management of work rosters, the provision of childcare for employees, the influencing of clients in choosing treatment options—all need to be considered in ethical terms if the individual nurse is to practise with integrity and fulfil his or her obligations to clients.

Most professional bodies have documented codes of ethics, and the nursing profession is no different. For example, the International Council of Nurses' *Code of Ethics for Nurses* (2021), which guides ethical practice for nurses, contains four elements that comprise acting as an ethical guide in relation to 'nurses' roles, duties, responsibilities, behaviour, professional judgment and relationships with patients, other people who are receiving nursing care or services; co-workers and allied health professionals' (2021:2). This will have meaning only as a living document' if applied to the realities of nursing and healthcare in a changing society. To achieve its purpose the Code must be understood, internalised and used by nurses in all aspects of their work. It must be available to students and nurses throughout their study and work lives.

Because it is a *guide* and needs to be *applied*, nurses need to develop skills to be able to think through these principles and evaluate various options for practice. Understanding ethical thinking as an argument can help in this task. Figure 9.8 illustrates the components of an ethical argument. Each of these components will now be examined in relation to critical thinking.

THE SITUATION

Ethical thinking is often taught using highly controversial case studies that involve situations where unethical decisions have been made. However, studies suggest that using simulated situations, role-playing and exposure to ethical situations may be more effective in supporting ethical decision making (Ghoozlu et al 2023:1093).

In reality, ethical thinking should underpin all nursing actions, and ethical questions about practice should be continually asked. Ethical thinking should be an everyday activity, which may not always be about problems.

We usually find ourselves in situations where a decision needs to be made about how to act towards another person. These situations continually occur for nurses. For example, a patient might require a sponge bath in bed. This may not appear to be a situation where ethical thinking needs to

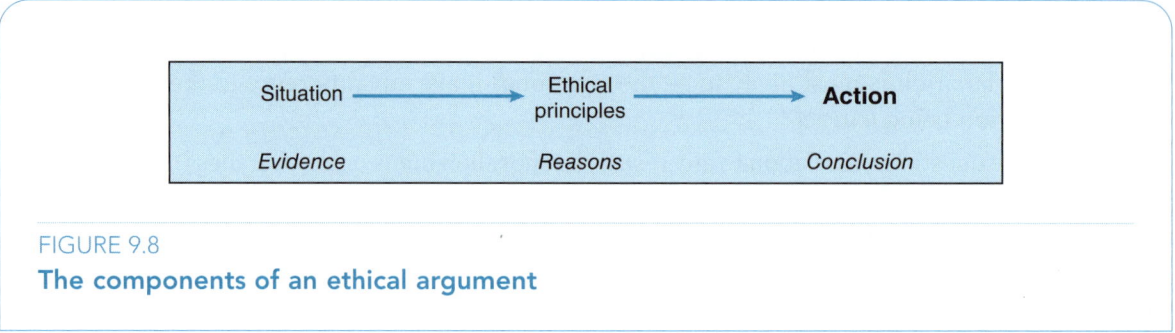

FIGURE 9.8

The components of an ethical argument

take place. But, as this example is explored below, it will be seen that ethical thinking is fundamental to ensuring that the best care is provided.

The first thing to do when thinking ethically is to be aware of as much about the situation as is possible. Too often assumptions are made based on past experience; but every person is different and has unique needs.

THE PRINCIPLES

Everyone has a system of principles (values) that guide their lives and how they act. Some of these will be conscious, others may be unconscious. In healthcare, four principles have been identified as an essential starting point for ethical thinking:

1. Autonomy: the right a person has to direct their own life and make their own decisions
2. Beneficence: the responsibility of actively doing good
3. Non-maleficence: the responsibility to actively avoid doing harm
4. Justice: the responsibility to be fair in the way we treat others.

After gaining knowledge of the situation, the next step is to ask which of the principles (values) are relevant to consider in the particular situation in which the nurse finds themselves. In the example of the person who needs to be washed in bed, the issue of autonomy is clearly relevant. How is autonomy to be ensured in this particular situation? How will the patient be empowered to make their own decisions about their hygiene and the way they wish to maintain it?

The principle of beneficence is also relevant. The whole reason for instituting the patient washing in bed is because it is believed it is good to promote hygiene. It is possible, however, that beneficence may spill over into a denial of the person's autonomy. When this happens, nurses are acting paternalistically—doing what they think is best for the patient—even if the patient does not agree with the nurse. Paternalism needs to be rigorously justified because it overrides a person's fundamental right to autonomy.

Many examples can be found of situations where paternalism occurs, imposing medication on a psychotic individual; or legally enforcing a blood transfusion for a child of a Jehovah's Witness parent. On many occasions paternalistic attitudes prevail without adequate ethical justification.

Depending on the specific circumstances, the other ethical principles (justice and non-maleficence) may also need to be considered.

ACTION

Once the situation is understood and the implications of the relevant ethical principles have been thought through, it is necessary to make a decision about how to act. Often this will not be easy. Sometimes, ethical principles conflict with each other (such as when beneficence and autonomy conflict). Nurses do not live and practise in an ideal world, and so it is necessary to be satisfied with the best decision that can be made under the circumstances. The point is not that perfect decisions have to be made; that is never possible. It is rather that whatever decisions are made and whatever actions are performed, they have been carefully thought through and can be justified by appeal to accepted ethical principles.

The ethics of critical thinking

Often, when people learn the tools of critical thinking, they become highly critical of others. It is important that critical thinking is viewed primarily as a set of tools applied to one's own thinking. When evaluating the ideas of others, critical thinking skills are used to decide whether an idea is acceptable or should be rejected. It is important to remember the distinction between an idea and the person who presents the idea. Usually, but not always, it is irrelevant who the other person is. When critical thinking skills undermine or attack other people, then the purpose of critical thinking is lost.

The critical thinker always needs to think critically within the framework of well-developed interpersonal relationship skills. Critical thinking skills are not weapons to be wielded to cut another person down to size. They are tools of personal growth, which allow one to travel through an often-confusing landscape and keep one's bearings, while providing the best possible quality care for those to whom one is responsible and accountable.

REFLECTION

Which of the above areas of nursing practice are most relevant to you in your own work? How will you begin to practise critical thinking skills in that area?

Developing critical thinking skills

There is no magical solution to developing critical thinking skills. An awareness of what critical thinking is and where it can be applied is an appropriate start. Like anything, it requires continual practice. Ultimately, it is about developing a conscious attitude of reflection during daily and professional life. We have discussed the need for habits of mind that are needed to continually apply and improve in critical thinking. It takes practice—and more practice. As Elder and Paul (2020:xxii) suggest:

> To make significant gains in the quality of your thinking, you will have to engage in a kind of work that most humans find unpleasant, if not painful—intellectual work… One doesn't become a skillful critic of thinking overnight, any more than one becomes a skillful basketball player or dancer overnight. To become a student of thinking, you must be willing to put the work into thinking that skilled improvement always requires.

This means you must be willing to practice special 'acts' of thinking that are initially at least uncomfortable, and sometimes challenging and difficult... Improvement in thinking, in other words, is similar to improvement in other domains of performance, where progress is a product of sound theory, commitment, hard work and practice.

Although it can be challenging to develop new skills in critical thinking, the time and energy are well worth the rewards that come with the ability to think clearly.

You may also find using some software useful in helping you think critically. There are quite a few software packages available that can help visualise arguments and aid in the process of analysis. One of the best of these is Rationale, which allows you to create diagrams of arguments and your evaluation. Figure 9.9 shows a diagram, produced by Rationale, of the argument about hair loss following chemotherapy, as described above. You can access information about this software and download a free account from https://www.rationaleonline.com/.

There are also an increasing number of apps available for iOS (Apple) and Android devices. Some popular apps include Luminosity and MindMeister. Have a go at searching for *critical thinking* in the app stores for your respective device.

> ### REFLECTION
> What resources are you going to follow up to learn more about critical thinking and how you can apply it in nursing practice?

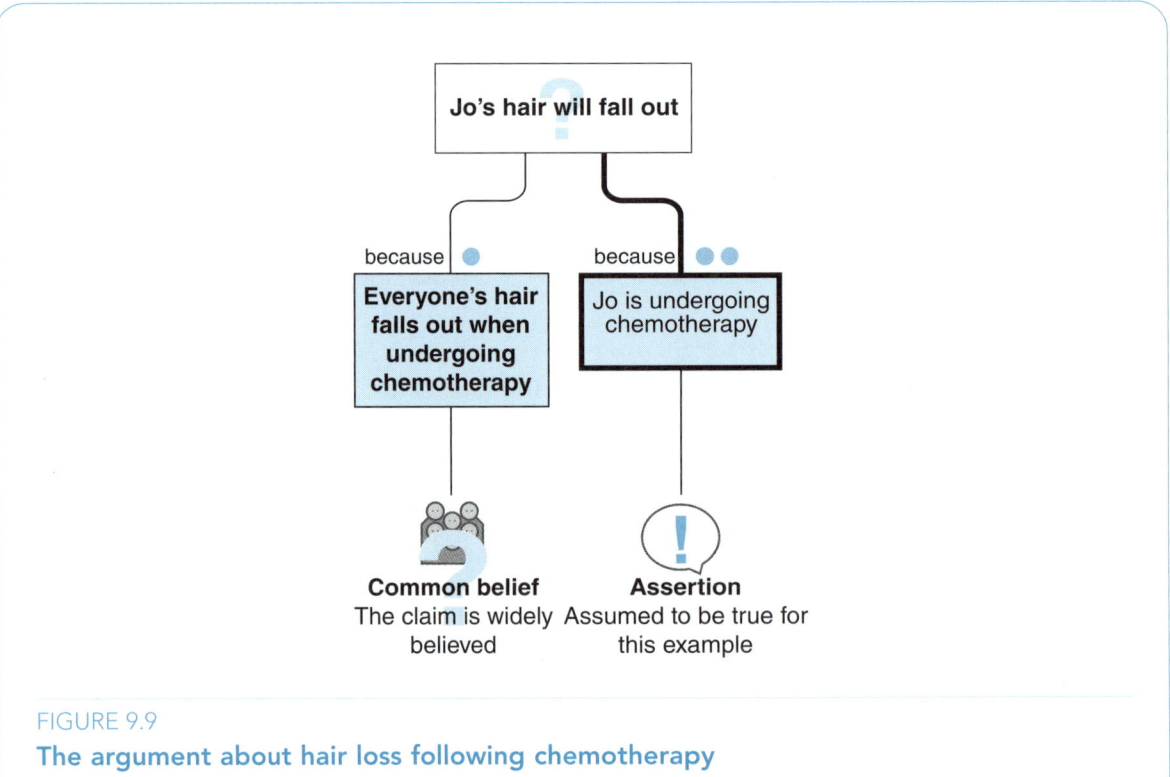

FIGURE 9.9

The argument about hair loss following chemotherapy

CONCLUSION

Critical thinking is a vital skill to have as a nurse. Nurses are engaged in providing care to people who have a right to high-quality professional conduct and health services. Nurses have a responsibility to make sure that their actions are based on rigorous evidence and can be justified with acceptable reasons. Although developing the skills to think critically may at times be challenging and demanding, thinking critically provides a greater level of confidence and satisfaction as nurses interact with colleagues, and it promotes high-quality, safe practice.

REFLECTIVE QUESTIONS

1. How has your understanding of thinking changed as a result of reading this chapter?
2. What areas of your professional life would benefit from applying the principles of critical thinking to them?
3. What will you do now to further develop your skill in critical thinking?

Recommended readings

Browne M N, Keeley S M 2020 Asking the right questions: a guide to critical thinking, 11th edn. Pearson Education, Essex

Levett-Jones T (ed) 2022 Clinical reasoning, 3rd edn. Pearson Australia, Frenchs Forest, NSW

Elder L, Paul R 2020 Critical thinking: learn the tools the best thinkers use. Foundation for Critical Thinking. Rowman & Littlefield, Lanham, MD

References

Costa A L, Kallick B 2008 Learning and leading with habits of mind. ASCD, Alexandria, VA

Elder L, Richard P 2020 Critical thinking: learn the tools the best thinkers use. Foundation for Critical Thinking

Ennis R H 2015 Critical thinking: a streamlined conception. In: Davies M, Barnett R (eds) The Palgrave handbook of critical thinking in higher education. Palgrave Macmillan, London

Falcó-Pegueroles A, Rodríguez-Martín D, Ramos-Pozón S et al 2021 Critical thinking in nursing clinical practice, education and research: From attitudes to virtue. Nursing Philosophy 22(1):e12332 https://doi.org/10.1111/nup.12332

Ghoozlu K J, Vanaki Z, Mohammad Khan Kermanshahi S 2023 Ethics education: nurse educators' main concern and their teaching strategies. Nursing Ethics 30(7-8):1083–1094 doi: 10.1177/09697330231153685

International Council of Nurses (ICN) 2021 The ICN code of ethics for nurses. Online. Available: efaidnbmnnnibpcaj pcglclefindmkaj/https://www.icn.ch/sites/default/files/2023-06/ICN_Code-of-Ethics_EN_Web.pdf

Johnson-Laird P N, Goodwin G P, Khemlani S S 2017 Mental models and reasoning. In: Ball L J, Thompson V A (eds) International Handbook of Thinking and Reasoning. Routledge, pp 346–365

Karaca A, Kaya G, Kaya L 2023 The relationship between critical thinking skills and caregiving roles of nurses. Journal of Education and Research in Nursing 20 (4):360–366. doi:10.14744/jern.2023.22354

Levett-Jones T 2022 Clinical reasoning: what it is and why it matters. In: Levett-Jones T (ed) Clinical reasoning: learning to think like a nurse, 3rd edn. Pearson Australia, Frenchs Forest, NSW, pp 61–95

Nursing and Midwifery Board of Australia 2016 Professional standards. Online. Available: https://www.nursingmidwiferyboard.gov.au/Codes-Guidelines-Statements/Professional-standards.aspx 9 Jan 2024

Nursing and Midwifery Board of Australia 2016 Registered nurse standards of practice.Online. Available: https://www.nursingmidwiferyboard.gov.au/Codes-Guidelines-Statements/Professional-standards/registered-nurse-standards-for-practice.aspx#

Urhan E, Zuriguel-Perez E, Harmancı Seren A K 2022 Critical thinking among clinical nurses and related factors: a survey study in public hospitals. Journal of Clinical Nursing 31(21–22):3155–3164 https://doi.org/10.1111/jocn.16141

Von Colln-Appling C, Giuliano D 2017 A concept analysis of critical thinking: a guide for nurse educators. Nurse Education Today 49:106–109 https://doi.org/10.1016/j.nedt.2016.11.007

Zmuda A, Costa A L, Kallick B 2023 Discovering and exploring habits of mind. In Altan S, Farber Lane J (eds) Mindfulness and Thoughtfulness: Leading and Teaching with Habits of Mind in Research and Practice, Rowman & Littlefield, MD, Ch 16, pp 1–16

Perez E Z, Lluch Canut M T, Falcó Pegueroles A et al 2015 Critical thinking in nursing: scoping review of the literature. International Journal of Nursing Practice 21(6):820–830 https://doi.org/10.1111/ijn.12347

CHAPTER 10
POWER AND POLITICS IN NURSING

Sharon Brownie and Letitia Del Fabbro

KEY WORDS

advocacy
empowerment
equity
power
politics
social justice
nursing

LEARNING OBJECTIVES

After reading this chapter, readers should be able to discuss:

- the nature of power and politics; the ways in which nurses possess power individually and collectively
- advocacy and agency and how these relate to power and nursing
- the relevance of social justice and equity to nursing
- the complexities of speaking up for safe practice and whistleblowing.

INTRODUCTION

In this chapter, we explore the concepts of power and politics in relation to nursing practice, including the political and structural influences that create unjust health systems and inequitable health outcomes. The need for nurses to claim and utilise political and collective professional power to influence and improve issues of social justice and support equitable access and outcomes is discussed. We consider the role of nursing in influence and agency enabling nurses to claim their legitimate power, to lead, to speak up for safe practice and to advocate for people's rights in a socially just and morally sound way. We also note that the COVID-19 pandemic significantly impacted the work of nurses; therefore, we highlight examples and outcomes arising from nurses working during this period.

Power and politics in the nursing context

Power, in the broadest sense of the word, is part of all nurses' lives and it is important to think about politics along with the associated concept of power. Nurses should understand that the health sector is a politicised environment at both micro- and macro-levels. It is not an apolitical or neutral context (Wilson et al 2020). Health, healthcare and workforce are dependent on the socioeconomic and political systems that guide the distribution of increasingly scarce resources (Fainman & Kucukyazici 2020). Power plays a central role in determining health systems' functioning and underpins health systems' governance, ideology, values, expectations and resource allocation (Friel et al 2023, Kickbusch 2015). Policies and legislation originating from leaders in power directly impact the day-to-day work of nurses and their patients and clients (Hajizadeh et al 2021, Willis et al 2017).

Although the World Health Organization (2021) recognises the key leadership roles that nurses have in achieving global health and social gains, nursing has a history of having a limited voice in policy making and political influence. This is despite being the largest regulated workforce (Rafferty 2018). In a highly complex, financially rationed context nurses are often excluded from conversations about resource allocation and subsequently are a 'soft target' for health system savings. The consequences can be seen in nurse retention, staffing levels, workload, patient/client ratios and workplace conditions with flow-on effects of negative patient/client outcomes (Rafferty 2018). The echoes of this history were evident in some places during the COVID-19 pandemic (Ramsay et al 2022). In contrast, the pandemic also elevated awareness of nurses and nursing, providing opportunity to capitalise on reputational gains and increase public awareness of the value and contribution of nurses (Gottlieb et al 2021, McDonald 2022) and to seek recognition (James et al 2024). The COVID-19 pandemic led to rapid resource re-allocation, to support health systems and vulnerable populations unprepared for such a large-scale event (Chiu 2023). While nurses received recognition and 'reputational gains' for their visible role in this crisis (Gottlieb et al 2021, McDonald 2022), the increased professional visibility came with a struggle and was not universally recognised (Abrams et al 2023). While some gains were made, the COVID-19 pandemic was challenging and exacerbated the global nursing shortage with inequitable impact across various communities and socioeconomic groups (International Council of Nurses 2022).

First Nations nurses are significantly under-represented in nursing workforces worldwide. Indeed, nursing education programs have been critiqued for promulgating whiteness in nursing (Jackson 2023). Recruitment and retention of First Nations nurses and midwives is also an ongoing priority in Australia and New Zealand (Aotearoa). In Australia, 1.4% of nurses and midwives are First Nations people (Congress of Aboriginal and Torres Strait Islander Nurses and Midwives 2022), and in New Zealand (Aotearoa) a disproportionally small percentage of Māori nurses are employed in comparison to the percentage of Māori in the total population (Komene et al 2023).

If success in politics is judged by control over resources, nurses have historically been unsuccessful in the political arena if factors such as constraints on expanded practice roles, low numbers of Indigenous nurses and pay parity with equivalent professional groups are considered. Some nurses have effectively engaged in politics in different domains with emerging imageries depicting nurses as strong and autonomous (James et al 2024). However, stereotypical views of nursing, along with the issues around the gendered nature of nursing, have limited the full realisation of the potential of nurses, and of nursing, in political action, influence and advocacy.

Historically, nurses have been disadvantaged by professional role divisions positioning the practice of nursing as subservient to the practice of medicine and physician-led care (Adams et al 2024). This positioning can inhibit nurses' sense of power and the capacity for productive action. Specific jurisdictional factors are reported as restricting practice, for example, the restricting role of medicine in respect to nurse practitioner roles and opportunities, including barriers to reciprocal licensing networks (Feyereisen & Goodrick 2021). While beliefs persist that healthcare provision must be led by the medical profession, obvious solutions to address health sector provision will not be realised.

Nurses have highlighted how austerity measures impact workload, resulting in missed care with some nursing interventions unable to be provided when resource allocations are inadequate (Bosley et al 2021). Health budget rationalisation, staffing levels based on patient/client numbers rather than acuity, casualisation of the workforce and non-regulated role substitution directly impact nursing roles and care (Willis et al 2017). Despite these challenges, nurses have considerable potential for action.

The World Health Organization (WHO) has recommended global directions for nursing development in education, jobs, leadership and service delivery (WHO 2021). Nurses can work together to maximise the capacity and potential through intra- and interprofessional collaborative partnerships and continuing professional development. They can mobilise political will, advocating for investment to build the nursing workforce to sufficient numbers and capacity to meet health service needs.

Taylor (2016) argues that nurses have a key role in active political advocacy to influence issues of social injustice, equity, access to healthcare resources and healthy working environments. Adams et al (2024:13) emphasise the importance of addressing 'oppressive and racist social health structures', and in their recent concept analysis of health equity, Lewis et al (2023) identify specific actions nursing can take in addressing power inequities. Friel and others (2021:282) refer to achieving health equity as 'a power-saturated long game' requiring continuous efforts. In the words of Moorley et al (2020:2450), 'Being a nurse … in 2020 must mean being aware of social injustices and the systemic racism that exist in much of nursing … and having a personal and professional responsibility to challenge and help end them'.

REFLECTION

Reflect on what you have read about nursing and political power. Worldwide, the COVID-19 pandemic amplified inequities in care delivery. Thinking of your own experience during the COVID-19 pandemic, did you feel a loss of power or a gain of power? Write a brief paragraph about this experience; you may want to use reflection tools from Chapter 11.

Agency relates to the actions taken by individuals or groups to influence people, processes and systems. Jones et al (2020) propose that nurses utilise their agency to effectively address 'endemic' problems such as missed nursing care. Nurses have a vital political role in creating practices and systems that support humane and just healthcare provision, and nurses' political and professional power has the potential to positively impact healthcare systems and patient/client outcomes (Dickman & Chicas 2021).

Health is fundamental to life, and nurses are intimately involved in caring for the sick and supporting the healthy, either directly or indirectly, wherever they are working. Nurses are in a privileged position in that millions of people every day put their trust in nurses and assume that nurses will always work on their (and the public's) behalf. Nurses accept the obligations and expectations that go with being in a responsible and respected (particularly by the public) role. With registration comes the commitment and accountability to work within a code of ethics, at the centre of which is the safety and wellbeing of those for whom nurses provide care. Key to the delivery of safe care is wise use of the power that nurses hold while being aware of the moral and ethical obligations entrusted to them (Jeong et al 2021).

The concept of personhood is central to any contemporary discussion related to power and obligations in nursing. This starts with the recognition and acknowledgment of the patient's personhood translated to person-centred care (Benner 2010, Chapman et al 2024). Every nurse possesses power (Sepasi et al 2016). Even newly registered nurses immediately have power over patients/clients, who are frequently in a less powerful position due to nurses' knowledge of health, illness and the healthcare system. Knowledge is linked to power, and the ability to impart or withhold information puts nurses in a privileged position in relation to the people and/or communities with whom they work. Working in partnership with patients and their families in a way that gives 'power to' the patient, or empowers the patient, is the most preferable and ethical way to work with your patients. However, the agency for a nurse to work this way is impacted by the structures and constraints of the organisations that nurses work in or for; for example, time constraints or lack of resources to provide optimal patient care.

Nurses require an understanding of power and its effects, and the way that they can use their power to enhance the health and wellbeing of people, along with their working conditions and professional status—an empowered nurse is able to provide more effective care and is more likely to be professionally fulfilled and retained in the workforce (Conroy et al 2023, Ko 2020). Power is often considered a negative and oppressive attribute. More recent definitions of the nature of power discussed in this chapter incorporate the notion of power as constructive and constitutive, as well as having the potential to be destructive and oppressive. These definitions also provide us with a way of considering power, where nurses can be viewed as being powerless in certain situations but very powerful in other circumstances. This representation frees nurses from the idea of inherent powerlessness and/or being victims, simply through being nurses. Rethinking and reshaping of nurses' positioning in terms of agency is important in this era of intense governmental scrutiny and concerns about controlling health sector costs. Appropriate resourcing of nursing care and workforce planning, and education are critical enablers of effective person-centred care (Conroy et al 2023, Gilmour et al 2016).

Understanding power

Power is a complex concept which impacts nursing roles and satisfaction (Sepasi et al 2016). Contemporary definitions of power are multi-faceted and traverse broad theoretical domains including structural and ideational approaches to power (Friel et al 2021). It is challenging to fully understand the complexities and interrelationship of power dynamics and the impact on healthcare systems, the nursing profession and health outcomes. Power can be negative and oppressive; but used intentionally and effectively, power can be used to positively influence, facilitate change and contribute to social good and improved health outcomes. Power is a useful tool for getting things done and achieving the goals and outcomes of an organisation. Such framing challenges negative notions associated with more traditional conceptions of power. Traditionally, power has been associated with wielding 'power over' other groups or individuals, or controlling others with the goal of achieving obedience or conformity (Hokanson Hawks 1991). Social theorists (Harris et al 2020, Topp et al 2021) have informed an understanding of power in nursing; for example, according to Foucault (2003), where there is knowledge there is power, and power is at play when individuals exercise action upon themselves and others. We can consider that this relationship between professional knowledge and the ability to act affords nurses the capacity and the responsibility to assume legitimate power and act accordingly to assert influence within the healthcare domain. Katriina et al (2013) propose that when power is viewed as the ability to achieve goals, it becomes a significant and necessary resource for nurses to harness and utilise. The 'Expressions of Power Framework' (Topp et al 2021, Veneklasen & Miller 2002) includes four categories of power including 'power to'. This framework continues to resonate with the nursing profession. Nursing has achieved a trusted social status that allows us the ability to act in a way that constitutes 'power to' influence individuals, communities and social systems. Nurses require power and agency to be effective in working within multidisciplinary teams and complex environments. It is important for nurses to understand how power can be used in a positive way because nurses who perceive themselves to be powerless are reported as being less efficacious and experience lower satisfaction with their work (Azizi et al 2023).

Positive perspectives of power provide nurses with an alternate way of considering power and its use. It is necessary to recognise that power dynamics will be ever present but can be employed to act and pursue goals of improving people's health and wellbeing outcomes and influencing systems of care to be more socially just and effective.

> ### REFLECTION
> Do you think you can influence your practice setting? If so, how do you exercise that influence? If not, what processes need to be in place to enable nurses the opportunity to voice concerns and ideas for change?

Politics and power

Politics permeates all aspects of life and is a concept associated and intertwined with many other terms such as power, influence, disempowerment and policy, each of which can have different meanings in different contexts. In the nineteenth century, politics related to the state and the mechanisms used by governments to shape and lead nations (Alexander 2014). Chaffee et al (2012:5) define politics as 'the process of influencing the allocation of scarce resources'. Politics at state and national levels are often thought of as only involving government. Governments are critical bodies for regulating behaviour in that 'government lays down the "rules of the game" in conflict and competition between individuals, organisations, and institutions within society' (Harrison 2014:166). But politics, seen as the exercise of power in the form of influence, is also part of everyday life. Definitions have broadened in recent years.

'Politics' is now considered to include a broad and multi-level concept by which government entities, business, professional groups, communities and individuals can establish power and gain resources (Alexander 2014, Boswell & Smith 2017, Mayne et al 2018, Wilson et al 2020).

Political effectiveness is linked with concepts of both power and disempowerment. It is commonly understood that power includes the freedom, ability and choice to act, whereas disempowerment is associated with lack of control in respect to life factors at home and work, including within professions (Lundin et al 2022, Tojamjan 2012a, 2012b). 'Influence' involves the capacity to facilitate and enact change, change beliefs, change behaviour and achieve results (Flaubert et al 2021, Scharlatt & Smith 2015). Engaging in political action—learning to be more influential in relation to matters that count—is therefore both possible and necessary for all nurses (Flaubert et al 2021).

Influence exists through relationships and is often more significant than authority (Gottlieb et al 2021, Sullivan 2013). Influence is earned through effort and the skills to exercise this can be learned, with the most crucial factor being the personal decision to become influential. Nurses sometimes consider that because they are good people doing a good job they should be valued and appropriately rewarded and, if that does not happen, they may blame themselves, the profession or their workplace (Alahiane et al 2023, Sullivan 2013). Nurses may be unrewarded if they have not engaged in an underlying political game, which requires adherence to a particular set of rules that they may not know exists. Critically, nurses must recognise the existence and reality of politics, the legitimacy and necessity of being involved in politics and learn skills to gain greater influence if personal and professional goals are to be achieved. Now more than ever, political and professional empowerment of the nursing workforce is central to healthcare access and quality care (Gottlieb et al 2021, Lundin et al 2022). Being influential and developing assertive and satisfying interdisciplinary relationships are essential contributors to nurses' agency in ensuring the provision of high-quality nursing care. Gottlieb et al (2021) identified workplace values to support empowerment and autonomy in nursing staff:

- systems thinking
- uniqueness
- health and healing
- multiple perspectives
- self-determination
- goodness of fit
- learning, timing and readiness
- collaborative partnership.

Nurses' collective political power

All people have political power as individuals, but nurses also have great potential as a collective body to exercise their power. This means that, in addition to an individual nurse's power in the patient/client relationship, nurses also have collective power. In many countries, nurses are the largest occupational group in the healthcare sector. In 2023 in New Zealand (Aotearoa) there were 77,634 nurses (enrolled, registered and nurse practitioners) (Nursing Council of New Zealand 2023) and in 2022, 372,759 registered nurses and 53,612 enrolled nurses were registered and employed in Australia (Australian Government 2023). Many of the reforms and restructuring that have taken place in Western health systems in recent years are focused on controlling nursing numbers and budgets. This is partially due to the cost of providing nursing services. However, these numbers provide nurses with critical mass and collective power that can be used to influence the health system and improve patient care.

Realising collective power requires formal ways to organise groups of people with a well-articulated position that appeals to broad segments of the population. In nursing, the protection, support and influence derived from the power of the collective is realised through trade unions and professional organisations. This power is shown clearly in legislation such as the *Safe Patient Care Act 2015* and 2019 amendment. This is landmark patient/client safety legislation to ensure in law the minimum number of nurses to care for patients/clients. As a result, 600 additional nurses and midwives were employed in areas such as the Australian state of Victoria (Victoria State Government 2019). The underpinning legislation has had a major impact on the working environment for nurses. Similar work has occurred in other Australian jurisdictions and in New Zealand (Aotearoa) with the mandated safe staffing fostering healthy workplace partnership between the nursing unions and the District Health Boards (New Zealand Nurses Association n.d.). The Care Capacity Demand Programme (CCDM) provides methods with which to match patient/client care requirements with the appropriate nursing resource and includes acuity measures in addition to ratios (New Zealand Nurses Association n.d.). The goal of these programs is to match the capacity to care with demand, improve the quality of care and the work environment, and make best use of health resources. Another example of collective bargaining power is the Multi-Employer Collective Agreements negotiated by the New Zealand Nurses Organisation. These agreements would be impossible to negotiate at an individual level. While trade union membership has been declining in Australia, it is notable that in the previous decade membership of the Australian Nursing and Midwifery Federation (and its affiliated branches) increased by 84% (Parliament of Australia 2018), realising some of the best wages and conditions ever achieved by the profession.

One of the most important choices a registered nurse makes is the decision to join a professional body. There are many organisations that primarily serve to advance the interests of the nursing workforce and the profession. As nurses there is the opportunity to be involved and shape the political activity of these organisations through contribution as a member or at governance level. While nurses are often considered a homogeneous group, in fact nursing is enormously diverse. As a result, while the overall goals of nursing may be shared by everyone in the profession, individual nurses will not always share worldviews at either the macro- or micro-level. Therefore, using the power nurses have means being highly skilled at working not only with diverse population groups, but also with diverse nurses and nursing groups. Nurses hold many different philosophical and political positions. One strategy for managing this diversity is through the focus that professional organisations can bring. In these contexts, individual difference can be accepted, but organisational power can focus on collective professional issues and goals.

An example of nurses successfully using their collective political power to advance practice through the legislative process is the gaining of medication prescribing authority. Australian and New Zealand (Aotearoa) nurses and their regulatory bodies advocated for changes in legislation and governmental processes to enable nurses (usually advanced practitioners) to prescribe medications within their scope of practice. In New Zealand (Aotearoa), extending prescribing rights to nurse practitioners was contentious, with some members of the medical profession, such as general practitioners, concerned about potential competition for funding or professional status and dominance (Adams et al 2024, Carryer & Yarwood 2015). The now well-established *Medicines (Designated Prescribers: Nurse Practitioners) Regulations 2005* provided a framework for nurse practitioner prescribing; this was the starting point in expanding the prescribing role of registered nurses to meet the treatment needs of specific population groups more effectively. Further developments since include the *Medicines (Designated Prescriber—Registered Nurses Practising in Diabetes Health) Regulations 2011* and the *Medicines (Designated Prescriber—Registered Nurses) Regulations 2016*, which enable suitably qualified registered nurses to act as designated prescribers of a specified range of medicines in primary health and specialty teams (Nursing Council of New Zealand 2016).

Table 10.1 lists some ways of developing influence through knowledge, communication skills and action.

TABLE 10.1
Developing influence through knowledge, communication skills and action

KNOWLEDGE AND CONTEXT	COMMUNICATION SKILLS	ACTION
Nursing knowledge		
Evidence-based clinical practice knowledge Person-centredness, patient/client and family knowledge/agendas/issues Policy/legislation knowledge at government, discipline and organisational levels	Articulate, respectful and assertive verbal communication Creates space for consumers to voice preferences Clear and appropriate written communication meeting academic/media/political/popular conventions, depending on context	Respond in a timely and coherent manner Document using appropriate channels Incorporates consumer preferences Take opportunities to be involved in shaping policy through submissions and committee work Use information technology competently for communication and information retrieval
Understanding power and political behaviours in your particular nursing practice. Knowledge of who has the most power and finding ways to achieve your desired sphere of influence		
Relationship of knowledge with power Power as a circulating force The capacity for resistance Differentiation of power relations and force relations	Professional introductions Title parity Adhere to professional code of dress Prepare accounts demonstrating importance of nursing work	Take leadership opportunities—formal and informal Accept responsibility Use knowledge to inform patients/clients and families Act as an advocate
Understanding the rules of the game What are the norms in your workplace or organisation? Are there unstated expectations? Can you find a trusted peer or mentor to talk with for support?		
Nursing Healthcare teams Organisations Communities	Network within and outside the profession Develop and use relationships with media and politicians	Develop respectful and communicative relationships within and outside nursing Be tenacious Enlist support from broader communities of interest in issues of concern to nursing

> **REFLECTION**
>
> Can you provide examples where the collective power of the nursing profession influenced healthcare system changes? In expanding your understanding, what can you find out about Ryan's Rule?

POWER IN PRACTICE

Knowledge carries with it power and authority, but not all forms of knowledge are created equally. In the preceding section on nurses' political power there was a discussion on the power that nurses have as a collective. However, there is ample evidence to suggest that nurses have been conspicuously silent (or been silenced) at times when it has been vital that patients/clients have had vocal, assertive and knowledgeable advocates (Rasmussen et al 2022, Zhang & Casas 2022).

There has been a long history of documented instances where the devaluation of nurses' knowledge and authority by the medical profession has resulted in lethal consequences for patients/clients. One example is where 12 children died during or shortly after undergoing cardiac surgery in a Canadian hospital in 1994. Medical peers of the surgeon dismissed the validity of claims by several nurses that there were competency issues because nurses did not have medical expertise (Ceci 2004). In another example where nurses were concerned about surgical competency, the hospital authorities did not act upon the repeated complaints of Queensland nurses about the actions of a surgeon, who was eventually implicated in at least eight patient deaths (Johnstone 2022).

When nurses themselves feel powerless, however, they may choose not to act, and this can have dire consequences (Zhang & Casas 2022). An example where nurses did not speak up is referenced in New Zealand's Cartwright Inquiry into cervical cancer, which investigated unethical medical research practices and the lack of informed consent about treatment options. Nurses working at this hospital throughout this period did not openly voice their concerns or ensure the women had been provided with the information necessary to make an informed choice about participation. Judge Silvia Cartwright stated that:

> ... nurses who most appropriately should be advocates for the patient, feel sufficiently intimidated by the medical staff (who do not hire or fire them) that even today they fail or refuse to confront openly the issues arising from the 1966 trial.
>
> (Committee of Inquiry into allegations concerning the treatment of cervical cancer at National Women's Hospital and into other related matters 1988:172)

Expressing agency is built upon the realisation of the importance of nurses' work and the confidence of nurses themselves. Making this agency explicit requires change at the fundamental level of day-to-day practice. Every encounter with patients/clients, families and other staff members is an opportunity to communicate, verbally and non-verbally, messages about the competency and the knowledge base underpinning nurses' decisions and practices.

Nurses are highly educated practitioners with both formal education in, and considerable informal knowledge of, the culture and processes of the health system within which clients and patients find themselves. This has important implications for power relationships between nurses and the people for whom nurses care. An example of the everyday exercise of power is the categorisation of people through the practice of assessment and the ensuing allocation of resources to them. Assessment requires recording a range of information and judging whether a person meets certain predetermined criteria for normality and/or abnormality. The distribution of a wide range of resources, including the time and expertise of nurses and other health professionals, medical equipment, pharmaceuticals and access to the care setting, can be determined by nursing assessment. Nurses can provide opportunities for patients/clients and their families to exercise control. This can be achieved by providing information about the purpose, scope and implications of the assessment in clear language, obtaining informed consent and validating the documented information with the person concerned. Similarly, nurses in inpatient/client hospital settings wield considerable power over family and friends' access to patients/clients (Flaubert et al 2021).

Practising from a person-family/whānau-centred approach aims to enable people with personal choice and control. Nurses can use their power to improve clinical practice and human experience. An individual nurse can utilise power by advocating for social justice and equity for people in their care and by speaking up for safe practice.

> ### REFLECTION
> How can you balance power between you and your patients/clients in everyday practice?

ADVOCATING FOR PARTNERSHIP AND SOCIAL JUSTICE

Advocacy consists of acting on behalf of a person, or supporting an individual or group to gain what they need from the system. The terms advocacy, activism and political participation are used interchangeably in the literature (Mundie & Donelle 2022). The advocacy role is now considered a fundamental element of practice at all levels (Laari & Duma 2023). The *Code of Ethics for Nurses in Australia* states from the outset that nurses must act when the standard of care is considered unacceptable: 'this includes a responsibility to question and report what they consider, on reasonable grounds, to be unethical behaviour and treatment' (Nursing and Midwifery Board of Australia 2018a). The increasingly overstretched and changing world of service delivery means that, more than ever before, nurses need to understand and enact an advocacy role at the micro- and macro-level.

Nurses may work on behalf of a person or group to advocate for resources or appropriate treatment and care. However, this approach could be seen as limiting the empowerment of individuals or groups; and so it is often more appropriate to support a person or community to advocate for themselves (Cole et al 2022). It is important to recognise that acting as an advocate does not involve taking over, which can result in a nurse acting out what he or she feels is best for the person, rather than acting to ensure that the person achieves what they want. According to the Nursing Council of New Zealand (2012a) *Code of Conduct*, partnership occurs when health consumers are given sufficient information, in a manner they can understand, to make an informed choice about their care and treatment and are fully involved in their care and treatment. Their independence, views and preferences are central to maintaining a person-centred approach. Nurses must be aware of the inherent power imbalance between themselves and health consumers, especially when the health consumer has limited knowledge, may be vulnerable or is part of a marginalised group. Supporting individuals or groups to act still involves the nurse in an act of advocacy, but one that reflects a social justice approach to power, in which everyone *has* power but may need support and information to *enact* that power. If a nurse is not able to speak up for equity and social justice, then the appropriate action is to ensure that the person or group has access to suitable advocacy support.

To be able to act effectively, speak up for equity and advocate for socially just outcomes for people using healthcare services, nurses need the following:

- understanding of the politics, culture and systems of health sector institutions and health service delivery
- understanding of the nature of power
- respect for the client or community and their rights
- understanding of relevant clinical issues
- understanding of ethical issues
- commitment to the client and/or group, and a professional obligation to act to ensure safe clinical care and health equity for people, and
- understanding of the need for evidence and the way it can be used to support decisions.

Advocating for equity and social justice can be used at all levels in the health system. It can be part of day-to-day practice in relationships with patients and clients, or it can involve influencing service delivery to enhance services for a client group or community. Advocacy at service delivery level aims to address health outcome disparities between different groups of the population. Nurses are well placed to detect access and treatment issues and advocate for services that provide equitable healthcare. Through membership of nursing associations, such as the Australian College of Nursing, nurses can participate in collective advocacy on a range of issues that affect nursing and service delivery (Wilson et al 2020).

Many nurses are also key players in groups working with people with health issues. Patient/client and family representative groups are effective lobbyists often accorded a voice in health policy development. Joint initiatives with these groups offer productive alliances to further nurses' and health consumers' agendas, focused on improving healthcare services. In New Zealand (Aotearoa), community voice led to a national inquiry into the state of mental health services (Health and Disability Commission 2018). The Australian National Disability Advocacy Program is focused on the rights of people with a disability to full community participation, and the promotion of choice and control in attaining personal goals and the use of support services. The program notes the range of disability advocacy models that can be employed, including systemic advocacy focused on long-term change addressing discriminatory policies and practices, and citizenship advocacy where people with a disability are matched with trained volunteer advocates (Department of Social Services 2018). It is important that nurses understand that there are limits to their advocacy skills, and that in some areas people may prefer external or non-health professional advocates. External advocates can be provided by special interest sector groups or be paid independent advocates. Part of nurses' advocacy role is to be aware of the form of advocacy that is preferred by the clients or patients concerned, and to be able to discuss this in an informed manner (Mundie & Donelle 2022).

Speaking up for safe practice is essential to achieving safe, effective, quality care (Ko 2020, Lee et al 2022, Morrow et al 2016). Nurses have a professional duty to put first the interests of the people they care for and act to protect them if they are at risk (Nursing and Midwifery Council 2019). Nurses can speak up even while still in the student role (Fagan et al 2016, 2021). However, organisational elements such as trust, hierarchies, whether concerns will be believed and moral courage impact on whether nurses raise their concerns (Ko et al 2020, Lee et al 2022, Morrow et al 2016, Yilmaz & Özbek Güven 2024).

Following the Francis (2013) report in the UK,[1] the Nursing and Midwifery Council (NMC) (2019) has developed guidance on nurses raising concerns. Speaking up for safe practice calls nurses to act without delay, escalating concerns to the appropriate authority. Several stages of escalation are recommended commencing with a direct line manager, escalating to a higher authority if concerns are not reduced and then utilising regulatory bodies if the concern continues and is sufficient to warrant continued concern for patients/clients or public safety (NMC 2019). In Australia and New Zealand (Aotearoa), there are programs that support speaking up for safety through the development of organisational cultures, systems and processes to support communication that effectively raises concerns. If these avenues fail, speaking up may involve whistleblowing, which is described as employee information disclosure about misconduct, illegal, unethical or illegitimate practices that are within the control of their employers, to a person or an organisation that has the authority or power to act (Johnstone 2022). Further, there may be public disclosure to authorities external to the organisational reporting processes. A key reason for whistleblowing is the belief that there is something significantly wrong that has or will cause serious harm that is not being paid attention to by the organisation, having raised it in appropriate channels (Johnstone 2022).

The reported concerns in the whistleblowing context about retribution (Francis 2013, Jackson et al 2014, Moore & McAuliffe 2012, Peters et al 2011, Yilmaz & Özbek Güven 2024) are not surprising given the substantial published nursing discussion and research focused on the concept of horizontal or lateral violence. These behaviours are also labelled as bullying, incivility, disruptive behaviour and hostile clinician behaviours (Hutchinson & Jackson 2013). If nurses perceive a lack of support in environments where communication is ineffective or where hierarchies and power dynamics negatively affect them, they are less likely to speak up for safety (McDonald 2022, Morrow et al 2016). Nurses who do use safety voices to raise evidence-based concerns are courageous and need the support of nurse leaders, colleagues, friends and family. Too often, those who choose to take a stand can feel isolated and are at risk of reprisal, such as harassment and loss of employment (Johnstone 2022, Yilmaz & Özbek Güven 2024).

When practising in complex and challenging work environments, nurses need to be resilient. The concept of 'personal resilience' is considered important in terms of being able to respond positively to adverse situations and advocate effectively. Resilience involves developing strategies such as productive professional networks and focusing on personal development in areas such as the maintenance of a positive attitude, work–life balance and emotional insight (Hart et al 2014, Li et al 2024). However, the moral obligation to act in instances of poor-quality care is not solely an individual nurse's concern—health professionals and other staff have a collective responsibility to create conducive environments for quality patient/client outcomes. The Nursing Council of New Zealand

---

[1] *In 2012, Sir Robert Francis was commissioned to Chair an independent inquiry into reported failures in care at Mid Staffordshire NHS Foundation Trust and lack of response to the concerns raised by nurses and others. The report confirmed that those who had raised concerns were not heard.*

(2012a:28) articulates in the *Code of Conduct for Nurses* the expectations for professional behaviour, including working respectfully with colleagues 'in a professional, collaborative and co-operative manner'. This code, like many others internationally, recognises that others have a right to hold different opinions. The public media has been used by some whistleblowers to draw attention to health issues. The media can serve a useful purpose in promoting accountability, but it also creates intense public scrutiny and critique, confidentiality concerns and may present an unbalanced picture. There are similar concerns about the role of social media as an instant but unmoderated communicative avenue. Major breaches of patient/client confidentiality have led to the development of social media guidelines for nurses and other health practitioners (Australian Health Practitioner Regulation Agency 2014, Nursing Council of New Zealand 2012b).

Not all nurses who have spoken up for unsafe practice have personally experienced workplace retaliation when reporting unsafe patient/client care. The nursing profession, in particular nursing leadership, holds a powerful influence to facilitate a culture of safety. Although not a new concept, leadership in fundamentals of care has emerged strongly post COVID-19 (Kitson et al 2023), with nursing leaders calling for all nurses to stand up for fundamental nursing care. This includes proactively addressing unsafe practices, fostering advocacy, and standing with nurses who speak up (Lee et al 2022). The need to legally protect people in whistleblowing situations is recognised with specific legislation aiming to ensure disclosures are investigated and to protect whistleblowers from retaliation.

Serious lapses in safe and humane healthcare are rooted in systemic organisational inadequacies; as individuals, nurses have been driven to bravely act against prevailing practices or, alternatively, have been part of the invisible forces enabling injustices to be perpetuated. Professional bodies have clearly articulated the criteria for monitoring and improving the quality and safety of healthcare, along with health professional accountability, to act effectively when patient/client safety is in jeopardy (Nursing and Midwifery Board of Australia 2018b, Nursing and Midwifery Council 2019, Nursing Council of New Zealand 2012a).

STORY

Joseph is a third-year nursing student on clinical placement in an orthopaedic rehabilitation unit that provides care for older people following falls-related fractures. Joseph has recently completed a class module related to the advocacy role of nurses. He has learned how nurses can help patients navigate complex health systems and understands his nursing responsibility to be a liaison point between his patient, the doctor, and the broader healthcare team. The doctor has just left after declaring that Mrs Ackers is physically fit for discharge; however, Mrs Ackers tells Joseph that she is frightened and doesn't feel she is ready to go home. She explains that she lives alone and there is no food in the house and is scared she will fall again.

Reflective questions

Reflect on the above scenario and consider the following questions and issues:

1. What actions should Joseph take in the first instance?
2. What needs to be in place to best support Mrs Ackers's safe discharge from hospital?
3. What advocacy role can Joseph undertake in this scenario?

CONCLUSION

Nursing services are pivotal in the provision of healthcare. Nurses are mediators between healthcare institutions, with their associated mysterious practices, language and technologies, and people and their families/whānau—translating and making the health system understandable and accessible for the individual or community. Nurses are a powerful group, expert in terms of their knowledge base, their practice, and their understanding of the impact of health on people and communities. This knowledge and experience places nurses in positions of power as they are well positioned to influence health service resourcing and quality and to speak up for an equitable and socially just healthcare system. Understanding and being consciously and purposefully political, at both a collective and individual level, is central to the role of the nurse. Embracing this responsibility empowers nurses to work with patients, families and communities in a person-centred way, improving healthcare quality outcomes.

REFLECTIVE QUESTIONS

1 Do you think you are influential as a nurse? If so, how have you become influential? If not, how could you be more influential?
2 What do you think patient/clients and families need to know to be effective advocates for themselves and others?
3 What do you think are the most important steps to take when raising concerns about healthcare issues?

Recommended readings

Chapman K, Dixon A, Ehrlich C et al 2024 Dignity and the importance of acknowledgement of personhood for people with disability. Qualitative Health Research 34(1–2):141–153

Kitson AL, Conroy T, Jeffs L et al 2023 'No more heroes': The ILC Oxford Statement on fundamental care in times of crises. Journal of Advanced Nursing 79(3):922–932

Mundie C, Donelle L 2022 Health activism as nursing practice: a scoping review. Journal of Advanced Nursing 78(11):3607–361

Rasmussen B, Holton S, Wynter K et al 2022 We're on mute! Exclusion of nurses' voices in national decisions and responses to COVID-19: an international perspective. Journal of Advanced Nursing, 78(7):e87–e90 https://doi.org/10.1111/jan.15236

Topp S M, Schaaf M, Sriram V et al 2021 Power analysis in health policy and systems research: a guide to research conceptualisation. BMJ Global Health 6(11):e007268

References

Abrams R, Conolly A, Rowland E, et al 2023 Speaking up during the COVID-19 pandemic: nurses' experiences of organizational disregard and silence. Journal of Advanced Nursing 79(6):2189–99

Adams S, Komene E, Wensley C et al 2024 Integrating nurse practitioners into primary healthcare to advance health equity through a social justice lens: an integrative review. Journal of Advanced Nursing 10.1111/jan.16093. 6 Feb doi:10.1111/jan.16093

Alahiane L, Zaam Y, Abouqal R et al 2023 Factors associated with recognition at work among nurses and the impact of recognition at work on health-related quality of life, job satisfaction and psychological health: a single-centre, cross-sectional study in Morocco. BMJ Open 13(5):e051933 https://doi.org/10.1136/bmjopen-2021-051933

Alexander J 2014 Notes towards a definition of politics. Philosophy 89(2):273–300

Australian Government 2023 Summary Statistics, Nursing and Midwifery Professions. Online. Available: https://hwd.health.gov.au/resources/data/summary-nrmw.html

Australian Health Practitioner Regulation Agency 2014 National Board policy for registered health practitioners: social media policy. Australia. Online. Available: https://www.nursingmidwiferyboard.gov.au/Codes-Guidelines-Statements/Codes-Guidelines/Social-media-guidance.aspx

Azizi T H, Begjani J, Arman A et al 2023 The concept analysis of helplessness in nurses during the COVID-19 pandemic: a hybrid model. Nursing Open 10:6782–93 https://doi.org/10.1002/nop2.1955

Benner P, Sutphen M, Leonard V, Day L (eds) 2010 Educating nurses: a call for radical transformation. Jossey-Bass, San Francisco

Bosley H, Appleton J V, Henshall C et al 2021 The influence of perceived accessibility and expertise of healthcare professionals, and service austerity, on mothers' decision-making. Health Soc Care Community 29(2):526–34. doi: 10.1111/hsc.13115. Epub 2020 Aug 3. PMID: 32744784.

Boswell C, Smith K 2017 Rethinking policy 'impact': four models of research-policy relations. Palgrave Communications 3(1):1–10

Carryer J, Yarwood J 2015 The nurse practitioner role: solution or servant in improving primary health care service delivery. Collegian (Royal College of Nursing, Australia) 22(2):169–174

Ceci C 2004 Nursing, knowledge and power: a case analysis. Social Science and Medicine 59:1879–1889

Chaffee M, Mason D, Leavitt J 2012 A framework for action in policy and politics. In: Mason D, Leavitt J, Chaffee M (eds) Policy and politics in nursing and healthcare, 6th edn. Saunders, St Louis, pp 1–18

Chapman K, Dixon A, Ehrlich C, Kendall E 2024 Dignity and the importance of acknowledgement of personhood for people with disability. Qualitative Health Research 34(1–2):141–153

Chiu P, Thorne S, Schick-Makaroff K, Cummings G G 2023 Lessons from professional nursing associations' policy advocacy responses to the COVID-19 pandemic: an interpretive description. Journal of Advanced Nursing 79(8):2967–79

Cole C, Mummery J, Peck B 2022 Empowerment as an alternative to traditional patient advocacy roles. Nursing Ethics 29(7–8):1553–1561

Committee of Inquiry into allegations concerning the treatment of cervical cancer at National Women's Hospital and into other related matters 1988. The report of the committee of inquiry into allegations concerning the treatment of cervical cancer at National Women's Hospital and into other related matters. The Committee, Auckland

Congress of Aboriginal and Torres Strait Islander Nurses and Midwives 2022 'gettin em n keepin em n growin em' (GENKE II) Strategies for Aboriginal and Torres Strait Islander Nursing and Midwifery Education Reform. Congress of Aboriginal and Torres Strait Islander Nurses and Midwives, Brisbane. Online. Available: www.catsinam.org.au

Conroy N, Patton D, Moore Z et al 2023 The relationship between transformational leadership and Staff Nurse retention in hospital settings: a systematic review. Journal of Nursing Management

Department of Social Services 2018 National disability advocacy program. Australian Government. Online. Available: https://www.dss.gov.au/our-responsibilities/disability-and-carers/program-services/for-people-with-disability/national-disability-advocacy-program-ndap

Dickman N E, Chicas R 2021 Nursing is never neutral: political determinants of health and systemic marginalization. Nursing Inquiry 28(4):e12408

Fagan A, Parker V, Jackson D 2016 A concept analysis of undergraduate nursing students speaking up for patient safety in the patient care environment. Journal of Advanced Nursing 72(10):2346–2357 https://doi.org/10.1111/jan.13028

Fagan A, Lea J, Parker V 2021 Student nurses' strategies when speaking up for patient safety: a qualitative study. Nursing & Health Sciences 23(2):447–455 https://doi.org/10.1111/nhs.12831

Fainman E Z, Kucukyazici B 2020 Design of financial incentives and payment schemes in healthcare systems: a review. Socio-Economic Planning Sciences 72:100901

Feyereisen S, Goodrick E 2021 Examining variable nurse practitioner independence across jurisdictions: a case study of the United States. International Journal of Nursing Studies 118:103633

Flaubert J L, Le Menestrel S, Williams D R et al (eds) 2021 The future of nursing 2020–2030: charting a path to achieve health equity. National Academies Press (US), 11 May 2021 doi:10.17226/25982

Foucault M 2003 What is an author? In: Rabinow P, Rose N (eds) The essential Foucault: selections from essential works of Foucault, 1954–1984: Volume 1. The New Press, New York, pp 377–391

Francis R 2013 Report of the Mid Staffordshire NHS Foundation Trust Public Inquiry. Volume 1: analysis of evidence and lessons learned (part 1). The House of Commons, United Kingdom. Online. Available: https://webarchive.nationalarchives.gov.uk/20150407084231/http://www.midstaffspublicinquiry.com/report

Friel S, Townsend B, Fisher M et al 2021 Power and the people's health. Social Science & Medicine 282:114173

Friel S, Collin J, Daube M et al 2023 Commercial determinants of health: future directions. The Lancet 401(10383):1229–1240

Gilmour J, Huntington A, Slark J, et al 2016 Newly graduated nurses and employment: a dynamic landscape. Online. Available: https://doi.org/10.1016/j.colegn.2016.02.004

Gottlieb L N, Gottlieb B, Bitzas V 2021 Creating empowering conditions for nurses with workplace autonomy and agency: how healthcare leaders could be guided by strengths-based nursing and healthcare leadership (SBNH-L). Journal of Healthcare Leadership 13:169–81

Hajizadeh A, Zamanzadeh V, Kakemam E et al 2021 Factors influencing nurses' participation in the health policy-making process: a systematic review. BMC Nursing (20):1–9

Harris P, Baum F, Friel S et al 2020 A glossary of theories for understanding power and policy for health equity. Journal of Epidemiology and Community Health 74(6):548–552

Harrison B C 2014 Power and society: an introduction to the social sciences, 13th edn. Wadsworth Cengage Learning, Boston

Hart P L, Brannan J D, De Chesnay M 2014 Resilience in nurses: an integrative review. Journal of Nursing Management 22:720–734

Health and Disability Commission 2018 New Zealand's mental health and addiction services: the monitoring and advocacy report of the Mental Health Commissioner. Online. Available: https://www.hdc.org.nz/media/m2wfw5vk/mental-health-commissioners-monitoring-and-advocacy-report-2018.pdf

Hokanson Hawks J 1991 Power: a concept analysis. Journal of Advanced Nursing 16:754–762 https://doi.org/10.1111/j.1365-2648.1991.tb01734.x

Hutchinson M, Jackson D 2013 Hostile clinician behaviours in the nursing work environment and implications for patient/client care: a mixed-methods systematic review. BMC Nursing 12:25

International Council of Nurses (ICN) 2022 International Council of Nurses policy brief. The global nursing shortage and nurse retention. https://www.icn.ch/sites/default/files/inline-files/ICN%20Policy%20Brief_Nurse%20Shortage%20and%20Retention_0.pdf

Jackson D, Hickman L, Hutchinson M et al 2014 Whistleblowing: an integrative literature review of data-based studies involving nurses. Contemporary Nurse 48(2):240–252.

Jackson D 2023 Perpetuating the whiteness of nursing: enculturation and nurse education. In: Lipscomb M (ed) Routledge handbook of philosophy and nursing. Routledge, pp 392–403

James A H, Kelly D, Bennett C L 2024 Nursing tropes in turbulent times: time to rethink nurse leadership? Journal of Advanced Nursing 80(1):8–10

Jeong H E, Nam K H, Kim H Y 2021 Patient safety silence and safety nursing activities: mediating effects of moral sensitivity. International Journal of Environmental Research and Public Health 18(21):11499 https://doi.org/10.3390/ijerph182111499

Johnstone M J 2022 Bioethics: a nursing perspective, 8th edn. Elsevier Health Sciences

Jones T, Drach-Zahavy A, Amorim-Lopes M et al 2020 Systems, economics, and neoliberal politics: theories to understand missed nursing care. Nursing & Health Sciences 22(3):586–92

Katriina P, Sari V, Anja R et al 2013 Nursing power as viewed by nursing professionals. Scandinavian Journal of Caring Sciences 2:580–588. https://doi.org/10.1111/j.1471-6712.2012.01069.x

Kickbusch I 2015 The political determinants of health—10 years on. British Medical Journal 350:h81

Kitson A L, Conroy T, Jeffs L et al 2023 'No more heroes': The ILC Oxford Statement on fundamental care in times of crises. Journal of Advanced Nursing 79(3):922–932

Ko Y, Yu S, Jeong S H 2020 Effects of nursing power and organizational trust on nurses' responsiveness and orientation to patient needs. Nursing Open 7(6):1807–1814 https://doi.org/10.1002/nop2.567

Komene E, Gerrard D, Pene B et al 2023 A tohu (sign) to open our eyes to the realities of Indigenous Māori registered nurses: a qualitative study. Journal of Advanced Nursing 79(7):2585–96 https://doi.org/https://doi.org/10.1111/jan.15609

Laari L, Duma S E 2023 Barriers to nurses health advocacy role. Nursing Ethics 09697330221146241

Lee E, De Gagne J C, Randall P S et al 2022 Effectiveness of speak-up training programs for clinical nurses: a scoping review. International Journal of Nursing Studies 136:104375

Lewis C L, Yan A, Williams M Y et al 2023 Health equity: a concept analysis. Nursing Outlook 71(5):102032

Li L, Liao X, Ni J 2024 A cross-sectional survey on the relationship between workplace psychological violence and empathy among Chinese nurses: the mediation role of resilience. BMC Nursing 23(1):85

Lundin K, Silén M, Strömberg A et al 2022 Staff structural empowerment—observations of first-line managers and interviews with managers and staff. Journal of Nursing Management 30(2):403–412

Mayne R, Green D, Guijt I et al 2018 Using evidence to influence policy: Oxfam's experience. Palgrave Communications 4(1):1–10

McDonald T 2022 Speak truth to power and consolidate the nursing visibility gained during COVID-19. International Nursing Review 69(3):25560

Moore L, McAuliffe E 2012 To report or not to report? Why some nurses are reluctant to whistle blow. Clinical Governance: An International Journal 17(4):332–342

Moorley C, Darbyshire P, Serrant L et al 2020 Dismantling structural racism: nursing must not be caught on the wrong side of history. Journal of Advanced Nursing 76(10):2450–53

Morrow K, Gustavson M, Jones J 2016 Speaking up behaviors (safety voices) of healthcare workers: a metasynthesis of qualitative research studies. International Journal of Nursing Studies 64:42–51

Mundie C, Donelle L 2022 Health activism as nursing practice: a scoping review. Journal of Advanced Nursing 78(11):3607–3617

New Zealand Nurses Association n.d. Safe staffing. Online. Available: https://www.nzno.org.nz/get_involved/campaigns/safe_staffing

Nursing and Midwifery Board of Australia 2018a Code of ethics for nurses in Australia. Online. Available: https://www.nursingmidwiferyboard.gov.au/documents/default.aspx?record=WD17%2f23849&dbid=AP&chksum=ki92NMPa9thp9f9ZhTQNJg%3d%3d

Nursing and Midwifery Board of Australia 2018b Code of professional conduct for nurses in Australia. Australia. Online. Available: https://www.nursingmidwiferyboard.gov.au/documents/default.aspx?record=WD17%2f23849&dbid=AP&chksum=ki92NMPa9thp9f9ZhTQNJg%3d%3d

Nursing and Midwifery Council (NMC) 2019 Raising concerns: guidance for nurses, midwives and nursing associates. United Kingdom. Online. Available: https://www.nmc.org.uk/globalassets/blocks/media-block/raising-concerns-v2.pdf

Nursing Council of New Zealand 2012a Code of conduct for nurses. Wellington. Online. Available: https://www.nursingcouncil.org.nz/Public/Nursing/Code_of_Conduct/NCNZ/nursing-section/Code_of_Conduct.aspx

Nursing Council of New Zealand 2012b Guidelines: social media and electronic communication. Wellington. Online. Available: https://www.nursingcouncil.org.nz/Public/Nursing/Code_of_Conduct/NCNZ/nursing-section/Code_of_Conduct.aspx

Nursing Council of New Zealand 2016 Tapuhi tūtohu kua rēhitatia Registered Nurse Prescribing. Wellington. Online. Available: https://www.nursingcouncil.org.nz/Public/Nursing/Nurse_prescribing/NCNZ/nursing-section/Nurse_Prescribing.aspx

Nursing Council of New Zealand 2023 Quarterly Data Report. New Zealand. Online. Available: https://www.nursingcouncil.org.nz/common/Uploaded%20files/Nursing%20Council%20Quarterly%20Data%20Report%20-%20December%202023%20Quarter.pdf

Parliament of Australia 2018 Trends in union membership in Australia – Parliament of Australia. Online. Available: https://www.aph.gov.au/About_Parliament/Parliamentary_Departments/Parliamentary_Library/pubs/rp/rp1819/UnionMembership#Reasons%20Fordecline%20in%20Union%20Membership

Peters K, Luck L, Hutchinson M et al 2011 The emotional sequelae of whistleblowing: findings from a qualitative study. Journal of Clinical Nursing 20(19–20):2907–2914.

Rafferty A M 2018 Nurses as change agents for a better future in health care: the politics of drift and dilution. Health Economics, Policy and Law 13:475–91

Ramsay A, Birks M, Hartin P 2022 Advocacy in nursing: speaking truth to power? Collegian 29(5):549–50

Rasmussen B, Holton S, Wynter K et al 2022 We're on mute! Exclusion of nurses' voices in national decisions and responses to COVID-19: an international perspective. Journal of Advanced Nursing 78(7):e87–e90. https://doi.org/10.1111/jan.15236

Scharlatt H, Smith R 2015. Influence: gaining commitment, getting results, 2nd edn (ESLA-e). Center for Creative Leadership, Greensboro

Sepasi R R, Abbaszadeh A, Borhani F et al 2016 Nurses' perceptions of the concept of power in nursing: a qualitative research. Journal of Clinical and Diagnostic Research 10(12):LC10–LC15

Sullivan E J 2013 Becoming influential: a guide for nurses, 2nd edn. Pearson Education Inc, New Jersey

Taylor M R S 2016 Impact of advocacy initiatives on nurses' motivation to sustain momentum in public policy advocacy. Journal of Professional Nursing 32(3):235–245 https://doi.org/10.1016/j.profnurs.2015.10.010

Tomajan K 2012a Advocating for Nurses and Nursing. Online Journal of Issues in Nursing 17:1–1

Tomajan K 2012b Advocating for Nurses and Nursing. Online Journal of Issues in Nursing, 17, Manuscript 4.

Topp S M, Schaaf M, Sriram V et al 2021 Power analysis in health policy and systems research: a guide to research conceptualisation. BMJ Global Health 6(11):e007268

Veneklasen L, Miller V 2002 A new weave of power, people & politics: the action guide for advocacy and citizen participation. World Neighbors, Oklahoma City

Victoria State Government 2019 Safe patient/client care (nurse to patient/client and midwife to patient/client ratios) Act 2015. Online. Available: https://www.health.vic.gov.au/nursing-and-midwifery/nursing-and-midwifery-legislation-and-regulation

Willis E, Carryer J, Harvey C, Pearson M et al 2017 Austerity, new public management and missed nursing care in Australia and New Zealand. Journal of Advanced Nursing 73(12):3102–10

Wilson D M, Anafi F, Kusi-Appiah E et al 2020 Determining if nurses are involved in political action or politics: a scoping literature review. Applied Nursing Research 54:151279

World Health Organization 2021 The WHO global strategic directions for strengthening nursing and midwifery 2021–2025. Online. Available: https://iris.who.int/bitstream/handle/10665/344562/9789240033863-eng.pdf?sequence=1 2025

Yılmaz Ş, Özbek Güven G 2024 The relationship between nurses' moral courage and whistleblowing approaches. Nursing Ethics: 09697330241230686

Zhang N, Casas B 2022 Professional discrimination toward nurses increases nurse silence threatening patient safety outcomes. Evidence Based Nursing 25(4):133. https://doi.org/10.1136/ebnurs-2021-103474

CHAPTER 11

REFLECTIVE PRACTICE: THE IMPORTANCE AND WAYS OF REFLECTION IN NURSING

Kim Usher

KEY WORDS
complex environments
critical incident analysis
critical thinking
ethics
journalling
moral distress
reflection
reflective practice

LEARNING OBJECTIVES
After reading this chapter, readers should be able to:
- understand the importance and benefits of reflective practice in a practice-based discipline such as nursing in the contemporary climate of health services
- have insight into the development of and the nature of reflection and be able to identify its leading theorists
- appreciate the link between reflection and professional nursing practice
- identify the strategies that assist with reflection
- have insight into the legal and ethical issues surrounding reflection.

INTRODUCTION

Changing levels of complexity in the healthcare environment, especially since the arrival of the COVID-19 pandemic, means nurses are faced with fast-paced, critical clinical environments and demands that often include ethical dilemmas, as well as clients with multiple health problems. Such situations require practitioners who are '...astute, measured, competent, and decisive' (Nguyen-Truong et al 2018:115). To function in these complex environments, practitioners are required to focus their attention on their clients amidst multiple competing demands that may impact the nurse's ability to remain attentive in their attempts to deliver quality, safe care to avoid ethical dilemmas that often result in moral distress – a rising problem in nursing (Storaker et al 2017). A study by Storaker et al (2017:560) reported how new graduates described their days at work as 'painful busyness', where they were left feeling out of control and responsible for poor quality care, including incidents of missed opportunities for care and where patients were being discharged too soon due to bed shortages. Events such as these may leave nurses experiencing moral distress as they try to come to terms with their inability to deliver the level of care they aspire to provide as a student or registered nurse (Storaker et al 2017). This situation has become the reality that educators must now prepare nursing students to face upon graduation. The contemporary healthcare environment that nurses face on a daily basis requires them to be capable of being reflective, adaptable and independent thinkers to manage the uncertainty of the environment. *Reflective practice* is one way to assist nursing students to learn in a fast-paced and dynamic healthcare environment where students learn to review and evaluate their actions with the aim of learning from their experiences (Naicker & van Rensburg 2018). The practice of reflection assists students and graduate nurses to review their own thoughts, biases, assumptions, feelings and behaviours to reconnect with their desire to deliver safe and competent care (Peterkin & Brett-MacLean 2016). Reflective practice is considered an effective way to help students and new graduates to adapt to the fast-paced and dynamic healthcare environment (Naicker & van Rensburg 2018) and has been supported as an essential component of nurse education and practice since the 1980s (Bulman et al 2012). For reflective practice to be effective, nurses must recognise the deliberate nature of identifying the knowledge and values that underpin their practice (Patel & Metersky 2021). Basically, reflective practice is a cognitive skill that requires nurses to address their own situation while also recognising individual beliefs, values and experiences (Patel & Metersky 2021).

This chapter introduces you to the need for reflective practice in the contemporary healthcare environment, describes and defines reflective practice, and explains why reflection is a useful strategy for undergraduate nursing students, as well as registered nurses. Finally, the chapter closes with discussion around tools and techniques, which may assist the reader in understanding strategies that can assist with engaging in reflection and reflective practice.

Why be reflective?

Every workplace presents a complex environment to the new graduate as well as to the experienced nurse. The environment is often difficult to understand and appears to abound with multiple decisions, each coupled to a host of different ways in which the desired outcomes could be achieved. When you first enter a nursing context, perhaps during your first clinical placement, you will be confronted by discrepancies, such as those between 'ideal' and 'real' practice. You may also experience or witness difficult interpersonal relationships. It is important that these unpleasant situations do not distract you from your nursing goals or from seeking to provide the best possible care you can provide for your clients.

Although systematic reflection may at first seem difficult to undertake when you are working in a demanding clinical situation, reflection will help you to recognise and set aside the emotional content and enable you to learn from otherwise negative experiences. Reflection can take on an even more important role when you find yourself faced with difficult working conditions and environments (Nguyen-Truong et al 2018). Proposed to make meaning out of complex situations (Naicker & van Rensburg 2018), reflection will help you identify alternative ways you could react in the future, hopefully resulting in more positive outcomes. Importantly, reflection helps to ensure that our practice does not become so routine that our actions begin to contradict our values (Storaker et al 2017).

Nurses need to take account of the relationship between reflective practice as a professional activity and as an opportunity to understand everyday practice. Meaningful reflection needs theoretical understanding of what we consider as everyday practice; it must include purpose, focus and questioning (Nicol & Dosser 2016). Others suggest the need for reflective practice to be related to an action orientation (Mohamed et al 2022), which indicates a focus on what rather than a focus on why. Reflection, which is assumed to enhance the learning process, is however recognised as a cognitive skill that demands conscious effort to look at a situation with an awareness of our own beliefs, values and practice, thus enabling us to learn from our experiences, and to incorporate that learning into the process of improving patient care outcomes (Patel & Metersky 2021).

Johns (2010) explains how reflection offers a way to bring to the surface the contradictions between what you intend to achieve in a situation and how you actually practise. In other words, being faced with contradiction opens the possibility for change and offers the practitioner the opportunity to achieve desired practice. One of the outcomes of reflection is thus a process of continuous monitoring and improvement of practice. It assists us to avoid taking situations at face value but rather to move beyond the taken-for-granted assumptions that may be informed by prejudice and discriminatory ideas (Patel & Metersky 2021).

Regulatory authorities in Australia have embraced the need for practitioners who are reflective practitioners and require that all nurses engage in some form of reflective activity. This is explicit in the Nursing and Midwifery Board of Australia's (NMBA's) *Registered Nurse Standards for Practice* (NMBA 2016). They comprise seven interlocking standards, the most relevant here being the first, which concerns critical thinking and analysis. One component of this standard states that the registered nurse 'develops practice through reflection on experiences, knowledge, actions, feelings and beliefs to identify how these shape practice' (NMBA 2016:6). The *National Competency Standards for the Midwife* (NMBA 2018c) also has reflective and ethical practice embedded throughout its seven domains. Furthermore, the *Code of Professional Conduct for Midwives* (NMBA 2018a) and the *Code of Conduct for Nurses* (NMBA 2018b) also require that they practise reflectively and ethically.

In addition, the Nursing Council of New Zealand (NCNZ) has also incorporated reflection as a key competency for registered nurses. In the New Zealand registered nurse competencies, reflection is a component of domain one, which focuses upon the professional responsibilities of the registered nurse (NCNZ 2022). Like the NMBA, the NCNZ also has information about codes of conduct and scope of practice for nurses. Further information about these competencies is available from the following websites:

- Nursing and Midwifery Board of Australia: https://www.nursingmidwiferyboard.gov.au/codes-guidelines-statements/professional-standards/registered-nurse-standards-for-practice.aspx
- Nursing Council of New Zealand: https://nursingcouncil.org.nz/Public/NCNZ/nursing-section/Standards_and_guidelines_for_nurses.aspx

As a result, all pre-registration nursing programs of study must ensure graduates have been provided with the opportunity to develop the skill of reflection. In other words, it is a requirement of your nursing education that you exit the program of study with the ability to be a reflective practitioner.

What is reflection or reflective practice?

Reflection comes from the Latin verb *reflectere*, which means to bend or turn backwards. This infers that reflection is a process of going back over something after it has already occurred. The reflection might include recalling thoughts and memories, in cognitive acts such as thinking or contemplation, or as a way of making sense of the situation so that necessary changes may be identified or made (Patel & Metersky 2021). We all reflect on what goes on around us to some extent. If you think about it, we do not generally just walk around in the world without noticing things or thinking about what has happened and how it has impacted on us. Similarly, we all reflect at some level on our practice, but it may only involve thinking about what happened rather than theorising or thinking deeply about what happened and looking for ways to improve it in the future.

Thus, the type of reflection to be discussed in this chapter is a much more purposeful activity that leads to action that is better informed than that which occurred before the reflection took place (Patel & Metersky 2021). Rolfe (2014) argues that the wicked problems that we encounter in nursing practice often are unable to be addressed by available theories and knowledge. Rather, nurses need to become more adept at developing their own theories and develop their own knowledge from experience (Patel & Metersky 2021). Reflection therefore provides the practitioner with access to the processes by which he or she makes clinical judgments, which can then be used to justify actions to others or pass on expertise to less experienced colleagues.

Nurses should recognise the importance of reflective practice as a purposeful professional activity. In other words, it must involve a sophisticated understanding of everyday practice (Thompson & Pascal 2012) that goes beyond the ordinary experience of the everyday life. In this way it requires a meaningful, focused reflection with the intent of developing new knowledge and understanding (Patel & Metersky 2021).

Much of the contemporary emphasis on reflective practice in nursing can be attributed to the work of the American educationalist Donald Schön (1983, 1987). Even though he was not the first to write about reflective practice, he coined the term 'reflective practice' and has been very influential in the way nursing has since embraced the notion of the concept. Schön (1983) argued that reflection is a strategy whereby professionals become aware of their implicit knowledge base. While he did not attempt to define reflection or reflective practice, he advocated two distinct types of reflection: *reflection-on-action* and *reflection-in-action*. The former, reflection-*on*-action, occurs after the event or action, and involves recalling and analysing details with the aim of reviewing practice.

Reflection-*in*-action occurs simultaneously or at the same time as practice. That is, reflection-*in*-action is said to occur when the practitioner engages in practice and adjusts because of relevant feedback. Reflection-*in*-action is a more advanced form of reflection and leads to more advanced practice. It is a process whereby the nurse is constantly testing theories and hypotheses in a cyclical process while simultaneously engaged in practice, which can also be referred to as a 'nursing praxis' (Patel & Metersky 2021). There is an additional step in the reflective process, that of *pre-reflection*, where individuals engage in reflection in anticipation of events. Reflection-before-action assumes learners reflect before entering clinical practice. Reflection-before-action assists students to acknowledge and identify the nature of learning from practice. This strategy helps students to identify strategies that may help to analyse situations prior to engagement (Edwards 2017). Given the greater complexity of healthcare services today, the clinical environment may require a skill set beyond the student's current capacity. In this case, clinical simulation-based activities are ideal preparation for practice and offer further opportunities for students to use reflection in a debriefing situation (Nascimento et al 2020).

> # REFLECTION
> Consider your personal experience with reflection. Perhaps beginning your nursing degree might be a good place to start.
> - What type of reflection did you engage in today if any?
> - It is important to recognise the importance of experiential learning where we seek to understand the ways in which students learn to be included and accepted in their discipline area
> - How does reflective practice help you to understand the complexities of the clinical environment?
> - Did you think about what this would mean to you and how it would impact on your life, your opportunity for a professional career or whether or how you would work with people in the clinical setting?
> - Did you engage in any reflection-on-action? Have you thought about an event or experience where you have identified that you would like to improve your practice? You may have done this individually or as a group, or even formally as an assessable item in your studies.
> - Did you engage in any reflection-in-action? Have you encountered a difficult event or situation where you have been required to think through the issues and how you might address them as they are occurring? You may have done this during an experience in the clinical setting.

The roots of reflective practice

The ancient Greek philosopher Plato declared that the unreflective life was a life not worth living. Plato was drawing attention to the view that reflection is a distinctively human activity and without it we would be no more than unthinking automatons, our lives governed by our biological instincts and forever subject to those forces, human and natural, exerting power over us. In other words, Plato saw reflection as vital to our identity as human beings and to our having a mind of our own, and thus vital to our personal freedom. We are free, he concluded, only to the extent that we are reflective beings.

This idea resurfaced and drove the huge change of thinking that occurred in seventeenth- and eighteenth-century Europe, which became known as the Enlightenment. Enlightenment argued that human beings are free to think and decide for themselves rather than simply accepting the prevailing norms, largely imposed by those in power and notably by the Christian churches. Today we just accept this as natural and probably do not think twice about it, but in those days, it was a radical and rather dangerous claim.

This history reminds us of several important principles concerning reflection. First, reflection is not an artificial technique that is being imposed by regulatory authorities or universities; rather, it is the refinement of a natural process that is part of being human, and which needs to be nurtured and encouraged. Second, we should always reflect upon, and if necessary, challenge prevailing ways of thinking and acting, even if it occasionally means being unpopular or thought foolish. When it involves 'big issues', this may be hard to do, but reflection and action working together (i.e. 'praxis') is the impetus for change, and ultimately for improvement. This applies in all arenas of human activity, including your local healthcare setting.

Although there are many ways of conceiving reflective processes, even within the same discipline, reflection as we refer to it here is not simply thinking, but rather thinking deeply, systematically, logically and deliberately. Political theorists have emphasised the role of reflection in challenging the status quo, and it plays an important part in the teachings of some political radicals and revolutionaries. Educationalists have emphasised the role of reflection in learning and problem solving and have explored how reflection is related to experience.

Reflection also played an important part in the development of psychology as a discipline during the nineteenth century, in the form of 'introspection'—that is, reflection focused upon oneself. Until the rise of scientific psychology in the 1880s, introspection was the primary source of data for the elucidation of human psychology. An especially important figure, who brings the political and educational aspects together, was the Brazilian Marxist Paulo Freire. His work is widely cited as the basis for the development of reflective processes in nursing, although nurses have mostly shied away from acknowledging the political revolutionary aspects of his work. Freire's concept of reflection was developed as part of a strategy for educating and politicising the impoverished and largely illiterate peasants of Brazil and has an explicit emancipatory intent. The key idea, which makes it 'emancipatory', is that reflection and action should work together, to generate new, enlightened and empowering ways of thinking and behaving.

This is an important way for you to think about reflection because, as a nurse, you will work in complex systems where you may feel powerless and unable to express your concerns, similar to those individuals discussed above. To create a sense of control and of having a worthwhile part to play, you can begin by engaging in reflective processes, and out of these should arise constructive courses of action.

The benefits of reflection

Some of the benefits derived from reflective processes have already been noted but let us now discuss these in more detail. It is essential that action and reflection work together, and for this reason action is seen as an important outcome of the reflective process (Johns 2017). However, 'action' can take many forms. For example, when you reflect upon your practice world and become sensitive to its inadequacies and injustices, you are most likely to want to do something about them, especially as you consider them in relation to individuals' rights. In contrast, action might involve improving your own clinical skills; your reflections having alerted you to shortcomings in your attitudes or skills, and you take action to bring them to a higher standard.

Thus, reflection has the effect of 'educating the emotions'. Reflective processes should be mutually encouraged, and there is an educative element as you help others by recognising and responding to their needs and sensitivities, as well as your own; reflective processes also help you come to terms with the uncertainty of clinical practice and with its inevitable injustices and inadequacies. Clinical practice is never perfect; it is always constrained by resource shortages and by the failings of the system and those who work in it. It is part of the human condition that we cannot do everything right all the time, and that things sometimes go wrong. Reflective processes enable us to face up to this reality, but at the same time challenge us to overcome the obstacles and aspire to the best possible standards of practice. They contribute to our development as thinkers, practitioners, and as people.

Another benefit of reflection is that it can help you elucidate the theory–practice relationship. Critical social theory insists that this relationship is 'reflexive'; in other words, theory feeds into your practice and practice informs your theory. Since critical social theory is closely tied to these conceptions of reflection, it is widely argued that any theory of nursing developed in this way should be consistent with critical social theory, and many nursing scholars have attempted to show how this can work. This link has become more difficult to sustain, however, as critical social theory has been the subject of criticism considering alternative ways of thinking about social structures and processes, including 'post-structuralism' and 'postmodernism'.

Another positive outcome of reflection, which follows on from its role in the 'education of the emotions' noted above, is that it encourages us to be sensitive to the needs of individuals from marginalised and vulnerable populations. We become more sensitive to the suffering, courage and determination of people who are faced with serious illness and to the problems faced by those who are oppressed, such as people experiencing mental illness or people with a disability, people from low socioeconomic backgrounds, people experiencing homelessness, and people who belong to ethnic and religious minorities. This increased sensitivity impels you towards greater engagement with such people and a willingness to become involved in their problems. Not only are you aiming to improve your clinical performance, but you will also develop your ability to support and advocate. You are not only motivated to question inadequate practices, but also to generate possible strategies for improvement. Even though it may be challenging, you will find that you cannot do otherwise, and you will enjoy increased levels of job satisfaction because this heightened level of engagement is intrinsically rewarding.

We might add that these benefits accrue not just in the context of your work, but also in your life generally. The big claim being made here is that because reflection educates your emotions and impels you to action, it helps to make you a better person, not just a better nurse. Let us now turn to consider the 'how' of reflection.

Strategies for reflection

Many strategies can be used for reflection, including debriefing, portfolios, paintings, storytelling (including writing, e.g. journalling and critical incident analysis), photography, drawing and other forms of creative expression (Scheel Schumann et al 2017). Many of these approaches are used collectively. A recent study found that student nurses who used reflection reported being able to recognise the attributes of a good nurse, disperse the emotional load of caring after a clinical experience, understand and challenge areas of professional overlap, and know themselves better as a nurse (Rees 2013). This is especially important to nursing as a caring discipline where nurses need to have in-depth understanding of their motivations and emotions.

WRITING

Reflective writing has long been advocated as a technique to aid reflection (Johns 2010). Writing for the purpose of reflection differs from other forms of writing in that it is undertaken primarily for the purpose of learning and to assist us to develop a deeper understanding of the subject of our reflection. Writing an account of an experience offers the opportunity to go back and reflect on what happened and why; in this way it provides the practitioner with a way to make sense of actions, identify clinical challenges and develop an in-depth understanding of related processes. In this way it can assist nurses to attain professional competencies (Choperena et al 2019).

Journalling and *critical incident analysis* are two well-known types of reflective writing, but clinical supervision, poetry, letter, story- and group-writing activities are also examples of reflective writing.

Guided reflective writing and journalling

Guided reflective writing is a strategy for the development of reflective practice as it promotes questioning and exploration (Smith 2020). Journalling is one example of reflective writing.

The journal becomes an ongoing critique of the practitioner's thoughts about an experience as well as their overall practice. Journals have also been described as cathartic because they offer an opportunity to 'work through' problems or difficult situations (Davies & Sharp 2000). Some students find starting a reflective journal a difficult task, but you should remember that there is no right or wrong way to do it. However, it is important to remember that journalling for reflection is different to the process of journalling for personal use. There is a need to put value upon the process of journalling if it is used for reflection, ensuring that you are thinking critically during and about the process. For journalling to be helpful it is recommended that you are spontaneous; express yourself freely; remain open to ideas; choose a time to suit you; be prepared personally; and choose a reflective method that best suits you. It is also important to avoid the use of abbreviations, and resist the temptation to censor your writing, as this is more likely to assist with the exposure of the 'isms' we hold as an individual. Box 11.1 lists some journalling techniques, which may be useful for all reflective practitioners.

A further strategy that may also be helpful is the notion of a *critical friend*. Sharing with others opens reflective journal entries to a different perspective. Dialogical conversations with another student/graduate can challenge you to think more deeply by the introduction of multiple perspectives that may help uncover your assumptions and biases (Miller et al 2012). It is important that the critical friend is someone you trust, as they will be reading your entries and discussing them with you.

Ethical and legal issues related to journalling

One aspect of journalling that became a problem in the early 1990s, and is still discussed in the contemporary setting, concerns its ethical and legal status. In short, these concerns were:
- whether journalling required the consent of institutions and individuals to whom it referred
- whether journalling was appropriately conducted in work time or in the clinician's own time
- who owned the journals, and who had a right of access to them, and
- what status the journals had in law; for example, whether they could be used as evidence in the court room.

With the formal recognition that registered nurses are required to be 'reflective practitioners', it is now widely accepted that journalling can be considered part of their professional practice.

BOX 11.1
Journalling techniques

- Select a quiet environment where you will not be interrupted
- Write vividly and as close to the event as possible
- Include your initial thoughts but leave space where you can add comments later
- Where possible, make use of diagrams, illustrations, photographs and drawings to aid your memory

However, intellectual property is a vexed issue in law, and there does not appear to be any precedent set in either Australian or New Zealand law as to the obligations of clinicians in relation to journals, but there does appear to be general acceptance that they belong to their authors, and that employers therefore normally have no right of access. Despite, or perhaps because of, these issues, you should ensure that your reflective journals conform to the usual ethical standards that apply in healthcare situations—namely, that they are securely stored and accessible only to authorised individuals, that you use pseudonyms when referring to individuals, and that they are strictly for your private professional use. Existing privacy provisions in Australia and New Zealand (Aotearoa) require that no information is gathered from an individual beyond what is required for the appropriate management of their health problem, and so you should not obtain additional information simply for the purposes of your journal.

Like all documents, journals may be ordered to be submitted as evidence in courts of law. Although this is extremely unlikely, and most of what appears in a journal may only have the status of 'hearsay evidence', it is wise to bear this possibility in mind. Another principle you should adopt, therefore, is that your journal should always refer to your colleagues and individuals in your care in a professional and respectful manner, even though it may express criticism. Your journal is, after all, not simply a vehicle for catharsis or unrestricted emotional expression. Rather, your reflective journal is the professional documentation of your deeply and carefully considered thoughts.

You may prefer to maintain a 'live' e-journal rather than a 'paper and pencil' document, and to engage in reflective writing online. In either case, you must be careful to observe all the legal, professional and ethical restrictions that apply. These refer principally to matters of privacy and accuracy as they concern colleagues, patients and others, and you should obtain relevant guidance or policy documents from your employer, education provider and professional organisation.

Critical incident or technique analysis

A critical incident is usually an event that is remembered as important to an individual or one that is provided to a learner for the purpose of reflection. The notion of a critical incident is considered problematic by some (Thompson & Thompson 2018) who suggest that the term is negative because it recalls something unfortunate or life-threatening. For others, however, this approach offers an opportunity to review an incident that may have had a negative connotation to develop a new understanding that enhances learning.

Critical incidents, or technique analysis, should be thought of as events that are meaningful or significant in some way; they need not necessarily be large or major occurrences, and they can be negative or positive experiences. Critical incident analysis is considered to refer to issues of patient safety in many clinical situations (Steven et al 2020). However, it is also a useful reflective learning technique as it offers an opportunity to review and explore alternative ways of acting. It is important that nurses (and other health clinicians) see the importance of reporting errors in practice, but we recognise that what occurs after errors are reported remains elusive (Gartmeier et al 2017).

Rees (2013), however, found that engagement with reflective practices helped nursing students to understand and better manage the distressing emotional challenges of their work. Participants in the study also reported that reflection helped them understand what it meant to them personally to be a nurse. Box 11.2 provides a framework for critical incident analysis.

> **BOX 11.2**
> **Framework for critical incident analysis**
>
> 1. Give a concise description of the incident (which relates to the learning outcomes)
> 2. Outline the rationale for choice of incident and its significance and relevance to you
> 3. Identify pertinent issues related to the incident
> 4. Reflect on and analyse the key issues focusing on: your own involvement; feelings and decision making; the involvement and role of others; identification of any dilemmas or ethical elements; and the rationale for action, drawing on relevant theory evaluation of the situation and the implications for practice and personal learning
> 5. Conclusion
>
> Source: Davies & Sharp (2000:67–68)

PHOTOGRAPHY, DRAWING AND OTHER FORMS OF CREATIVE EXPRESSION

Art as a precursor to clinical experiences has been identified as an effective strategy to assist the new graduate incorporate aspects of clinical practice to understand the nuances of the situation (Bailey & Davis 2011). Some have been inspired to draw or write poetically because of events they have experienced, while others have used art forms, such as photography, drawing, painting or music to express their reactions or to use with students to assist them become more aware of their own emotions and able to reflect on ethical issues (Nguyen-Truong et al 2018). These techniques are described as creative because they use the imagination to transform experience away from the use of metaphor as a way to create insights and facilitate learning. Their value is nicely illustrated in a study by Nhguyen-Truong et al (2018): participants reported positive benefits from the use of poetry in reflective writing and preferred it to formal methods of reflective writing because it freed them up to express their emotions.

SELF-AWARENESS AND CLINICAL SUPERVISION

In essence, self-awareness is the foundation skill upon which reflective practice is based. It offers individuals the opportunity to see themselves in certain situations and to observe how they affected the situation, and the situation affected them. In fact, this is what differentiates reflection from other types of mental activity such as logical thinking or problem solving (Boud et al 1985). Reflection is also a very personal experience, as it opens the self up to scrutiny (Johns 2010, 2017). As a result, reflection can be disconcerting to the individual, as taken-for-granted competence and ways of coping are exposed as inadequate.

Self-awareness is also an essential skill for professional monitoring. As a professional you are required to be aware of yourself, and the influence you have on the person and the healthcare context. Consequently, constant and vigilant self-monitoring is an important skill that every nurse needs to develop. Registered nurses need to come to an understanding of any preconceptions and attitudes and identify how these impact on their practice. An awareness of your own frailties and susceptibilities is crucial to maintaining high standards of practice.

Many nurses find it difficult to adequately care for their own psychological and physical wellbeing, and yet are under pressure from their work and their domestic lives. For example, it is important to consider whether you are going to work tired and distracted; whether you are overanxious, depressed or angry; whether you are going to work with a hangover. Many nurses find that the stress of their lives leads them to overuse medications, smoke heavily or resort to illicit drugs (Happell et al 2013). The reflective practitioner is aware of these tendencies and will take remedial action, seeking appropriate advice and support.

A similar argument applies to any tendency that may ultimately lead to professional misconduct, including inappropriate preconceptions and other prejudiced attitudes. A reflective practitioner becomes aware of these possibilities, takes action and thus maintains high standards of practice. This self-monitoring role leads us almost seamlessly into the issue of clinical supervision.

Reflective processes have been linked by many authors to the process of clinical supervision. The clinical supervisor incorporates the processes of reflective practice in the clinical supervision experience to assist the supervisee to deepen their understanding of their behaviour and thus create important spaces for workplace learning (Koh et al 2022).

Reflective practice groups

Reflective practice groups are a form of group clinical supervision based on the premises of reflective practice. These group have reported increased work satisfaction, lower levels of burnout and improved work engagement for participants (Tims et al 2013). A recent study found that nurses who participated in these groups reported greater personal and job resources and that they experienced greater social support, autonomy and increased skill discretion (Sundgren et al 2020).

Problems, criticisms and responses to reflective practice

Despite its endorsement by regulatory authorities and encouragement by educators, the use of reflective processes in nursing is not without critics. The empirical evidence for their effectiveness in increasing critical thinking, promoting learning and improving practice remains weak (Mann et al 2009), but the reasons for supporting them are strong:

- Although little research has been conducted on its value to nursing, the concept of reflective practice is supported by empirical research conducted and elaborated over many years, notably in education, and the accumulated evidence as to its value in a variety of disciplines (e.g. science, social work, medicine, law, education) cannot be ignored
- The research results, although limited, are favourable, and there is no evidence that clinicians taking time to engage in critical reflection has any detrimental effects
- There are strong *a priori* (logical) arguments in its favour, such as the argument that a problem is unlikely to be acted upon unless it is recognised as a problem, and that learning entails reflection, and not merely experience or the absorption of facts

- Reflective processes acknowledge the value of the experiences and beliefs of all members of a discipline in contributing to its knowledge base and practice development; the alternative is that the views of a privileged group are allowed to dominate
- Reflective processes happen naturally, and one cannot simply stop them without denying an integral part of one's personal identity; the alternative is to be robotic.

Finally, for the sake of balance, we should add that there are also several theoretical arguments that can be levelled at reflective processes in nursing. Some of these are:
- Despite its championship by many nursing authorities, reflection remains ill-defined and elusive
- There is also a lack of scales to identify differences in individual capabilities of critical reflection in clinical nursing care situations.

These are important issues that need to be considered by those who champion reflection, but none of them are necessarily fatal to that cause. The alternative considerations to these criticisms are that:
- the meaning of words is a matter of convention, and agreement takes time to emerge
- self-scrutiny is a positive feature of professional life; indeed, 'profession' is often characterised by such self-regulation
- the aim is to open the practitioner's mind to possibilities, not to impose rules, and reflective practitioners are therefore more likely to be creative, to challenge the status quo and to be independent thinkers, and
- the problems of reflective practice may have been underestimated, but they are increasingly acknowledged; in any case, this means only that we need to be better at reflective processes, not that they should be abandoned.

As a reflective practitioner you should consider carefully, and reflect upon, the claims made in this chapter, and come to a reasoned and practical personal arrangement for your own development. To help you do this, consider the questions below, and undertake some further reading on the subject.

CONCLUSION

In summary, reflection is a useful learning and professional development strategy that helps the practitioner to monitor their practice, recognise the link between practice and theory, remain in touch with their values, develop awareness of their impact on their work and on relationships with others and remain in touch with the needs of the vulnerable in society. Reflective practice, while still considered to be a developing area by some scholars, is now considered of sufficient importance to be mandated by the regulatory authorities that oversee the practice of nurses and midwives. There are many strategies to enhance reflective practice such as writing, journalling, critical incident analysis, creative techniques and clinical supervision. Given the rapidly changing and challenging nature of healthcare services, it is important to continue to reflect on your practice and develop reflection as a routine part of your day.

REFLECTIVE QUESTIONS

1 How will you use reflective practice to help you manage the reality of clinical practice in the current dynamic healthcare environment?

2 Write a paragraph about how you will use reflective processes during your clinical practice. In the paragraph address the following:

   a the technique you think would be best suited to you and why

   b whether a framework would help you, and

   c the benefits you might receive.

3 How will you use reflective processes to enhance your self-awareness and ensure you practise at the highest possible standard?

Recommended readings

Nguyen-Truong C K Y, Davis A, Spencer C et al 2018 Techniques to promote reflective practice. Journal of Nursing Education 57(2):115–120

Patel K M, Metersky K 2021 Reflective practice in nursing: a concept analysis. International Journal of Nursing Knowledge 33:180–187 doi 10.1111/2047-3095.12350

Storaker A, Nåden D, Saeteren B 2017 From painful busyness to emotional immunization: Nurses' experiences of ethical challenges. Nursing Ethics 24(5):556–568 https://doi.org/10.1177/0969733015620938

References

Bailey C, Davis C A 2011 It's the physical versus the emotional: using poetics to represent the power of art in the nursing clinical experience. Adult Education Research Conference. Online. Available: https://newprairiepress.org/aerc/2011/papers/4

Boud D, Keogh R, Walker D 1985 Reflection: turning experience into learning. Kogan Page, London

Bulman C, Lathlean J, Gobbi M 2012 The concept of reflection in nursing: qualitative findings on student and teacher perspectives. Nurse Education Today 32(5):e8–e13. https://doi.org/10.1016/j.nedt.2011.10.007

Choperena A, Oroviogoicoechea C, Salcedo A Z et al 2019 Nursing narratives and reflective practice: a theoretical review. Journal of Advanced Nursing 75:1637–1647 doi: 10.1111/jan.13955

Davies C, Sharp P 2000 The assessment and evaluation of reflection. In: Burns S, Bulman C (eds) Reflective practice in nursing: the growth of the professional practitioner, 2nd edn. Blackwell Science, Oxford, pp 52–78

Edwards S 2017 Reflecting differently. New dimensions: reflection-before-action and reflection-beyond-action. International Journal of Development Practice No. 1, Article 2 https://doi.org/10.19043/ipdj.71.002

Gartmeier M, Ottl E, Bauer J, Berberat PO 2017 Learning from errors: critical incident reporting in nursing. Journal of Workplace Learning 29(5):343–356 http://dx.doi.org/10.1108/JWL-01-2017-0011

Happell B, Reid-Searle K, Caperchione C M et al 2013 How nurses cope with occupational stress outside of their workplace. Collegian 20(3):195–199

Johns C 2010 Guided reflection: a narrative approach to advancing professional practice, 2nd edn. Blackwell, Oxford

Johns C 2017 Becoming a reflective practitioner, 5th edn. Wiley-Blackwell, Oxford

Koh D, McNulty G, Toh-Heng H L 2022 Reflective practice through clinical supervision: implications for professional and organisational sustainability. British Journal of Guidance and Counselling 50(6) https://doi.org/10.1080/03069885.2021.1978056

Mann K, Gordon J, MacLeod A 2009 Reflection and reflective practice in health professions education: a systematic review. Advances in Health Science Education: Theory and Practice 14(4):595–621. doi: 10.1007/s10459-007-9090-2. Epub 2007 Nov 23. PMID: 18034364

Miller L R, Nelson F P, Phillips E L 2021 Exploring critical reflection in a virtual learning community in teacher education. Reflective Practice 22(3):363–380 https://doi.org/10.1080/14623943.2021.1893165

Mohamed M, Rashid R A, Alqaryouti M H 2022 Conceptualizing the complexity of reflective practice in education. Frontiers in Psychology 13 https://doi.org/10.3389/fpsyg.2022.1008234

Naicker K, van Rensburg G H 2018 Facilitation of reflective learning in nursing: reflective teaching practices of educators. Africa Journal of Nursing and Midwifery 20(2):14 pages https://doi.org/10.25159/2520-5293/3386

Nascimento J D S G, Costa A B F, Sangiovani J C et al 2020 Pre-simulation, pre-briefing or briefing in nursing simulation: what are the differences? Revista Eletronica de Enfermagem 22.60171, 1-10. https://doi.org/10.5216/ree.v22.60171

Nicol J S, Dosser I 2016 Understanding reflective practice. Nursing Standard 30(36):34–42 https://doi.org/10.7748/ns.30.36.34.s44

Nguyen-Truong C K Y, Davis A, Spencer C et al 2018 Techniques to promote reflective practice. Journal of Nursing Education 57(2):115–120

Nursing and Midwifery Board of Australia (NMBA) 2016 Registered nurse standards for practice. Online. Available: https://www.nursingmidwiferyboard.gov.au/Codes-Guidelines-Statements/Professional-standards/registered-nurse-standards-for-practice.aspx

Nursing and Midwifery Board of Australia (NMBA) 2018a Code of conduct for midwives. Online. Available: http://www.nursingmidwiferyboard.gov.au/Codes-Guidelines-Statements/Professional-standards.aspx

Nursing and Midwifery Board of Australia (NMBA) 2018b Code of conduct for nurses. Online. Available: http://www.nursingmidwiferyboard.gov.au/Codes-Guidelines-Statements/Professional-standards.aspx

Nursing and Midwifery Board of Australia (NMBA) 2018c National competency standards for the midwife. Online. Available: https://www.nursingmidwiferyboard.gov.au/Codes-Guidelines-Statements/Professional-standards/Midwife-standards-for-practice.aspx

Nursing Council of New Zealand (NCNZ) 2022 Competencies for registered nurses. Registered nurse. Online. Available: https://nursingcouncil.org.nz/Public/ncnz/nursing-section/registered_nurse.aspx

Patel K M, Metersky K 2021 Reflective practice in nursing: a concept analysis. International Journal of Nursing Knowledge 33:180–187 doi: 10.1111/2047-3095.12350

Peterkin A, Brett-MacLean P 2016 Keeping reflection fresh: a practical guide for clinical educators. Kent OH, The Kent State University Press

Rees K L 2013 The role of reflective practices in enabling final year nursing students to respond to the distressing emotional challenges of nursing work. Nurse Education in Practice 13:48–52

Rolfe G 2014 Rethinking reflective education: what would Dewey have done? Nurse Education Today 34:1179–1183

Scheel Schumann L, Peters M D J, Móbjerg M et al 2017 Reflection in the training of nurses in clinical practice settings: a scoping review protocol. JBI Database of systematic reviews and implementation reports 15(12):2871–2880 doi: 10.11124/JBISRIR-2017-003482

Schön D A 1983 The reflective practitioner: how practitioners think in action. Basic Books, New York

Schön D A 1987 Educating the reflective practitioner: towards a new design for teaching and learning in the professions. Jossey-Bass, San Francisco

Smith T 2020 Guided reflective writing as a teaching strategy to develop nursing student clinical judgement. Nursing Forum 56:241–248 https://doi.org/10.1111/nuf.12528

Steven A, Wilson G, Turunen H et al 2020 Critical incident techniques and reflection in nursing and health professions education: systematic review. Nurse Educator 45(6):E57–E61

Storaker A, Nåden D, Saeteren B 2017 From painful busyness to emotional immunization: nurses' experiences of ethical challenges. Nursing Ethics 24(5):556–568 https://doi.org/10.1177/0969733015620938

Sundgren M K M, Millear P M, Dawber C et al 2020 Reflective practice groups and nurse professional quality of life. Australian Journal of Advanced Nursing 38(4):355 https://doi.org/10.37464/2020.384.355

Thompson N, Pascal J 2012 Developing critically reflective practice. Reflective Practice: International and Multidisciplinary Perspectives 13(2):311–325 https://doi.org/10.1080/14623943.2012.657795

Thompson S, Thompson N 2018 The critically reflective practitioner, 2nd edn. Palgrave Macmillan, London

Tims M, Bakker A B, Derks D 2013 The impact of job crafting on job demands, job resources, and well-being. Journal of Occupational Health Psychology 18(2):230–40

CHAPTER 12

INTERPROFESSIONAL LEARNING AND WORKING

Ann Bonner and Jacqueline Bloomfield

KEY WORDS

collaborative care
communication
integrated care
interprofessional education
interdisciplinary team
multidisciplinary team
person-centred care
teamwork

LEARNING OBJECTIVES

After reading this chapter, readers should be able to:

- describe what is meant by interprofessional education and why it is an important part of learning to be a nurse
- explain the dynamic relationship between interprofessional education, interprofessional teamwork, collaboration and person-centred care
- describe the role of nurses in multidisciplinary and interdisciplinary teamwork
- identify and describe the importance of communication in the context of effective delivery of integrated care for patients and their families.

INTRODUCTION

This chapter will describe what is meant by interprofessional education and will explore why it is essential for the development of effective teamwork and collaboration across different healthcare disciplines to ensure the provision of high-quality, safe, person-centred care. The chapter also provides nurses with guidance around integrated work and the contribution of nurses to healthcare teams. It clarifies the different ways of integrated working through examining multidisciplinary, interdisciplinary and transdisciplinary healthcare teams. In doing so, it emphasises the development of a suite of core skills to support integrated working for nurses, and the importance of effective communication.

What is interprofessional education and why is it important?

Nurses rarely work alone but typically spend much of their time working within teams of other nurses, and with other healthcare professionals. While nursing education traditionally focuses on the development of the clinical skills and theoretical knowledge required for patient care, the increasing complexity of contemporary healthcare now also requires that nurses and other healthcare professionals work together seamlessly across disciplines (Zenani et al 2023). The World Health Organization (WHO) Framework for Action on Interprofessional Education and Collaborative Practice (2010) states that 'Interprofessional education occurs when two or more professionals learn about, from and with each other to enable effective collaboration and improve health outcomes.' Interprofessional education is viewed as a fundamental aspect of learning to be a healthcare professional and is gaining prominence in all healthcare curricula including nursing. During your time as a nursing student, it is likely that you will participate in several interprofessional learning activities with students from other healthcare disciplines.

> ### REFLECTION
> 1. Have you participated in any interprofessional learning activities as part of your nursing studies?
> 2. What were your thoughts about these and how have they impacted your future role as a member of the interprofessional healthcare team?

By engaging in authentic interprofessional education opportunities both on campus and during practice placements, nursing students can acquire the competencies needed to thrive in interprofessional healthcare teams, ultimately contributing to improved patient outcomes and quality of care.

Why learning with, from and about others is important

Importantly, interprofessional education provides nursing students with the opportunity to communicate and engage with peers from various healthcare professions, such as medicine, pharmacy, social work and allied health. This helps to foster a deeper understanding of each profession's roles, responsibilities and expertise. As you will read more about later in the chapter, interprofessional education is also important for dispelling myths and traditional stereotypes that historically placed doctors at the top of the health hierarchy, with nurses and allied health members positioned at a much lower level. Historical healthcare stereotypes can represent a barrier to the provision of collaborative healthcare. Interprofessional education can, however, help to reinforce accurate clarification of healthcare roles and responsibilities and, in doing so, help to develop an understanding and mutual respect among students from different health disciplines (Wilbur et al 2022).

Interprofessional education is crucial in health profession education for several reasons:

3. **Improved patient outcomes:** interprofessional education equips students with the competencies to navigate teamwork challenges and make evidence-based decisions in real-world healthcare settings. This preparation contributes to improved patient outcomes through coordinated care and person-centred treatment plans
4. **Coordinated patient care:** healthcare is increasingly complex, requiring health professionals from different disciplines to work together to address the diverse needs of patients.

Interprofessional education ensures that students understand how their role fits within the broader healthcare team and how to collaborate effectively to deliver holistic patient care

5 **Enhanced communication and collaboration:** by learning alongside students from a range of other healthcare disciplines, nursing students develop effective communication skills and learn to appreciate the unique perspectives and expertise of each profession. This fosters respect and trust among team members, which is essential for effective collaboration in clinical practice

6 **Professional socialisation:** interprofessional education facilitates professional socialisation, where students from different disciplines learn about professional roles, responsibilities, and discipline-specific ethical considerations. This process helps students develop a shared identity as healthcare professionals committed to person-centred care

7 **Preparation for interprofessional practice:** as healthcare systems evolve towards interprofessional practice models, interprofessional education prepares students to work effectively in diverse healthcare teams. It cultivates a culture of collaboration and continuous learning, essential for navigating the complexities of modern healthcare delivery.

You may now be starting to see how interprofessional learning prepares nursing students to navigate the intricacies of teamwork in dynamic healthcare environments. By engaging in collaborative activities, such as interprofessional learning workshops, case-based discussions, simulations, and joint clinical placements, students develop critical thinking abilities and learn to appreciate the value of diverse perspectives in problem solving.

STORY

Jed Pan is a second-year nursing student. He notes that his timetable includes an interprofessional workshop that includes other undergraduate students from different health disciplines. At the workshop Jed is allocated to a small group that includes students studying dietetics, pharmacy, medicine, physiotherapy and occupational therapy. The students are instructed to work together through a patient care scenario that focuses on Mrs Twee, an 81-year-old widow who lives alone in a small house. Mrs Twee was admitted to hospital following a fall at home that resulted in a fractured right hip. She has a history of arthritis, which has decreased her mobility and limited her ability to go shopping for groceries. On admission her body mass index (BMI) was 18.

Mrs Twee is to be discharged home and the students are to develop a discharge plan for Mrs Twee.

Reflective questions

Reflect on the scenario and answer the following questions.

1 What are the benefits of students from different health disciplines working together to complete the interprofessional workshop activity?
2 What knowledge would each student contribute to the development of the discharge plan for Mrs Twee?
3 As a nursing student, what could Jed contribute to the group?

What is interprofessional working and why is it important?

The increasing age of the population, chronic conditions, climate change, urbanisation, technological advancements and globalisation are rapidly transforming the way healthcare is required. Interprofessional working is a group of healthcare professionals who form collaborative partnerships with each other and with patients to deliver person-centred care (Stucky et al 2022). Often the term interprofessional working is used alongside integrated care or collaborative practice. All these terms indicate that teamwork across and within different health disciplines is key to developing effective interventions in various healthcare settings, and key to modern service delivery. Interprofessional teams are an approach to overcome care fragmentation, especially where there is a disconnection among the different healthcare providers, and it is this disconnection that leads to an adverse impact on people's care experiences and health outcomes. In Australia, this fragmentation tends to occur because the federal government is responsible for primary care and aged care, whereas the states/territories are responsible for acute hospital services. Interprofessional working is particularly important for those with multiple chronic conditions or complex healthcare needs. By reducing the fragmentation (and often duplication) between healthcare providers, societies have improved access to healthcare, better health outcomes, reduced hospitalisations and improved patient satisfaction (Ski et al 2023).

Historically, nurses (and other health professions) have encountered reduced status on healthcare teams due to the dominance of medicine; however, these traditional hierarchical relationships are changing towards a greater focus on collaboration (Bonner et al 2020). Breaking these traditions leads to innovative models of healthcare and joint decision making. Interprofessional collaboration is critical to the effective organisation of the tasks required to provide specific patients and/or populations with the best evidence-based healthcare (Wei et al 2022). Collaboration among healthcare professionals has also improved the work environment, workloads, and increased job satisfaction for those who work in these teams (Carney et al 2019, Labrague et al 2022).

Schot et al (2020), in a systematic review on interprofessional working, described it as: 1) bridging professional social, physical and task-related gaps; 2) negotiating overlaps in roles and tasks; and 3) creating spaces to do work this way. The goal of interprofessional working is to increase efficiencies and improve patient outcomes by organising care in accordance with the patient's needs and preferences, and by reducing fragmentation. Research suggests that a patient's functional status and length of hospital stay; a health professional's adherence to recommended practices and prescription of drugs; and the use of healthcare resources and costs can be positively impacted by interprofessional teams (Wei et al 2022).

Indeed, the lessons learned during the COVID-19 pandemic and the rapid changes to healthcare delivery sees the need for greater emphasis to be placed on adequately preparing the next generation of health professionals. Interprofessional and/or transprofessional education will assist in preparing undergraduate health professionals to enter the workforce with the skills and knowledge required to work collaboratively to improve care outcomes (Spaulding et al 2021).

Interprofessional working is best described as care that:
- is explicitly shaped by the patient's perspective and needs
- is linked to the needs of a specific patient population group as defined by the life cycle (i.e. adolescents and young people with mental health needs, older people living at home, or people with palliative care needs)

- is arranged to ensure continuity of care across time, which is provided by multiple providers (i.e. the patient's general practitioner [GP], community health nurses, chronic disease teams, and home care services) from different organisations (i.e. acute, community or aged care) and services (i.e. home nursing, diabetes education, wound care and community transport)
- requires interprofessional collaboration, whereby the healthcare service/team/nurse identifies and establishes linkages with the appropriate sector(s)/organisations (i.e. health, education and welfare) essential to improving the patient's care outcomes (Schot et al 2020).

Due to the complexity of care required, the care needs of patients with one or more chronic conditions often cannot be met by one single professional as different areas of expertise are necessary to optimise care. The interprofessional team consists of different professionals, such as nurses, general practitioners, pharmacists, dietitians, social workers and others, who work side by side and rely on each other's expertise. Integrated care does not mean all services required by an individual are combined into one 'care' package, but rather, the services required across various organisations and departments are coordinated and tailored to meet each patient's unique care needs. Integrated care is a way of coordinating the existing services to optimise patient outcomes. It has many forms and approaches, including:

1. 'horizontal integration', which links together relevant health and social services and requires healthcare professionals to optimise care at the patient level
2. 'vertical integration', which enables a person's care to be integrated across primary, community, acute care and tertiary healthcare services/settings
3. care integrated within one sector (e.g. mental health or palliative care), or across prevention and curative services
4. linking healthcare professionals and patients to optimise shared decision making and self-management
5. a 'whole of population approach', which requires the integration of public health, population-based and patient-centred approaches to optimise population health outcomes (Heeringa et al 2020).

Provision of integrated care that is flexible, personalised and seamless, which addresses the health and social needs of individual patients, requires significant change at the healthcare systems, health provider and patient levels. However, implementing these changes is complex as it requires action at multiple levels, engagement of health professionals and managers, as well as a sustained commitment from healthcare organisations and policymakers (Bhat et al 2022). These changes also challenge the traditional supply-driven models of care provision and require health professionals to have the foundation skills necessary for them to collaborate effectively with other disciplines involved in the person's care. If these challenges can be overcome, integrated care offers significant benefits for the patient, healthcare provider(s) and healthcare organisations, funding bodies and government (Bhat et al 2022).

What is the role of the nurse in multidisciplinary, interdisciplinary and transdisciplinary teamwork?

Optimal integrated care is dependent upon well-coordinated and effective teamwork involving multiple disciplines and services. There is good evidence that healthcare teams provide much better care than autonomous health professionals working in parallel and separate to one another (Wei et al 2022).

Integrated care teams can take many forms and operate in different care settings and with diverse populations (i.e. rapid response medical emergency teams, disaster response teams, chronic care teams, mental health teams, primary and/or acute care teams). The most effective integrated care team is non-hierarchical and utilises a collaborative, consensus-building approach to care delivery, which is delivered via a multidisciplinary, interdisciplinary, transdisciplinary or collaborative community-led team, which is often preferred by Indigenous populations (Peake et al 2019). While these terms are often used interchangeably and inconsistently in practice (and literature), each have different meanings and applications (Flores-Sandoval et al 2021). An integrated care team is:

- **multidisciplinary**, if it is composed of members from more than one discipline (hence multiple) who work on addressing a patient problem in parallel or sequentially without challenging or going outside of their disciplinary boundaries. These team members usually work independently to assess, plan and formulate goals for the patient. They interact formally at a multidisciplinary team meeting. These teams are usually hierarchically organised with a designated team leader. While working collaboratively with one another, these health professionals act autonomously. The cancer treatment team that meets to determine the optimal course of cancer treatment for each woman diagnosed with breast cancer is a good example of a multidisciplinary team

- **interdisciplinary**, if it is composed of a group of professionals from several different disciplines who are trained to use different tools and apply different concepts, working interdependently in the same care setting, and who interact both formally and informally to achieve a common goal. Interdisciplinary teamwork is defined as a dynamic process between two or more healthcare practitioners who use a concerted approach to assess, plan and evaluate patient care, using open communication, shared decision making and interdependent collaboration. Each team member contributes their own professional expertise but collaborates to interpret findings and negotiate priorities to develop an agreed plan of care for the patient. These members exhibit collaborative communication and interdependent practice. In this team, there is reciprocal interaction (hence 'inter') between the disciplines, leading to a blurring of disciplinary boundaries to optimise patient care outcomes. Interdisciplinary teams are considered to have a heightened ability to enhance and promote cooperation, coherence, shared responsibility, internal organisation, and communication

- **transdisciplinary**, if it involves a range of stakeholders and disciplines outside of health who transcend (hence 'trans') disciplinary boundaries and share role functions to optimise care outcomes. In addition to collaborating, team members entrust, prepare and supervise the sharing of disciplinary functions while retaining ultimate responsibility for services provided in their place by other team members. The emphasis is on sharing team responsibilities and the traditional hierarchies no longer exist. A transdisciplinary team is based on the premise that one person can perform several professional roles by providing services to the patient under the supervision of individuals from other disciplines. It requires cross-training and flexibility in accomplishing tasks. Transdisciplinary teams are most observed in environments where flexibility with roles and responsibilities is required, such as in rural, remote and humanitarian healthcare.

> **STORY**
>
> You are attending your first PEP (Professional Experience Placement) on a palliative care ward. During the shift you attend the interprofessional team meeting where you observe the team discussions of each patient on the ward. The team consists of a social worker, palliative care physician, palliative care nurse practitioner, dietitian, nurse unit manager and nurse navigator.
>
> **Reflective questions**
>
> Reflect on the above scenario and consider the following questions:
> 1. What is the role of each team member?
> 2. What is the difference between each of the nurses on the team and why would each be on the team?

What attributes do nurses require to be effective interprofessional team members?

It is challenging to define optimal team-based healthcare, including specific guidance on the best structure and functions for teams, because of the heterogeneity of their focus, tasks, patient types and settings. However, as health professional education advances, there are opportunities to improve interprofessional learning and practice whereby each discipline learns with, from and about each other. While there is not necessarily a recipe on how to create an effective interprofessional team, the Australian Health Practitioner Regulation Agency (Ahpra 2024) identifies shared values that exhibit:

- **Respect:** valuing each other's contributions, work and views
- **Commitment:** being committed to working together to achieve the vision and goals
- **Collaboration::** recognising that more can be achieved for patients when working jointly with others and together
- **Leadership:** leading consistently with integrity, fairness, and clear and honest communication
- **Innovation:** introducing new ideas and ways of working to change existing approaches in education, training and practice.

In addition to these personal values, effective interprofessional teams are also underpinned by the following key team principles:
- training and development
- appropriate resources and procedures
- appropriate skill-mix
- supportive team climate
- individual characteristics that support interprofessional teamwork
- clarity of vision
- quality and outcomes of care.

Developing interprofessional team practices

Regardless of the team's focus (i.e. chronic care, palliative care, primary care and/or acute care) and model (i.e. multidisciplinary, interdisciplinary or transdisciplinary), collaboration between team members is an essential element (Ho et al 2023). However, collaboration is a complex phenomenon, which requires individual team members and/or the service to forgo a competitive approach and be prepared to negotiate to optimise patient care outcomes.

Fostering collaborative practices is challenging, largely because of the numerous systemic conditions outside of the organisation (e.g. cultural, social, educational and professional systems), organisational conditions within the organisation (e.g. team structure, philosophy, resources and administrative supports) and interactional factors (interpersonal relationships with other team members, such as willingness to collaborate, trust, communication and mutual respect) at play (Schot et al 2020).

Creating clearly defined roles

The creation of clearly defined roles ensures the knowledge and skills that individual team members have from different disciplines are effectively harnessed. Differentiating the function of each team member, their responsibilities and accountabilities enables the integrated care team to take advantage of the division of labour and accomplish more than the sum of its parts (Farchi et al 2023). Achieving this requires team agreement about how discipline-specific roles and responsibilities will be optimised to improve care outcomes for individual patients and families (Wood et al 2022). It also requires an understanding of the legal parameters of each discipline's scope of practice and the reimbursement models that govern fee-for-services clinicians, such as medical practitioners.

Foster mutual trust

Individual team members' commitment to upholding the values of honesty, discipline, creativity, humility and curiosity build the trust required for the creation of a high-performance team essential for constructing more patient-centred and effective healthcare delivery (Ho et al 2023). Mutual trust creates an environment that allows for continuous learning and ensures team norms are upheld. However, it requires team leaders who are committed to creating a safe and trusting environment where everyone has a voice, regardless of role, and that members' ideas and concerns are welcomed and addressed. Healthcare organisations can foster the establishment of mutual trust by investing in strategies that enable the team to get to know one another at a personal level, embedding the personal values for high-functioning teams into the organisational recruitment and selection processes, and building the team's communication, negotiation and conflict resolution capabilities.

Effective communication

Mutual trust and effective communication are interlinked and are essential elements of interprofessional teams. Along with trust, the quality and timeliness of communication between members of the healthcare team is consistently cited as one of the main factors impacting on their experiences, satisfaction and the success of integrated care (Gleeson et al 2023). Inadequate team communication across and within care settings contributes to clinical errors, inefficient care delivery and compromises patient safety. An effective interprofessional team prioritises and continuously refines their communication skills and practices. In the digital age, communication is not only limited to face-to-face and written communication but also to telephone, email, text messages, virtual and electronic health records. The establishment of good communication systems and mechanisms to support the timely transfer of information is crucial for team functioning and to optimise care outcomes.

The adoption of standards, policies and interprofessional protocols, combined with interprofessional team meetings, are all strategies designed to support effective communication (Australian Commission on Safety and Quality in Health Care [ACSQHC] 2020). Setting a high standard for team communication, ensuring consistent, clear and professional communication among team members is essential. Team members are encouraged to speak clearly and succinctly, drawing upon their professional knowledge but avoiding jargon, discuss verifiable observations and use evidence rather than personal opinions and actively listen. Effective team communication requires a commitment to continual reflection and identifying and testing strategies for improvement. It also requires an organisational commitment to investment in building team members' communication capabilities (ACSQHC 2020).

Authentic collaboration

Interprofessional teams require persistence, continuous monitoring and improvement practices to address the elements that appear to deteriorate over time and impact on the team's capacity to provide healthcare. The domains of successful interprofessional teams that appear to improve over time are bridging professional, social, physical and task-related gaps, negotiating (and renegotiating) overlap in roles and tasks, and creating the time to collaborate (Schot et al 2020).

REFLECTION

1. Collaboration is a complex, voluntary and dynamic process that is dependent upon individual team members having the necessary leadership, communication and relationship-building skills
2. Respecting and trusting other members of the interprofessional team are key elements of all effective collaborations
3. As the discipline that spends the most time with patients and their families, nurses are ideally positioned to take a lead role in coordinating and facilitating communication between other team members.

The benefits of interprofessional working

The benefits for the patient, healthcare provider and organisations of interprofessional teams are summarised below:

- **Patient:** for the patient, care is coordinated and focused on long-term wellbeing and not episodic care. Care is provided by well-informed health professionals, who understand the patient's condition(s) and care needs and communicate effectively with other members of their care team. The patient experiences a seamless, smooth and easy-to-navigate healthcare system with shorter waiting times, better outcomes and quality of life
- **Healthcare providers:** working collaboratively with other members of the interprofessional team ensures that all technical/care services are provided in a coordinated and efficient way, so the patient gets the right care, in the right place at the right time. By working collaboratively with other health professionals from different fields, the team can coordinate services and tasks across traditional professional boundaries

▸ **Organisations:** there is a potential reduction in healthcare costs due to less duplication of medical tests (i.e. pathology and radiological tests), better information sharing and a reduction in avoidable or unnecessary hospitalisations. Interprofessional teamwork requires all the necessary processes, policies, and funding arrangements to be in place. Effectively managing strategic alliances and partnerships between different institutions helps optimise care outcomes and results in better use of scarce health resources.

CONCLUSION

Collaboration between health professionals improves healthcare outcomes and enhances patient and professional satisfaction while reducing healthcare costs. Given the global health workforce shortage, now more than ever, interprofessional working through effective collaboration is needed. Interprofessional learning across disciplines is fundamental to the preparation of the current and future health workforce so that they can work together to better meet the needs of different groups in our society. The defining features of interprofessional teams are: 1) the organising principle of service delivery is the patient's perspective (i.e. person-centred care); 2) it is linked to the needs of a specific patient population group as defined by the life cycle; 3) it involves the arrangement of multiple providers; and 4) it often requires inter-sectoral collaboration. As the largest health professional group, nurses have a unique role in providing interprofessional healthcare within multidisciplinary and interdisciplinary teams.

REFLECTIVE QUESTIONS

1. Explore the differences in the nurse's role if the team functions as multidisciplinary, interdisciplinary or transdisciplinary.
2. How do nurses retain their professional identity when working in interprofessional teams?

Recommended readings

Australian Health Professional Regulation Agency (Ahpra) 2024 Interprofessional collaborative statement of intent. Online. Available: https://www.ahpra.gov.au/News/2024-03-13-Interprofessional-Collaborative-Practice-Statement-of-Intent.aspx

Cucolo D, Oliveira J, Rossit R et al 2024 Effects of interprofessional practice on nursing workload in hospitals: a systematic review. International Journal of Health Planning and Management 39:824–843

Saragih I D, Hsiao C-T, Fann W-C et al 2024 Impacts of interprofessional education on collaborative practice of healthcare professionals: a systematic review and meta-analysis. Nurse Education Today 136:106136

References

Australian Commission on Safety and Quality in Health Care (ACSQHC) 2020 Communicating for safety: improving clinical communication, collaboration and teamwork in Australian health services. ACSQHC, Sydney

Australian Health Professional Regulation Agency (Ahpra) 2024 Interprofessional collaborative statement of intent. Online. Available: https://www.ahpra.gov.au/News/2024-03-13-Interprofessional-Collaborative-Practice-Statement-of-Intent.aspx

Bhat K, Easwarathasan R, Jacob M et al 2022 Identifying and understanding the factors that influence the functioning of integrated healthcare systems in the NHS: a systematic literature review. BMJ Open 12:e049296

Bonner A, Havas K, Stone C et al C 2020 An integrated chronic comorbid disease clinic: outcomes of nurse practitioner led service model. Collegian 27(4):430–436.

Carney P A, Thayer E K, Palmer R et al 2019 The benefits of interprofessional learning and teamwork in primary care ambulatory training settings. Journal of Interprofessional Education & Practice 15:119–126

Farchi T, Dopson S, Ewan F 2023 Do we still need professional boundaries? The multiple influences of boundaries on interprofessional collaboration. Organization Studies 44(2):277–298

Flores-Sandoval C, Sibbald S, Ryan B L et al 2021 Healthcare teams and patient-related terminology: a review of concepts and uses. Scandinavian Journal of Caring Sciences 35(1):55–66

Gleeson L L, O'Brien G L, O'Mahony D et al 2023 Interprofessional communication in the hospital setting: a systematic review of the qualitative literature. Journal of Interprofessional Care 37(2):202–213

Heeringa J, Mutti A, Furukawa M F et al 2020 Horizontal and vertical integration of health care providers: a framework for understanding various provider organizational structures. International Journal of Integrated Care 20(1):1–10

Ho J T, See M T A, Tan A J Q et al 2023 Healthcare professionals' experiences of interprofessional collaboration in patient education: a systematic review. Patient Education and Counseling 116:107965

Labrague L J, Al Sabei S, Al Rawajfah O et al 2022 Interprofessional collaboration as a mediator in the relationship between nurse work environment, patient safety outcomes and job satisfaction among nurses. Journal of Nursing Management 30(1):268–278

Peake R M, Jackson D, Lea J, Usher K 2019 Investigating the processes used to develop and evaluate the effectiveness of health education resources for adult Indigenous people: a literature review. Contemporary Nurse 55(4–5):421–449.

Schot E, Tummers L, Noordegraaf M 2020 Working on working together. A systematic review on how healthcare professionals contribute to interprofessional collaboration. Journal of Interprofessional Care 34(3):332–342

Ski C F, Cartledge S, Foldager D, Thompson D R et al 2023 Integrated care in cardiovascular disease: a statement of the Association of Cardiovascular Nursing and Allied Professions of the European Society of Cardiology. European Journal of Cardiovascular Nursing 22(5):e39–e46

Spaulding E M, Marvel F A, Jacob E et al 2021 Interprofessional education and collaboration among healthcare students and professionals: a systematic review and call for action. Journal of Interprofessional Care 35(4):612–621

Stucky C H, Wymer J A, House S 2022 Nurse leaders: transforming interprofessional relationships to bridge healthcare quality and safety. Nurse Leader 20(4):375–380

Wei H, Horns P, Sears S F et al 2022 A systematic meta-review of systematic reviews about interprofessional collaboration: facilitators, barriers, and outcomes. Journal of Interprofessional Care 36(5):735–749

Wilbur K, El-Awaisa A, El-Hajj M S 2022 Reducing health provider stereotypes through undergraduate interprofessional education. Journal of Taibah University Medical Science 17(6):991–999

Wood A, Copley J, Hill A, Cottrell N 2022 Interprofessional identity in clinicians: a scoping review. Journal of Interprofessional Care DOI:10.1080/13561820.2022.2086222

World Health Organization 2010 Framework for action on interprofessional education and collaborative practice. World Health Organization, Geneva. Online. Available: http://apps.who.int/iris/handle/10665/70185

Zenani N E, Sehularo L A, Gause G, Chukwuere P C 2023 The contribution of interprofessional education in developing competent undergraduate nursing students: integrative literature review. BMC Nursing 22:315

CHAPTER 13

ENGAGING WITH SOCIAL MEDIA: OPPORTUNITIES AND CHALLENGES FOR NURSING PROFESSIONALS

Matthew Barton, Michael Todorovic and Jessica Stokes-Parish

KEY WORDS
digital communication
digital nursing
e-professionalism
ethics
professionalism
social media
social networking

LEARNING OBJECTIVES

After reading this chapter, readers should be able to:

- define social media and describe the utility of various social platforms
- describe how social media can be used across nursing practice, education, research and policy
- apply regulatory policies and guidelines for social media use and discuss their implications for nursing
- describe ethical and professional issues for nurses to consider when using social media.

INTRODUCTION

Communication is vital to human interaction. Within today's society, the internet is a critical piece of communication infrastructure and, therefore, denying or restricting access—while hospitalised for example—is failing to address people's needs. The internet has replaced more traditional mediums as the main source of communication and information sourcing. The face of the internet is constantly evolving, and social media platforms are rapidly changing society. As of January 2024, there were 5.35 billion internet users worldwide and 5.04 billion, or 62.8%

of the world's population, using social media—this number is projected to rise to around 5.85 billion users by 2027. Most social media consumers do not remain on one platform. On average, users engage with between six and seven different social media platforms (Statista 2024a). Social media platforms have a wide scope, with categories ranging from social networking, video sharing, professional networking, audio streaming, and chat messaging, to name a few. Users of these platforms can actively create their own content by posting and uploading, sharing content, 'liking' or blogging information and ideas.

Compared with other industries, the nursing profession has been relatively slow to utilise social media; however, the potential applications within nursing practice are immense. Social media offers a unique opportunity to challenge and improve healthcare practices, enable nurse professionals to connect with diverse individuals and build networks, create collaborative research projects, disseminate research and education, solve clinical issues, share solutions, provide professional development, and share workplace opportunities (Fedele 2019). However, social media should be approached with some caution. Nursing remains one of the most risk-averse professions, and rightly so, as nurses are charged with caring for vulnerable individuals. Therefore, it is important that when applying social media to the nursing profession, this is carefully risk managed and assessed for appropriateness in its application.

There is a vast array of novel examples of social media applications in nursing. These include online support blogs for individuals living with brain cancer, stroke survivor support groups on Facebook, educational videos on YouTube, professional networking on LinkedIn and X (formerly Twitter), and chat groups for nursing researchers and clinicians, to name a few. An extensive and diverse range of platforms continues to emerge. However, it is important that nurses have a basic understanding of social media and its implications for nursing practice within the context of the contemporary healthcare system.

What is social media?

Social media is a term that is constantly evolving. The Australian Health Practitioner Regulation Agency (Ahpra) defines social media as 'internet-based tools that allow individuals and groups to communicate, to advertise or share opinions, information, ideas, messages, experiences, images and video or audio clips' (Ahpra 2019). Meanwhile, the New Zealand Nurses Organisation (NZNO) states that social media encompasses web-based technologies that facilitate real-time connections, communication, and information exchange, allowing users to generate and share content instantly, distinguishing it from traditional internet usage (NZNO 2019). Social media can be categorised into five groups: 1) collaborative projects (e.g. Wikipedia); 2) micro-blogging (e.g. X [Twitter]); 3) content communities (e.g. YouTube); 4) social networking sites (e.g. Facebook); and 5) virtual gaming or social worlds (e.g. Second Life) (Rukavina et al 2021).

In healthcare, social media plays an important role in education, health promotion, research, recruitment and policy dissemination. Unfortunately, many health professionals lack the skillset or experience to engage with social media to its potential. A survey of 397 nurses found that 87% use some form of social media, but only 57% of respondents reported receiving formal training on how to use social media in the workforce (Lefebvre et al 2020). Within these social media platforms exists an unprecedented ability to expand access and communication, with the potential to revolutionise the way medical professionals interact with peers, patients and the public. Although most social media platforms share common features such as free registration, public and private communication, and fast content upload and retrieval, each platform is unique and has distinctive uses (Fig. 13.1).

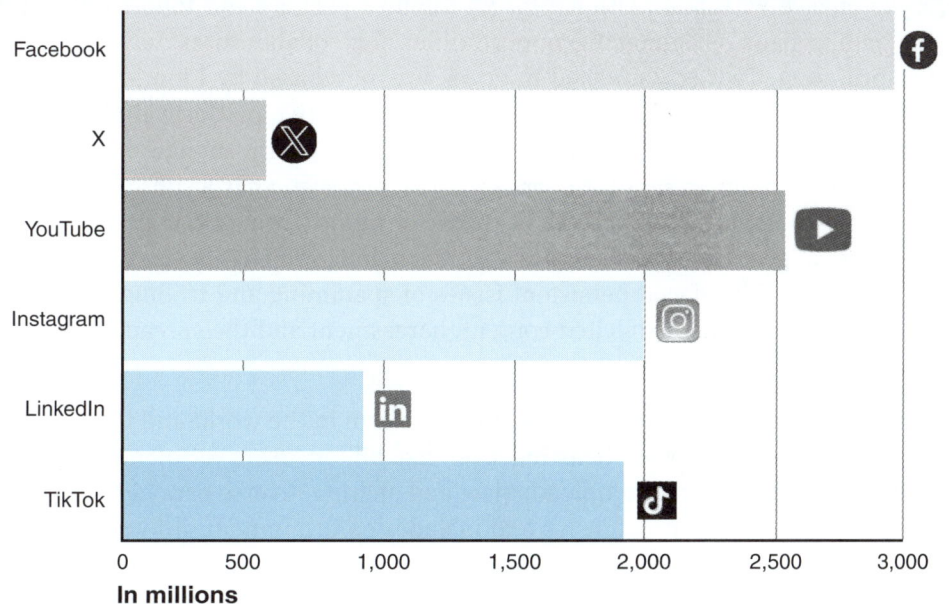

FIGURE 13.1

Social media platform characteristics and statistics

FACEBOOK

Facebook is the most popular social media platform in the world, with over 2.9 billion users as of 2023 (Statista 2024b). It is a social networking platform that serves as a hub for news, collaboration and multimedia content sharing among friends, family and broader communities. The platform is engaged with a variety of age groups, although those aged between 25 and 34 years are the heaviest users of this platform. On average, users engage with Facebook for 30 minutes per day (Statista 2024b). Globally, Facebook reaches a wide audience and connects users through its platform, allowing individuals, businesses and communities with similar interests to connect, share information and content, and engage in discussions. In addition to text, users can share a variety of multimedia content, including photos, videos and live streams, enhancing the richness of communication. Facebook has faced scrutiny recently over privacy issues, with concerns about data collection and data safety. Facebook's use of an algorithmic feed that prioritises certain content over others can potentially lead to biased information. Maintaining relevance and influence on Facebook demands a significant time investment due to the continual need for content creation and audience engagement.

X (FORMERLY TWITTER)

X is a micro-blogging platform with just over 500 million users in 2023 (Statista 2024c), allowing users to engage in real-time communication, share news and media, and express opinions in short messages called tweets. X's user base spans various age groups, with a significant presence among those aged between 25 and 34 years. Its dynamic nature and ability to quickly facilitate widespread dissemination of information has made X a go-to platform for real-time updates and discussions. On average, users engage with this platform for 35 minutes per day and follow influencers, industry leaders and public figures, enhancing opportunities for collaboration and networking (Statista 2024c). In April 2023, Twitter, launched in 2006, was purchased by Elon Musk and merged with X Corp. to become X. Historically, Twitter served as an effective platform for businesses and individuals to promote products, services and personal brands. Several changes have been made to the platform since transitioning to X. As of February 2024, users who pay a subscription fee have access to X Premium, which includes an increase in character limits (from 280 characters to 25,000 characters), the ability to post longer videos (up to ≈3 hours long or 8GB file size), and the ability to edit posts once published. X has faced persistent issues of spamming and trolling, where automated or malicious accounts engage in unsolicited content, harassment and the spread of misinformation.

YOUTUBE

YouTube stands as the number one video-hosting platform in the world and the second most popular search engine behind Google—boasting over 2.5 billion users as of 2023 (Statista 2024d). YouTube offers users a platform to upload, view and share a diverse array of videos. The range of content available on YouTube is extensive and includes entertainment, information and education, music videos and vlogs (video blogs). While catering to various age groups, users aged between 25 and 34 years emerge as the most active users. On average, users spend 45 minutes per day engaging with the platform (Statista 2024d). YouTube offers users the ability to create a personal account and, for content creators, the ability to host a 'Channel'. A YouTube Channel serves as the hub, or homepage, where creators can showcase their work and connect with their audience. Notably, video creators can monetise their content, providing an opportunity to earn income. YouTube videos are indexed by search engines like Google, enhancing their visibility in Google search results. Given the high competitiveness of YouTube, new creators face challenges in gaining visibility amidst the vast amount of content. The YouTube algorithm plays a crucial role in enhancing video visibility and discoverability, emphasising the importance of creating desirable and engaging content. This may compel creators to invest in professional-grade equipment to ensure their videos are of high quality.

INSTAGRAM

Instagram is a multimedia-sharing platform that allows users to post, share and discover visual content—primarily used for showcasing images and short videos. With just over 2 billion users in 2023 (Statista 2024e), it has become a popular platform for individuals, influencers and businesses to express themselves creatively and build an audience. Acquired by Meta (the parent company of Facebook) in 2012, the platform mostly attracts a younger audience, with 85% of users younger than 45 years of age, with the 18–24 age group being the most active (Statista 2024e). Users spend, on average, 30 minutes per day on Instagram (Statista 2024e), engaging with visually appealing content presented either transiently in the stories of the content creator or permanently in their feed. Instagram has stronger data privacy compliance compared with many other social media platforms, instilling tools to help users protect their data and comply with privacy regulations. These tools give users more control over their personal information and ensure strengthened data privacy management. Unfortunately, the visual nature of Instagram has been accused of perpetuating a state of perfectionism, with reports indicating that some users may feel pressured to curate an idealised version of their lives. Moreover, the platform's design encourages endless scrolling, which can contribute to addictive usage patterns, potentially affecting mental health and wellbeing. Meanwhile, the abundance of advertisements on the platform risks overshadowing content, potentially diminishing the positive aspects of the platform.

LINKEDIN

LinkedIn, a professional networking platform tailored for career development and business connections, distinguishes itself from other social media platforms by aligning with users' career-oriented objectives. In 2023, the platform had 875 million users who utilised LinkedIn to share professional profiles, connect with colleagues, seek job opportunities and provide industry insights (Statista 2024f). Predominantly used by adults in the 25–34 year age group, users typically—in comparison to other social media platforms—spend a moderate amount of time (7.5 minutes) on the platform daily (Statista 2024f). LinkedIn's drawbacks include a smaller audience, potentially leading to limited visibility and reduced audience interaction compared to larger platforms. Broadly speaking, LinkedIn provides users with a dynamic platform to showcase their digital curriculum vitae and build a network in their desired field of work.

TIKTOK

TikTok is a short-form video-sharing platform that saw 1.9 billion users actively engage with the platform in 2023 (Statista 2024g). Users are drawn to TikTok for its ability to empower creativity through engaging and highly entertaining short-form videos, often set to music. The platform has gained significant popularity among younger demographics, with young adults aged between 18–24 years forming the most active user base. On average, users spend 95 minutes on TikTok per day (Statista 2024g), immersed in viral videos that have been shared or recommended. TikTok has faced recent scrutiny over data privacy concerns, prompting questions about their handling of user data. Like other social media platforms, TikTok users are prone to cyberbullying and negative comments, while the short-form nature of TikTok videos may contribute to a shortened attention span among users.

Relevance to nursing and modern healthcare
CONTEMPORARY APPLICATION IN NURSING

It is important to highlight nurses' e-professionalism and regulatory obligations in relation to social media use, which will be explored later in this chapter. Now, it is essential to highlight some of the innovative approaches to integrating social media across the nursing profession. Figure 13.2 outlines four broad domains where social media is being successfully embedded: 1) patient support and health promotion; 2) professional networking and recruitment; 3) professional education and development; and 4) research, policy and procedures. This chapter will explore these four domains in more detail.

Domain 1: patient support and health promotion

Social media can be applied in a variety of care contexts. These can include using Instagram to promote health campaigns, Facebook for patient support, TikTok for medical education, and using X to report disease surveillance data.

One common use of social media is building online communities of support—often for people living with disease, particularly during or after treatment. Support groups use social media platforms to connect and share survivors' and caregivers' experiences—with one study reporting that

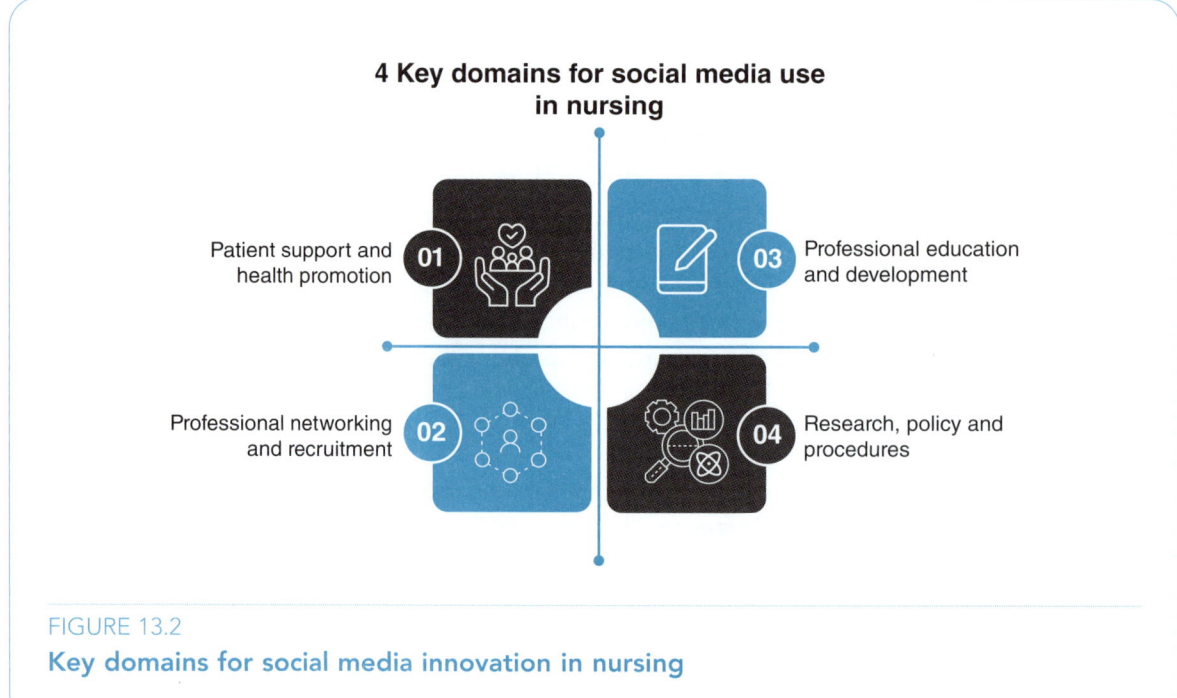

FIGURE 13.2

Key domains for social media innovation in nursing

> **BOX 13.1**
> **Domain 1: Examples of patient support and health promotion delivered via social media**
>
> **HEALTH PROMOTION**
> - Providing ad hoc supportive care for patients and family members via a digital forum
> - Maintaining a personal health diary (e.g. posting via MyFitnessPal to Facebook)
> - Connecting patients with similar conditions (National Stroke Foundation Australia's EnableMe—online patient community for stroke http://www.enableme.org)
> - Providing smoking cessation assistance (ability for real-time feedback from smoking cessation counsellors)
> - A platform to engage with exercise training and management
> - Receiving 'daily health tips' from credible sources (e.g. secondary stroke prevention)
>
> **PATIENT SUPPORT**
> - Obtaining weight management support (e.g. 'Lark' smartphone application)
> - Assisting with diabetes management (such as blood glucose tracking)
> - Engaging with epilepsy support groups (such as consumer-driven or NGO-led Facebook page initiatives)
> - Engaging with stroke survivor support groups
> - Engaging with brain tumour support groups (such as Nurse Consultant-led Facebook groups after discharge post-surgery)

80% of cancer patients connect with others about their cancer using social media (Beltrán Ponce et al 2023). We have provided some examples of how social media platforms are currently being used successfully to enhance patient support and facilitate health promotion.

More examples of patient support and health promotion delivered via social media are described in Box 13.1.

Facebook to build online communities

Facebook, as a platform for building online communities, has significantly impacted the landscape of healthcare engagement. Online communities, particularly within Facebook groups, can provide information on a wide range of health-related topics, catering not only to patients, but also to caregivers, clinicians and policy makers. Often dynamic and lively, these forums provide a rich insight into the experiences of patients and caregivers—providing a resource that has yet to be fully utilised for informing and shaping healthcare design and delivery.

In these online spaces, individuals find increased connectedness and less isolation, support in coping with challenges, learn from others' experiences, and can access important resources. Unlike traditional face-to-face focus groups, closed Facebook groups for patients provide an uncensored environment for individuals to share their concerns and experiences freely (Partridge et al 2018). They can also serve as a valuable resource, stepping in to offer information and support to patients in instances where traditional health services may fall short (Gaddy & Topf 2021).

However, it is important to consider that certain types of medical advice offered on these platforms, without appropriate health professional-led guidance, may result in the spread of misinformation and be subject to ethical and legal considerations. To address these concerns, developing guidelines and incorporating training programs for administrators and moderators of these platforms may help improve the quality and reliability of the support provided in these groups—helping maximise the benefits and minimise the risks.

Increasingly, nurses are approached by patients and caregivers in clinical practice to recommend online healthcare information and informal support after hospitalisation. There is a need for greater continuing education of nurses and credible tools to support the quality appraisal of these innovations. Furthermore, nurses working within clinical specialties have a responsibility to stay updated on credible and endorsed applications, blogs and webpages that have high relevance to patient care so they can recommend these to patients and caregivers in practice.

YouTube for health promotion

YouTube is a powerful tool to reach and educate a diverse audience on health-related topics. However, some studies advise caution as they have found that sometimes it can lead to the provision or reinforcement of inaccurate information to patients and caregivers (Osman et al 2022). Regardless, YouTube can be an effective platform to help target populations (e.g. young adults) with key public health campaigns such as cancer prevention strategies and cardiovascular risk reduction messages (Bottorff et al 2014). In 2021, the Australian medical education-based YouTube channel, Dr Matt & Dr Mike (https://www.youtube.com/@DrMattDrMike), hosted by two Australian academics and medical educators, collaborated with the Australian Medical Association to produce several evidence-based videos to combat COVID-19 vaccine myths. The six videos reached more than 300,000 viewers from 49 countries. By age, the largest audience was 25–44 years (48%), 45–64 years (25%), <24 years (14%), and over 65 years (12%). This underscores the utility of YouTube as a platform to reach and educate a diverse audience. A study of 165 young adults (18–24 years) reported that YouTube was considered a '… useful source for learning about everything …' (Lim et al 2022). The study noted that participants deliberately searched for health-related content on the platform and often consulted multiple videos to compare the information provided. Interestingly, the perceived trustworthiness of the YouTube personality influenced the perceived quality of the information in the videos. This highlights the importance for health professionals to consider their approach—ensuring their health-related content is designed for their target population. Furthermore, selecting the appropriate digital platform is crucial to maximise impact, especially considering the age and demographics of the users.

Domain 2: professional networking and recruitment

Social media is being used to build personal and professional networks and to streamline health service management processes. Social media can support the health workforce by providing electronic text reminders from clinics (e.g. WhatsApp), facilitate recruitment (e.g. LinkedIn), and enable in-house communication (e.g. Yammer). Yammer, a closed platform that only employees within an institution can access, is being used to help share information and build culture across small to large organisations. Further examples of patient services and workforce interventions that are delivered by social media are provided in Box 13.2.

> **BOX 13.2**
> **Domain 2: Examples of professional networking and recruitment delivered via social media**
>
> EXAMPLES OF SOCIAL MEDIA-DELIVERED WORKFORCE INTERVENTIONS
> - Transmitting critical laboratory values to nurses and physicians
> - Augmenting telemedicine
> - Remote wound care assistance
> - Shift bidding for nurses and other healthcare professionals (e.g. ShiftMatch, which is an online open shift-bidding platform for casual staff that can be accessed via smartphone and desktop devices)
> - Recruitment of healthcare staff (advertising on LinkedIn for job opportunities and vacancies)
> - Communicating with nursing supervisors

Healthcare recruitment agencies are using sites such as LinkedIn and X to source potential candidates for nursing vacancies. It is increasingly important for student nurses in Australia and New Zealand (Aotearoa) to develop and maintain a LinkedIn profile, showcase achievements during their studies and connect with peers and potential employers. Building professional relationships on social media can connect you with likeminded peers, facilitate professional development or employment opportunities, and provide access to experts and established professionals.

Social media is also being used to connect nurses with established professionals and to promote a network of evidence-based practice. One example of this is the *European Journal of Cardiovascular Nursing* (*EJCN*) Journal Club (see http://cnu.sagepub.com/site/additional/JournalClub/Articles.xhtml). This is a social media-based journal club facilitated by an expert moderator (usually a journal editor) and co-hosted by an author of a recent publication from that journal. The social media journal club is hosted on Google+ Hangout. This provides a unique opportunity for clinicians and the journal readership to directly engage with the researchers and authors of clinical studies (Ferguson et al 2017). At the time of writing, the *EJCN* hosted 25 sessions, which were also recorded and then uploaded onto YouTube at a later stage for people to view if they were unable to attend the live session. This innovative approach to a technology-enhanced journal club is exciting and removes geographical challenges to engaging in such scholarly activities.

Domain 3: professional education and development

The number of nurses, clinicians and other professional healthcare associations and bodies using social media has grown over the years, with one study reporting that 65% of physicians use social media sites for professional reasons (Ventola 2014). For nurses, social media can be an effective tool for fulfilling continuing professional development (CPD) regulatory requirements (Moorley & Chinn 2015). Historically, the 'WeNurses' X page (@wenurses) (see http://www.wecommunities.org) has been a successful way of engaging other nurses in professional discussion via social media on a regular basis, with discussions focusing on contemporary issues regarding clinical practice and discussing challenges in evidence-based care. Originally developed by Teresa Chinn (an agency nurse from the UK) in 2012, WeNurses has now amassed over 115,000 followers on X, demonstrating the ability of social media to connect and educate a diverse audience.

Increasingly, nurse teachers recognise that students learn outside traditional learning environments such as the physical classroom and the clinical environment. New pedagogical approaches to nurse education, including blended and flipped models, are increasingly common and driving greater integration of social media and other digital technologies within nurse education. The ease of access and instantaneous nature of social media make it an adaptable learning resource. An emergent area of interest among clinical teachers is its application in the development of clinical skills in novice nurses, with students also referring to YouTube as a quick way to refresh knowledge on elements of clinical skills (Burton 2022). A key driver is the rapid access to visual and video information, yet academics recommend caution and assessment of online resources to check for their quality and credibility (Duncan et al 2013). Further examples of professional education and development initiatives that are delivered by social media are provided in Box 13.3.

Tweetorials

Social media posts can be helpful to engage clinicians with a community of practice around particular issues or topics. Wright et al (2020) recently developed and evaluated an X chat focused on raising awareness of antimicrobial resistance among research students. X was selected as the optimal platform due to its outward-facing nature, and given that it has been successful in creating communities of practice such as #WeNurses. The X chat was hosted and convened over a 24-hour period. After 72 hours, the team identified that the chat obtained an impressive reach and engagement, with over 2.6 million accounts reached and over 10 million impressions achieved. Such studies highlight the utility of platforms like X to create conversation, promote awareness, and shine a light on topics of popularity. Another successful use of X, in the context of professional development, is the 'tweetorial'—a term created from combining tweet and tutorial. Designed to overcome the constraints (e.g. word count) of a post, a tweetorial is a collection of threaded tweets that succinctly and iteratively convey an educational

---

BOX 13.3

Domain 3: Examples of professional education and development delivered via social media

PROFESSIONAL EDUCATION

- Example NCLEX (National Council Licensure Examination) test questions for preparation for nursing registration in the USA
- Reviewing evidence-based byte-size education for clinicians

PROFESSIONAL DEVELOPMENT

- Clinician opinion-sharing via short tweets and X conversations
- Providing an avenue for nurse–mentor relationships and collaboration
- Live-tweeting surgical procedures for education (Watch: https://www.youtube.com/watch?v=LZycUg4OGhI)
- Live-tweeting nursing conferences and meetings (Example #PCNA2016; Preventative Cardiovascular Nurses Association 2016 Conference, Orlando, April 2016)
- Connecting genetic and basic science/bench researchers with clinicians

narrative. Breu et al (2021) nicely outline the anatomy of a tweetorial in their paper, highlighting that the first tweet is the 'hook' or premise of the thread. The middle tweets are the core of the narrative, and may include images, polls and links in addition to text. Finally, the closing tweet summarises the key messages and provides the learner with additional resources they can access for more information (Breu et al 2022). Creating chats and tweetorials have the potential to bring a global nursing community into a digital classroom to engage, reflect and discuss key nursing-related issues (Wright et al 2020).

Domain 4: policy, procedure and research

Many researchers are also reaping the benefits of social media as a tool for enabling and conducting nursing research. The global reach and viral ability of social media make it an adept tool for recruiting research participants and enabling the link to information about upcoming studies and disseminating research findings. Mannix et al (2014) described their experience of using social media for research participant recruitment and data collection via an online survey. Their work, alongside more recent research, highlights that social media can be useful for research purposes and can be helpful in large-scale data collection, recruiting hard to reach populations, and provides a cost-effective and efficient strategy for overall participant recruitment (Darko et al 2022).

Social media is embedded within health policy and adopted for public health procedures. Its utility to disseminate information, provide a platform for policy makers to engage with the public, advocate for specific policies, and monitor real-time public opinion is being increasingly recognised. Other examples of how social media is being adopted in the areas of policy, procedure and research are outlined in Box 13.4.

STORY

You are working as a new graduate registered nurse in a busy acute surgical ward in a major metropolitan teaching hospital. You are caring for Hayley, a 23-year-old female patient who has recently been involved in a road traffic accident and has fractured her neck of femur. You are administering an injection to her. While obtaining Hayley's consent for a subcutaneous injection, and checking the six rights of medication administration, Hayley asks you if she can record a short TikTok video of her injection using her smartphone. Hayley's mum is also present at the bedside and thinks this would be pretty 'cool' to do, too, and is keen to assist in recording this video.

Reflective questions

Reflect on the scenario and answer the following questions:

1. What would your nursing actions be in this scenario?
2. What are some ethical implications of recording and sharing medical procedures on social media platforms like TikTok?
3. What could the professional repercussions of your actions be if you allow Hayley to record and broadcast this procedure?
4. How does the request to record a TikTok video align with the principles of patient autonomy, privacy, and obtaining informed consent?

> **BOX 13.4**
> **Domain 4: Examples of health policy, procedures and research delivered via social media**
>
> **POLICY AND PROCEDURE**
> - Adverse event reporting in the clinical setting
> - Drug safety alerts from the Therapeutic Goods Authority (TGA) or new listings on the Pharmaceutical Benefits Scheme (PBS)
> - Tweeting updates on facility policies and safe operating procedures (local health districts and hospitals dissemination to employers via platforms such as Yammer)
> - Issuing emergency updates to hospital services to the general public
> - Clinical education coordination (updates to employees about upcoming educational events, such as opportunities to achieve mandatory training requirements)
>
> **NURSING RESEARCH**
> - Clinical trial awareness (updates to clinicians on clinical trial recruitment targets)
> - Research finding dissemination
> - Sharing peer-to-peer reviews of articles of interest
> - Generating streams of authoritative healthcare content online
> - Discussing public healthcare policy
> - Developing stronger patient–provider–researcher relationships

Social media ethics

Social media use is ubiquitous in nursing practice. Whether for building networks or seeking community, most nurses use social media—for both professional and personal use. And while poor social media practices are highlighted frequently by organisations and the media alike, the positive power of social media is often ignored. We argue that social media use can improve the public profile of nurses and create opportunities for sharing knowledge and community. There are numerous examples of the positive impact of social media:

- Tyler, 'The Visual Nurse' on Instagram, creates educational resources on ECG interpretation
- Penny, 'SickHappens', provides paediatric nursing education for parents and health providers on Instagram
- Pat, 'PatMacRN', provides commentary on research and nursing theory on TikTok.

However, there is no doubt that nurses must be trustworthy both online and offline, so how can we best guide practice?

E-PROFESSIONALISM

E-professionalism is a term that is used to describe professional conduct and integrity that encompasses the traditional definition and values of professionalism and extends to the digital environment (Cleary et al 2013). Today, the ethical principles of beneficence, non-maleficence, justice, respect for

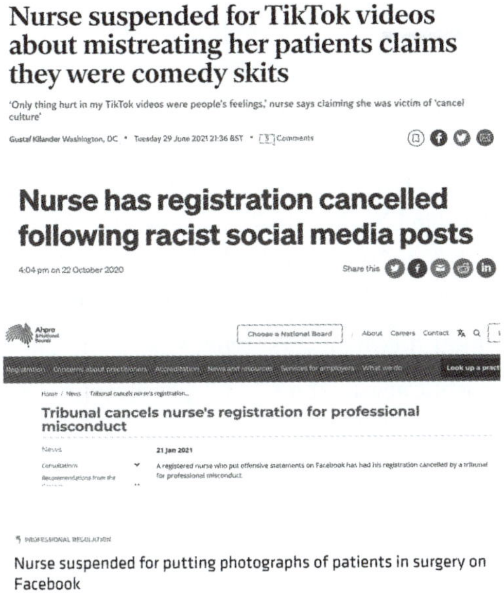

Nurse suspended for TikTok videos about mistreating her patients claims they were comedy skits

'Only thing hurt in my TikTok videos were people's feelings,' nurse says claiming she was victim of 'cancel culture'

Gustaf Kilander Washington, DC • Tuesday 29 June 2021 21:36 BST • Comments

Nurse has registration cancelled following racist social media posts

4:04 pm on 22 October 2020

Share this

Choose a National Board | About | Careers | Contact

Look up a pract

Home / News / Tribunal cancels nurse's registration...

Tribunal cancels nurse's registration for professional misconduct

News

21 Jan 2021

A registered nurse who put offensive statements on Facebook has had his registration cancelled by a tribunal for professional misconduct

Nurse suspended for putting photographs of patients in surgery on Facebook

FIGURE 13.3

News reports of nursing misconduct related to social media

autonomy, fairness, truthfulness and justice (as outlined in Chapter 3 'Ethics in nursing') extend far beyond the hospital walls and into the digital world. Nurses must be cognisant of this and maintain professionalism when identifying as a nurse within the digital world (Fig. 13.3). The boundaries between professional and personal are challenging to navigate, and in the eyes of the regulator, there may be no difference. In addition to ethical considerations, there are three domains a nurse could consider regarding social media practice:

- professional codes
- adjacent legislation
- employer requirements.

Professional codes

Globally, nurses are bound by their professional codes of practice. For example, in Australia, nurses are governed by the Australian Health Practitioner Regulation Agency (Ahpra) nursing Code of Conduct (Ahpra 2022), and in New Zealand (Aotearoa), nurses are governed by the Nursing Council of New Zealand (NCNZ) nursing Code of Conduct (NCNZ 2012a). These codes outline expectations regarding professionalism, confidentiality and privacy, evidence-based practice and more. More specifically, Ahpra advises on social media use, outlining that nurses should adhere to the following:

- complying with confidentiality and privacy obligations
- complying with your professional obligations as defined in your Board's Code of Conduct

- maintaining professional boundaries
- communicating professionally and respectfully with or about patients, colleagues and employers, and
- not presenting information that is false, misleading or deceptive, including advertising; only claims that are supported by acceptable evidence.

This policy clearly outlines that the obligations of nurses are not restricted to confidentiality but mandates that nurses must not contribute to misinformation.

NCNZ provides advice to nurses using social media and other forms of electronic communication to adhere to the following principles (NCNZ 2012b):
- Respect health consumers' privacy and confidentiality
- Work respectfully with colleagues to best meet health consumers' needs
- Act with integrity to justify health consumers' trust
- Maintain public trust and confidence in the nursing profession.

Adjacent legislation

Frequently an afterthought, legislation relevant to engaging on social media should be considered by the modern nurse. This includes federal advertising and consumer laws, such as the Therapeutic Goods Association (TGA) and Medsafe (New Zealand Medicines and Medical Devices Safety Authority) Advertising Codes, the Australian Consumer Law Ad Standards and the Advertising Standards Authority Ad Standards. For instance, nurses are not permitted to endorse or provide testimonials of therapeutic goods. What does endorsement mean? Any content or conversation that provides explicit or implicit recommendations of a good. This includes inadvertently having a picture of a therapeutic good in the background of an image. The TGA and Medsafe codes also provide explicit instructions on restricted representations, therapeutic claims, and discussing cosmetic procedures.

Employer requirements

Last but not least, nurses should be aware of their employer's policies on social media use. This often has similarities to the professional codes (such as confidentiality, privacy, etc.), but in some cases it provides explicit instructions as to what is not acceptable practice. For example, many policies explicitly note that the employee must not identify the place of work, post on social media while on the clock, and not talk negatively about their employer online.

Beyond these legislative requirements, it is important to think about the unintended consequences of what our presence on social media might do. Does your content have the potential to negatively affect the reputation of you, your employer or your profession? This can happen through things that may not occur to you. This is because reputation is all about perception and not intention. For example, you might comment on a bad experience you had at work with your colleagues—if framed carelessly, this might be perceived as a negative.

Finally, be aware that what you do in your personal capacity on social media may be judged as if you were engaging in a professional capacity. While this highlights the blurred lines between personal autonomy and professional identity, in the eyes of the regulator some content may be considered as professional. For example, if you were to comment on a news story with your personal profile, but you made discriminatory comments (about sex, gender, age, ethnicity or religion), you are likely to be held to account at your professional standard. Also, see Box 13.5.

BOX 13.5
Recommendations for nurses using social media

- Be aware of the terms and conditions of each of the social media sites that you use. This can often be challenging, given the frequency with which these are updated, but it is important to keep abreast of these updates and review these and their privacy settings on a regular basis
- Be aware of the unintended consequences of what you might post. Your digital footprint is lasting, and can have negative consequences for professional relationships and career prospects
- Never consider posts to be anonymous
- It is essential to regularly monitor and evaluate your digital presence. At a minimum, a yearly digital presence personal review is recommended
- Ensure that you are up to date with your professional standards for practice and employer code of conduct
- 'Stay in your lane'—do not post content outside your area of expertise
- Do not endorse therapeutic goods or share clinical testimonials

STORY

You have been working for 3 years in the general medical ward of a regional hospital. During this time, you have received many 'friend requests' on Facebook from your nursing colleagues in the ward, which you have accepted. You have had a busy morning shift and were short of staff and the acuity of patients was unexpectedly high. That evening, you log onto Facebook at home and see a post from a colleague that you were working with that morning. She is venting about the terrible shift she has experienced, makes note of the intensity of the workload and is insulting and offensive to other colleagues from your unit.

Reflective questions

Reflect on the scenario and answer the following questions.

1. What reaction would you have to your colleague's post?
2. How would you approach your colleague both online and offline?
3. How do the content and tone of the colleague's Facebook post align with professional ethics and standards of conduct in the nursing profession?
4. Would you report this behaviour to your nurse unit manager?

CONCLUSION

Social media is highly relevant to nursing practice, policy, education and research. It provides a platform for patients to engage with health professionals and seek support or outreach for centres with limited access to expert input from specialist centres and professionals. Nurses must consider social media as a method to remain abreast of nursing science and as an approach to continuous professional development. All nurses have a professional obligation to report unprofessional use and misconduct. Novel methods of communication and information sharing will allow nurses to apply evidence to practice without some of the technological barriers that exist today. Nurses must leverage social media and learn to adapt to its complexities. Social media platforms can be highly effective for healthcare when used appropriately. It is important that all nurses are adept in the appropriate use and application of technology within the contemporary healthcare system.

REFLECTIVE QUESTIONS

1. What application do you think social media has for nursing in modern society? What are the potential advantages and disadvantages for the discipline and profession?
2. How do you think social media may be used in patient and caregiver education and in making decisions related to healthcare choices?
3. What constitutes unethical professional conduct on social media for nurses?
4. How would you respond to professional misconduct if you witnessed a friend or colleague use social media in an unprofessional manner?
5. What guidance or policy documents are available to support you in using social media as a nursing tool in a safe and effective manner?

Recommended readings

AHPRA 2019 Social media: how to meet your obligations under the National Law. Online. Available: https://www.ahpra.gov.au/Resources/Social-media-guidance.aspx

National Council of State Boards of Nursing n.d. A nurse's guide to the use of social media. Online. Available: https://www.ncsbn.org/public-files/NCSBN_SocialMedia.pdf

Nursing and Midwifery Council (NMC) Guidance. Social media do's and don'ts. Online. Available: http://www.nursingtimes.net/roles/nurse-managers/nmc-guidance-dos-and-donts-for-social-media/5032912.fullarticle

New Zealand Nurses Organisation (NZNO) 2019 Social media and the nursing profession: a guide to maintain online professionalism for nurses and nursing students. Online. Available: https://www.nzno.org.nz/Portals/0/publications/Guideline%20-%20Social%20media%20and%20the%20nursing%20profession,%202019.pdf

Cleary M, Ferguson C, Jackson D, Watson R 2013 Social media and the new e-professionalism. Contemporary Nurse 42(2)

Moorley C, Chinn T 2015 Using social media for continuous professional development. Journal of Advanced Nursing 71(4):713–717

Ventola C L 2014 Social media and health care professionals: benefits, risks, and best practices. P & T: A Peer-Reviewed Journal for Formulary Management 39(7):491–520

American Nurses Association 2018 Social networking principles. Online. Available: https://www.nursingworld.org/social/

References

Beltrán Ponce S, McAlarnen L A, Teplinsky E 2023 Challenges of reaching patients with cancer on social media: lessons from the failed. #CancerRealTalk Experience. JCO Oncology Practice 19(2):63–65

Bottorff J L, Struik L L, Bissell L J et al 2014 A social media approach to inform youth about breast cancer and smoking: an exploratory descriptive study. Collegian 21(2):159–168

Breu A C, Cooper A Z 2022 Tweetorials: digital scholarship deserving of inclusion in promotion portfolios. Medical Teacher 44(4):450–452

Burton R 2022 Nursing students perceptions of using YouTube to teach psychomotor skills: a comparative pilot study. SAGE Open Nursing 8:23779608221117385.

Cleary M, Ferguson C, Jackson D et al 2013 Social media and the new e-professionalism. Contemporary Nurse 45(2):152–154

Darko E M, Kleib M, Olson J 2022 Social media use for research participant recruitment: integrative literature review. Journal of Medical Internet Research 24(8):e38015

Duncan I, Yarwood-Ross L, Haigh C 2013 YouTube as a source of clinical skills education. Nurse Education Today 33(12):1576–1580

Fedele R 2019 8 reasons why nurses and midwives should embrace social media. Australian Nursing and Midwifery Journal 26(6):14–16

Ferguson C, DiGiacomo M, Gholizadeh L et al 2017 The integration and evaluation of a social-media facilitated journal club to enhance the student learning experience of evidence-based practice: a case study. Nurse Education Today 48:123–128

Gaddy A, Topf J 2021 Facebook groups can provide support for patients with rare diseases and reveal truths about the secret lives of patients. Kidney International Reports 6(5):1205–1207

Lefebvre C, McKinney K, Glass C et al 2020 Social media usage among nurses: perceptions and practices. JONA: The Journal of Nursing Administration 50(3):135–141

Lim M S, Molenaar A, Brennan L et al 2022 Young adults' use of different social media platforms for health information: insights from web-based conversations. Journal of Medical Internet Research 24(1):e23656.

Mannix J, Wilkes L, Daly J 2014 Pragmatism, persistence and patience: a user perspective on strategies for data collection using popular online social networks. Collegian 21(2):127–133

Moorley C, Chinn T 2015 Using social media for continuous professional development. Journal of Advanced Nursing 71(4):713–717

Nursing and Midwifery Board of Australia 2022 Code of conduct for nurses. Online. Available: https://www.nursingmidwiferyboard.gov.au/documents/default.aspx?record=WD17%2f23849&dbid=AP&chksum=ki92NMPa9thp9f9ZhTQNJg%3d%3d

Nursing Council of New Zealand (NCNZ) 2012a Code of conduct for nurses. New Zealand, Wellington

Nursing Council of New Zealand (NCNZ) 2012b Guidelines: social media and electronic communication. New Zealand, Wellington

New Zealand Nurses Organisation (NZNO) 2019 Social media and the nursing profession: a guide to maintain online professionalism for nurses and nursing students. Wellington: New Zealand Nurses Organisation

Osman W, Mohamed F, Elhassan M et al 2022 Is YouTube a reliable source of health-related information? A systematic review. BMC Medical Education 22(1):382

Partridge S R, Gallagher P, Freeman B et al 2018 Facebook groups for the management of chronic diseases. Journal of Medical Internet Research 20(1):e21

Rukavina V T, Viskić J, Machala Poplašen L et al 2021 Dangers and benefits of social media on e-professionalism of health care professionals: scoping review. Journal of Medical Internet Research 23(11):e25770

Statista 2024a Digital population worldwide from 2010 to 2025. Online. Available: https://www.statista.com/statistics/617136/digital-population-worldwide/

Statista 2024b Facebook: global daily active users 2011–2023. Online. Available: https://www.statista.com/statistics/346167/facebook-global-dau/

Statista 2024c X (formerly Twitter) – statistics & facts. Online. Available: https://www.statista.com/topics/737/twitter/#topicOverview

Statista 2024d YouTube – statistics & facts. Online. Available: https://www.statista.com/topics/2019/youtube/#topicOverview

Statista 2024e Number of Instagram users worldwide from 2020 to 2025. Online. Available: https://www.statista.com/statistics/183585/instagram-number-of-global-users/

Statista 2024f LinkedIn – statistics & facts. Online. Available: https://www.statista.com/topics/951/linkedin/#topicOverview

Statista 2024g TikTok – statistics & facts. Online. Available: https://www.statista.com/topics/6077/tiktok/#topicOverview 15 Jan 2025

Wright R, Ferguson C, Bodric M et al 2020 Social media and drug resistance in nursing training: using a Twitterchat to develop an international community of practice for antimicrobial resistance. Journal of Clinical Nursing 29(13-14):2723–2729

CHAPTER 14

USING DIGITAL HEALTH TO ENHANCE PATIENT CARE AND CLINICAL QUALITY

Debra Jackson, Rikki Jones and Kim Usher

KEY WORDS

artificial intelligence
digital health interventions
telehealth
clinical decision support systems (CDSS)
mHealth (Mobile Health)
electronic health records (EHRs)

LEARNING OBJECTIVES

After reading this chapter, readers should be able to:

- define key terms in digital health
- critically reflect on the role of artificial intelligence in current and future healthcare
- discuss the growing role of digital health technologies in healthcare to improve patient outcomes and the quality of nursing care
- describe the ethical use of digital technologies.

INTRODUCTION

Digital health is an evolving field that encompasses the use of digital technologies to improve health outcomes, enhance the efficiency of healthcare delivery, and empower patients in managing their own health. It is defined as 'the field of knowledge and practice associated with the development and use of digital technologies to improve health' (World Health Organization 2021). The term 'digital health' encompasses a variety of technologies used to monitor, manage, and improve health, including mobile applications, telemedicine, EHRs, wearable devices and clinical decision support systems (CDSS). As healthcare systems become increasingly complex and resource-limited, digital health interventions are emerging as a crucial solution to address these challenges.

The role of technology in healthcare is expanding rapidly (Zhao et al 2024) and the need for digital health interventions has never been more urgent. With an ageing population, rising chronic disease burdens, healthcare inequity and increasing healthcare costs, the healthcare system faces significant challenges. Digital health tools can assist in addressing these issues, providing solutions to improve accessibility, affordability, and quality of care. Digital tools like telemedicine offer significant benefits in extending healthcare access to underserved populations, particularly in rural or remote areas where medical resources may be limited (Usher et al 2024).

One of the primary advantages of digital health is its ability to provide real-time, data-driven insights that inform patient care. For example, wearable devices like heart-rate monitors and fitness trackers can continuously collect real-time patient data, which can be used to monitor health status and inform healthcare decisions. This allows for more proactive and personalised care, as healthcare providers can adjust treatment plans based on data collected in real time. Digital health interventions can also enable better care coordination among healthcare teams, enhancing communication to improve patient outcomes. With telemedicine, people can access timely consultations from healthcare providers without the need for travel (Usher et al 2024), reducing both time and costs for patients while improving overall health outcomes.

In this chapter we introduce digital healthcare for nursing, the opportunities associated with digital healthcare, contemplate the use of technology to enhance patient safety and clinical quality, discuss how digital interventions and tools can meet gaps in patient care, consider barriers to the use of digital technologies in nursing practice and discuss ethical use of digital technologies.

Nursing and digital literacy

Digital literacy refers to the ability to use digital technology to find, evaluate, apply and generate information (van Kessel et al 2022). In nursing, this means being 'able to use technology to maximum effect for patients, service users and carers' (Martzoukou et al 2024:656). Nurses have a critical role in healthcare, and it is essential for nurses to understand and integrate digital health interventions within their practice, especially given the increasing presence of digital applications in clinical settings. By incorporating digital health tools into clinical practice, nurses can also improve the efficiency of care delivery. Technologies like electronic health records (EHRs) enhance availability of data, reduce errors in documentation and facilitate better communication among the healthcare team (Forde-Johnston et al 2023). Mobile health applications can be used to provide patients with information and reminders for various health-related issues such as post-discharge care, medication adherence or follow-up appointments, and they also empower patients to take an active role in their own care, which can lead to early detection of issues and improve outcomes (Dalcól et al 2024). For nurses, being well-versed in digital health is not just a professional advantage—it is increasingly becoming an essential component of delivering safe and effective care in today's technology-driven healthcare environment (Martzoukou et al 2024).

REFLECTION

As healthcare continues to adopt digital solutions, nurses must stay current with technological advancements to ensure that they are providing the highest standard of care. Embracing digital health interventions enhances nurses' ability to deliver safe, high-quality care and support a person-centred approach to healthcare.

Artificial intelligence (AI) is transforming digital health by enabling advanced data analysis, predictive modelling and personalised care, which are reshaping how healthcare providers deliver services and improve patient outcomes. AI algorithms can very quickly analyse vast amounts of medical data from multiple sources, including electronic health records, imaging studies and wearable devices to detect patterns that might be missed by human observation alone. AI-based technology enhances diagnostic accuracy, supports clinical decision making, and helps identify high-risk patients who may benefit from early interventions. Additionally, AI-powered tools, such as virtual health assistants and natural language processing systems, streamline administrative tasks and can improve communication between providers and patients. By integrating AI into digital health, healthcare systems are better equipped to provide efficient, proactive and person-centred care.

So, what is AI? AI is an umbrella term that refers to the capability of machines or software to perform tasks that typically require human intelligence, such as learning from experience, recognising patterns, understanding language and making decisions. AI has several core components that enable machines to perform increasingly complex tasks. Machine learning (ML), a key element, allows systems to learn from data and improve over time without explicit programming (Zhou & Liu 2020). Natural language processing (NLP) enables AI to understand and generate human language, essential for applications like chatbots and language translation. Large language models (LLMs), which are highly advanced NLP models, can generate text, answer questions and assist in research by analysing complex language patterns (Kamath et al 2024). Other important components of AI (at the time of writing) include computer vision for interpreting visual information, and robotics, where AI algorithms guide machines to perform tasks in the physical world. Together, these components form the foundation of AI, enabling diverse applications across healthcare. However, AI is a rapidly growing field and so other components and capabilities will continue to be developed over the course of your nursing careers.

STORY

Think about any digital health tools you have used in your own life, such as fitness devices, health-tracking apps, wearable devices (e.g. smartwatches, heart-rate monitors), or telehealth services (e.g. virtual appointments with a healthcare professional). Consider the following:

1. How have these tools helped you manage your health or wellness?
   a. For example, did they encourage you to exercise more, track your sleep patterns, or monitor your heart rate or blood sugar levels?
2. In the case of telehealth, how did the experience compare to in-person consultations?
   a. Were you able to access care easily?
   b. Did it feel efficient, or were there any technical issues?
3. Reflect on the positive aspects of using these digital health tools. Consider both the personal benefits to your health and wellness, as well as the potential benefits for patients in your future nursing practice. In doing this consider:
   a. Did the tools make it easier to manage your health?
   b. What aspects have you found particularly useful?

Continued

> c Did the use of these tools empower you to take control of your own health? How?
> d How do you think these tools help patients manage their health more effectively in a clinical setting?
> 4 Reflect on any challenges or negative aspects of using digital health tools. This could include issues like technical difficulties, accessibility, privacy concerns, or personal feelings about using technology for health
> 	a Were there any frustrations with using the tools (e.g. device malfunctions, difficulty interpreting data, poor connectivity during a telehealth consultation)?
> 	b Did you ever feel overwhelmed by the data provided by fitness trackers or health apps? How did you manage this?
> 	c Were there any concerns about privacy or data security while using telehealth services? Did you feel your personal information was protected?
> 	d For telehealth: How did you feel about the lack of in-person contact with healthcare providers? Did it affect your trust or satisfaction with the care you received?

Opportunities associated with digital healthcare

Digital health offers significant opportunities to enhance access to healthcare, particularly for underserved populations and regions (Gagnon et al 2024, Walker et al 2021). Telehealth platforms, mobile health apps and remote monitoring tools can bridge the gap for individuals and populations living in rural or remote areas, where access to healthcare services is often limited. These technologies allow patients to consult with healthcare providers without the need for extensive travel, reducing barriers related to geography, transportation and time (Usher et al 2024). Moreover, digital health can provide more equitable access to specialist care, allowing individuals in underserved communities to receive consultations from experts that may not be available locally. By reaching patients who might otherwise have not been able to access care, digital health tools have the potential to reduce health disparities and improve overall access to necessary healthcare services, promoting more inclusive and person-centred care delivery.

In addition to improving access, digital health technologies enable personalised care, allowing healthcare providers to tailor interventions based on individual patient data. Using EHRs, wearable devices and mobile health applications, clinicians can gather real-time data on patients' health status, preferences and needs, which can be used to develop personalised care plans. Digital health also offers the potential for cost savings in healthcare by reducing hospital admissions and readmissions through more effective monitoring of chronic conditions (Long et al 2023, Kilfoy et al 2024). Remote monitoring tools allow for ongoing patient assessment, which can help identify potential health issues early and prevent complications that, if untreated, would eventually require hospitalisation (Gagnon et al 2024). Furthermore, digital health solutions can alleviate administrative burdens for nurses and other healthcare providers by automating routine tasks, streamlining documentation and enhancing decision making through CDSS (Ameri et al 2024), not only freeing up time for direct patient care but also supporting more efficient and informed decision making, ultimately improving both patient outcomes and provider satisfaction.

REFLECTION
Digital health technologies also offer a significant opportunity to reduce the carbon footprint of healthcare services.

Digital and telehealth technologies also offer significant yet often overlooked opportunities to reduce the carbon footprint of healthcare services. By reducing the need for both patients and healthcare providers to travel for in-person consultations, telehealth can contribute to reduced transportation-related gas emissions (Usher et al 2024). Moreover, telehealth services such as video consultations, telephone appointments and remote monitoring tools not only reduce emissions but also improve care accessibility and chronic disease management, aligning with sustainability goals. Beyond travel reduction, telehealth minimises the need for physical resources like paper and medical supplies, further decreasing healthcare's environmental footprint. Wearable devices and mobile health apps that enable at-home monitoring further support this by reducing in-person visits and reliance on disposable materials. The COVID-19 pandemic highlighted the effectiveness of virtual health services in limiting unnecessary travel, reducing fossil fuel consumption, and improving access to care (Purohit et al 2021, Tsagkaris et al 2021, Usher et al 2024). The global decrease in carbon emissions during the early stages of the pandemic underscores the potential of telehealth to contribute to a cleaner and more sustainable healthcare system (Usher et al 2024). Despite challenges in accessibility and technology adoption, the growing use of virtual healthcare is a positive step towards a greener, more sustainable future, benefiting both patient outcomes and the environment.

Using technology to improve patient safety and clinical quality

Patient safety refers to the prevention of harm to patients during healthcare delivery, ensuring that the care provided does not cause injury or adverse outcomes (see Chapter 8 for a fuller discussion on patient safety). Clinical quality is a broader term that refers to the effectiveness, efficiency and consistency of care, aiming to achieve optimal health outcomes through evidence-based practices.

Technologies such as EHRs, CDSS and real-time monitoring tools such as wearable devices improve communication among healthcare providers, reduce human error and ensure that patients receive timely and appropriate care. For instance, EHRs help to consolidate patient data in one place, making it easier for nurses and members of the multidisciplinary health team to track treatment plans and avoid duplicate tests or conflicting prescriptions. Digital tools also facilitate adherence to clinical guidelines, ensuring that care decisions are based on the latest evidence, which enhances both safety and quality (see Table 14.1).

Digital health technologies can help mitigate common threats to patient safety, such as medication errors, falls and infections, by providing real-time data and alerts. Medication errors, for example, can be reduced through barcode medication administration (BCMA) systems and CDSS, which flag potential drug interactions or dosage errors before they occur (Sloss & Jones 2021). Fall prevention can be enhanced through remote monitoring tools that track patients' mobility alerting healthcare

TABLE 14.1
Digital technologies to support patient safety

TECHNOLOGY	DESCRIPTION	PATIENT SAFETY BENEFITS
Electronic health records (EHRs)	Digital systems for storing and managing patient data	Improve communication, reduce errors through accessible patient history, enhanced care coordination
Barcode medication administration (BCMA)	Barcode scanning system to verify medications before administration	Aims to minimise medication errors by confirming patient identity and correct dosage
Clinical decision support systems (CDSS)	Software that assists healthcare providers by alerting them to potential issues	Alerts nurses to safety risks such as drug interactions, abnormal laboratory results, or allergies, supporting informed decision making
Telehealth and remote monitoring	Technologies for remote patient interaction and continuous health monitoring	Enables early detection of health changes, supports chronic condition management and reduces hospital readmissions
Automated dispensing cabinets (ADCs)	Secure, computerised storage systems for medications in healthcare facilities	Reduces medication dispensing errors and limits unauthorised access to medications
Smart infusion pumps	Infusion devices with programmable drug libraries to control medication dosage	Ensures accurate dosing and prevents overdoses by automatically adjusting and stopping infusion if settings are incorrect
Wearable health devices	Devices like heart-rate monitors and glucose sensors worn by patients	Provides real-time data to healthcare providers, supporting timely interventions, especially for high-risk patients
Patient portals	Online access points for patients to view their health information and communicate with providers	Improves patient engagement and reduces risks of miscommunication, as patients can verify and understand their treatment plans

providers to intervene before an incident occurs (Moore et al 2023). Infections, another major threat to patient safety, can be mitigated through digital health tools (Dalcól et al 2024). Additionally, predictive analytics can identify patients at higher risk of developing complications or adverse events, enabling proactive interventions to prevent harm. By integrating these digital health solutions into healthcare settings, the risks associated with patient care can be reduced, leading to improved safety and higher-quality outcomes for patients.

Digital health tools can contribute to standardising care quality by promoting adherence to evidence-based practices and clinical guidelines, ensuring that patients receive consistent, high-quality treatment across various settings. These technologies facilitate quality improvement initiatives, as they enable healthcare providers to collect and analyse data continuously, allowing close monitoring of key factors such as infection rates, medication errors, patient falls, occurrences of pressure injuries and patient satisfaction measures, to quickly identify areas requiring improvement and implement necessary changes effectively.

Digital health interventions

Digital health interventions (DHI) refer to any technology-based solutions designed to improve health and healthcare delivery (such as accessibility, efficiency, effectiveness, safety and person-centred approaches). They can play a pivotal role in both patient safety and clinical quality by enhancing the accuracy and reliability of healthcare processes; for example, clinical decision support systems (CDSS) can alert nurses and other health professionals to potential safety risks, such as adverse drug interactions or abnormal laboratory results, enabling prompt action to prevent harm. These systems can also provide services in underserved populations, particularly in rural or remote areas where there are limited staff and resources (Kwasnicka et al 2022). Specifically, telehealth tools can help nurses monitor patients remotely, ensuring timely interventions when needed, which is particularly important for patients with chronic conditions who require ongoing care and patients in rural and remote locations. Similarly, DHI can circumnavigate barriers to help-seeking and improve individuals' and communities' engagement in health. For example, mental illness and being the survivor of sexual violence often come with a sense of shame and stigma that prevents the individual engaging with healthcare services and accessing treatment (Jones et al 2024).

With improving technology and the use of AI, DHI are continually being developed and becoming more robust and sophisticated, ensuring they are more able to capture the key 'social, behavioural and environmental determinants of health' (Abernethy et al 2022:6) allowing healthcare professionals to better identify individual and population need as a priority. DHI can be utilised in this way to improve inequality, allowing for equitable service delivery to populations currently underserved and reduce the impact of racism and stigma by increasing accessibility of services. This is particularly important for vulnerable populations, minority groups and First Nations, Māori and migrant communities.

Chronic condition management is a key example of how digital interventions can be utilised to improve patient safety, care outcomes and empower individuals. The burden of chronic disease is significant to both the patient and the healthcare providers, straining healthcare delivery and resources, with large costs associated with exacerbation of conditions often resulting in hospital stays and repeat attendance at emergency departments (Ferreira et al 2024). DHI can empower populations and individuals to better manage their own chronic conditions and have the potential to reduce exacerbations and improve patients' quality of life while also supporting communication between healthcare professionals and patients/families (Ferreira et al 2024, Wannheden et al 2022). For example, telehealth can be used for regular patient follow-up, specialist consultations (particularly important for rural patients with no access to face-to-face services) and case management; patient diaries can be used for self-monitoring of symptoms, diet and exercise and disease progression; medication monitoring for compliance, dosage and reminders; wearable devices can be used to collect real-time data by continually monitoring patients' conditions, making it easier to recognise deterioration and worsening symptoms, allowing for early interventions, thus reducing emergency presentations and hospital stays (Ferreira et al 2024).

However, there are issues of which health professionals should be aware. Not all DHI are evidence-based or evaluated, some are costly to access, difficult to use or not accessible in some rural and remote locations (Ban et al 2024). Tailoring interventions to specific populations can ensure maximum effectiveness, usability, acceptability and engagement; however, it may limit generalisability of the intervention to the broader population. Similarly, not all interventions are suitable to populations who have limited experience engaging with digital technologies or find technology hard to use, such as the elderly population and those with disabilities. Hence, there needs to be a rigorous evaluation process that ensures the tools we use as health professionals are based on evidence, have a positive impact on the population and include key stakeholder perspectives (including the patient, healthcare providers and developers) to fully ensure they are fit for purpose (Kwasnicka et al 2022, Table 14.2).

Patient engagement technologies

The integration of digital technologies into healthcare has accelerated rapidly in recent years and offers exciting possibilities due to advances in digital health, health informatics, genomics, AI and robotics (Scott & Hart 2024). These advancements have enabled the electronic collection and recording of patient information, commonly known as *electronic health records (EHRs)* or eHealth records. EHRs have replaced the need for paper-based patient records and offer other advantages such as management of appointment requests and access to educational materials. Additionally, electronic health services also provide electronic prescribing and telehealth (Smith & Magnani 2019). In many countries, patients are now being given access to their EHRs. The benefits of patient access to EHRs include lower levels of anxiety, better patient–carer relationships, improved awareness and adherence to medications, better patient safety and improved outcomes (e.g. enhanced glycaemic control in people with diabetes and improved LDL-cholesterol levels; Tapuria et al 2021, Neves et al 2020). Importantly, EHRs also improve the continuity of patient information as everything is collected and held on one digital platform. Access to EHRs is considered of greatest importance to people with chronic health conditions as EHRs can be used to trace disease trajectory and for patients with health issues that require greater information or communication (Tapuria et al 2021). EHRs have been reported to enhance patient-centred care in several recent studies (Benjamins et al 2021), but not in others (Neves et al 2020). More research is needed in this area to gain a better understanding of this outcome. Critics have suggested that providing access to EHRs could potentially undermine the patient–doctor relationship (Benjamins et al 2021), while others suggest the aim of EHR access is to transfer the costs and responsibility of healthcare to patients (Tapuria et al 2021). Regardless of the critics, patient access to EHRs is considered the first step towards patient empowerment and shared decision making (Tapuria et al 2021). Patient empowerment can also be enhanced using wearable health information devices.

Wearable sensor technology is a rapidly expanding area of technology. Electronic devices provide real-time feedback on an individual's health conditions. These devices provide rehabilitation outside of the acute care setting and have the potential to reduce the costs of health services significantly in the future (Vijayan et al 2021). For example, wearable devices can track sleep, exercise, pulse rate, oxygen saturation, stroke recovery, diabetes management, nerve conduction, tremors, joint limitations and heart rhythms (Jouffroy et al 2020, Vijayan et al 2021). These devices are now also being used to help in the transition from acute in-service healthcare to the community setting. Devices can offer constant quantification of patient outcomes and provide feedback to health providers. They are usable in varied locations, including rural and remote settings, and help to reduce the need for patients to return to a central location for follow-up (Vijayan et al 2021). Wearable devices like smart watches have been successfully used for the assessment of independence of older people (García-Moreno et al 2022), and for the collection of intricate physiologic data from people with chronic conditions such as ECG information, body temperature, blood glucose, blood pressure and

TABLE 14.2

Common digital health interventions

INTERVENTION	GENERAL USE	SPECIFIC POPULATIONS
Mental health screening	Digital tools designed to screen for mental illness in populations	General population
MindSpot, sTherapy, Head to Health	Online support and resources for mental illness, resilience and counselling services	General population
13YARN, Beyond Blue, Blue Knot Foundation, GriefLine, Lifeline, Headspace, Head to Health helpline	Online support and counselling services for people with anxiety, depression, suicidality or other mental illness, grief and those experiencing trauma	General population
Eye movement desensitisation reprocessing (EMDR), cognitive behavioural therapy (CBT)	Designed to treat posttraumatic stress disorder (PTSD) and trauma-related mental illness	General population with PTSD and mental illness related to trauma such as first responders, and survivors of violence
My Fitness Plus	App designed to monitor diet and exercise	General population
I-DECIDE, iSAFE, myPlan	Websites or apps that provide safety decision aids and safe relationship tools to manage and prevent domestic violence, intimate partner violence and sexual assault/violence	At-risk populations such as young women, and women in unsafe relationships
Remote blood glucose level (BGL) monitoring	Implant that continuously monitors BGL	People diagnosed with diabetes
Insulin pumps	Devices that monitor BGL and administer insulin	People diagnosed with diabetes
Manage Medication, MedicineWise, MedAdvisor, Medisafe Pill Reminder	Applications designed to monitor medications, dosages, times and important medication information	General population
CareKit, CareMonitor, Virtual care	Digital health platforms that provide real-time access to information, tools and healthcare professionals to manage chronic conditions	People diagnosed with a chronic disease
Health, Asthma, My Asthma portal (MAP), Breath, AsthmaCare, ASTHMAXcel	Applications that can monitor and track symptoms, medication use and compliance, peak flow, general information on environmental or trigger warnings	People diagnosed with asthma
TENS machine	Device that uses electric impulses to reduce the pain signals sent from the body to the brain	People who suffer from chronic pain
Internal cardiac monitoring, pacemakers and defibrillators	Designed to monitor and regulate cardiac rhythm and function	People with cardiac conditions
Remote ECG and heart-rate monitoring via wearable device		People with cardiac condition and general population
Online counselling and theory	Designed to provide counselling/therapy services for a range of issues	General population
Activity trackers	Wearable devices that monitor activity and heart rate	General population
Embrace2, SMP, Seer	Applications or wearable devices to support self-management of epilepsy and to predict seizures	Epilepsy
Motion monitoring	Monitors motion for elderly patient at risk of falls at home	Falls-risk elderly

respirations (Benjamins et al 2021). These devices offer an efficient means to remotely monitor the patient's condition when in their own environment and hence reduce the need for the person to be maintained in a hospital environment. As well as reducing the need to return to an acute centre for follow-up assessments, this strategy enhances reduced carbon emissions related to travel for follow-up appointments (Usher et al 2024).

For digital technology to be effective in healthcare, it is essential that people can access, understand and apply the information available in a digital format. This is known as **digital health literacy** (Fitzpatrick 2023). Essentially, digital health literacy involves individuals accessing and evaluating information using digital tools. While the uptake of digital access has been slow in some members of the community, this is mainly due to limited health literacy (Jimenez et al 2020). A scoping review conducted in 2020 found that much of the evidence related to digital health competencies is over a decade old and was focused on issues of little relevance in today's healthcare world (Jimenez et al 2020). Limited digital health literacy has been linked to poorer health outcomes (Fitzpatrick 2023), so digital health literacy is an important goal to which health clinicians and researchers should aim to improve health communication practices, design culturally appropriate health information and strengthen health systems to adjust to the needs of people with low levels of digital health literacy (Fitzpatrick 2023).

Digital health literacy is also essential for health professionals and must be included in all health professional undergraduate and postgraduate education courses to ensure that health professionals are able to access and analyse digital data and appraise digital health technologies and resources for accuracy and relevance (Scott & Hart 2022). A recent study of health professional students at a leading Australian university found that only 39% of students reported having the required digital technology skills to enter the workforce (Cham et al 2022). This problem needs to be addressed as a matter of urgency to ensure the health professionals of the future are adequately prepared for the use of available digital technologies to improve health outcomes.

Barriers to the use of digital health technologies

As with all technologies, there are barriers to use and engagement. The implementation of digital health faces several significant barriers, beginning with technological challenges. A major issue is the ***lack of adequate infrastructure***, particularly in rural and underserved areas, where internet connectivity and access to modern technology can be limited or unreliable (Gagnon et al 2024). This digital divide disproportionately affects low-income communities, where access to smartphones, computers and high-speed internet may be restricted, hindering patients' ability to engage with DHI (Walker et al 2021). Additionally, digital literacy remains a barrier, as many patients, particularly people with literacy issues or those from disadvantaged backgrounds, may struggle to gain access to or to navigate new technologies.

A recent review suggested barriers to the use of digital technologies in nursing could be categorised in four main areas: 'perceived risks, negative impact on workflow/workload, limited opportunities for involvement at policy and development levels and unsupportive organizational cultures' (Janes et al 2024). Integrating new digital technologies into everyday clinical practice does require ongoing learning on the part of healthcare providers: poor lead-in times and insufficient training can impact implementation in practice. It can also be challenging to effect change in any large organisation, and the widespread adoption of digital health technologies into healthcare involves changes in how health professionals work. Resistance to change among healthcare providers can also be a barrier to the uptake of digital technologies as nurses and other clinical staff may be hesitant to adopt DHI due to concerns about workflow disruptions, the potential for increased workload, or unfamiliarity with new tools. This reluctance may be compounded by a sense of change that is imposed without proper consultation, and a lack of confidence in the reliability or efficacy of digital solutions.

Privacy and security concerns also play a role in hindering adoption of digital technologies (Janes et al 2024). With the growing use of digital platforms to store and transmit sensitive patient data, data protection and ensuring compliance with privacy regulations are critical. Concerns about data security and the potential misuse of personal health information have also been identified as areas of concern and these can erode trust in digital health systems (Janes et al 2024). The development, adoption and deployment of digital health solutions can be expensive, and so financial constraints are a barrier to implementation by healthcare organisations, especially those with limited budgets. Health leaders may face difficulties justifying or supporting the investment needed to integrate digital health solutions effectively. The costs of implementation not only include the initial cost of technology but also the updating of systems, ongoing expenses related to maintenance, staff training and ensuring the continued functionality of these systems. So, while the benefits may be great, the initial and ongoing costs can be substantial.

Ethical use of digital technologies

AI and digital technology are growing faster than law and legislation can regulate (The Lancet Digital Health 2024). These rapid changes are having a negative impact on society; for example, pervasive misinformation and biased decision making, cyber-security issues and increasing use of technology to assist criminal activity. AI can develop false and misleading content, which patients and some clinicians use to guide the way they manage their health (The Lancet Digital Health 2024). AI models and some digital tools are currently not assessed, evaluated or even monitored once they are released, and this can lead to misleading and false information being shared. As AI and digital health technologies are being used to assist with decision making in healthcare, this can have a negative impact on patient safety if they are not evaluated or monitored correctly (Haydon et al 2023, The Lancet Digital Health 2024). What is needed are evidence-based frameworks, critical evaluation of the AI and digital technologies clinicians use and education of the new healthcare workforce to utilise AI and digital health in positive, ethical ways (Haydon et al 2023). Digital technologies are also increasingly being used by perpetrators of image-based abuse, domestic violence, intimate partner violence, sexual violence and childhood sexual assault (CSA) to access and control victims, as well as for intimidation, stalking and coercion (Usher et al 2023).

So, while digital health can have a positive impact on health outcomes, enhance the efficiency of healthcare delivery, and empower patients, there are several ethical principles that need to be considered when advocating for digital health tools. These are discussed below:

▸ *Autonomy*—there are issues with digital health that can threaten informed consent and patient awareness around the data that is collected, how the data is used and who has access to the data (Rezaei et al 2021). Similarly, digital tools/interventions may limit treatment options (creating a bias towards certain interventions) and may control who has access to medical results (Rezaei et al 2021). Generally, consent for data usage is open-ended without a clear explanation of how the data will be used now and into the future, and how long the data will be stored.

- *Privacy and confidentiality*—this is considered one of the most concerning ethical issues related to digital health, specifically data security and cyber-attacks. With AI-driven cyber-attacks successfully breaching current security and giving access to health information that can be used against patients (The Lancet Digital Health 2024), it creates mistrust in digital health and impacts patients' engagement with EHRs, digital interventions and other digital tools. Similarly, transparency around data storage, data use, how data are shared, who is accountable for the data and data ownership can help make digital health trustworthy (Vayena et al 2018).
- *Justice*—the ethical concerns with justice and digital health are around access, equity, discrimination and empowering people to manage their own health (Rezaei et al 2021). Digital health tools and technology should be readily available to all populations, and minority or ethnic groups.
- *Beneficence*—the cost of digital health to government organisations, maintaining cyber-security, evaluation and lack of research that clearly outlines the value of the tool to patients means it is often difficult to determine if the cost is outweighed by the benefits (Zarif 2022). Similarly, not all areas have the same access to the internet and the cost of devices and digital tools can result in inequality, which further widens the gap for underserved populations.

CONCLUSION

In conclusion, digital technologies hold immense potential to completely transform patient care, enhance patient safety, and drive improvements in clinical quality. This chapter has provided an overview of digital health, its growing role in modern healthcare, and the critical ways in which nurses can engage with these technologies to improve patient outcomes. As we navigate this dynamic and rapidly evolving field, it is essential to recognise that the integration of new technologies will be an ongoing process throughout your nursing education and career. As nurses, it is our responsibility to remain current with emerging innovations, embracing them as tools to enhance the quality and safety of care. Moreover, as nurses it is important to engage in continuous learning, and actively participate in the co-design of future healthcare interventions. In doing so, nurses will not only stay at the forefront of technological advancements but also have a vital role in shaping the future of patient care.

DHI offer exciting opportunities to improve patient outcomes, streamline clinical workflows, and increase efficiency within healthcare settings. However, it is important to remember that digital technologies are not a substitute for the expertise, empathy and clinical judgment that define nursing practice. These tools, when used ethically and appropriately, are meant to support—and never replace—the compassionate, empathic and person-centred care that nurses provide. As we incorporate these technologies into our practice, we must continue to uphold our responsibility for their ethical use, ensuring these are deployed with the highest regard for patient safety and wellbeing.

Recommended readings

Janes G, Chesterton L, Heaslip V et al 2024 Current nursing and midwifery contribution to leading digital health policy and practice: an integrative review. Journal of Advanced Nursing 81(1):116–139 https://doi.org/10.1111/jan.16265

Park J, Jeon H, Choi E K 2024 Digital health intervention on patient safety for children and parents: a scoping review. Journal of Advanced Nursing 80:1750–1760 https://doi.org/10.1111/jan.15954

Silveira Thomas Porto C, Catal E 2021 A comparative study of the opinions, experiences and individual innovativeness characteristics of operating room nurses on robotic surgery. Journal of Advanced Nursing 77:4755–4767 https://doi.org/10.1111/jan.15020

References

Abernethy A, Adams L, Barrett M et al 2022 The promise of digital health: then, now, and the future. NAM Perspectives https://doi.org/10.31478/202206e

Ameri A, Ameri A, Salmanizadeh F et al 2024 Clinical decision support systems (CDSS) in assistance to COVID-19 diagnosis: a scoping review on types and evaluation methods. Health Science Reports 7:e1919 doi:10.1002/hsr2.1919

Ban S, Kim Y, Seomun G 2024 Digital health literacy: a concept analysis. Digital Health 10 https://doi.org/10.1177/20552076241287894

Benjamins J, Haveman-Nies A, Gunnink M et al 2021 How the use of a patient-accessible health record contributes to patient-centered care: a scoping review. Journal of Medical Internet Research 23(1):e17655, 10.2196/17655

Cham K M, Edwards M-L, Kruesi L et al 2022 Digital preferences and perceptions of students in health professional courses at a leading Australian university; a baseline for improving digital skills and competencies in health graduates. Australasian Journal of Education Technology 38(1):69–86

Dalcól C, Tanner J, de Brito Poveda V 2024 Digital tools for post-discharge surveillance of surgical site infection. Journal of Advanced Nursing 80:96–109 https://doi.org/10.1111/jan.15830

Ferreira M A M, Dos Santos A F, Sousa-Pinto B et al 2024 Cost-effectiveness of digital health interventions for asthma or COPD: systematic review. Clinical and Experimental Allergy 54(9):651–668 https://doi.org/10.1111/cea.14547

Fitzpatrick P J 2023 Improving health literacy using the power of digital communications to achieve better health outcomes for patients and practitioners. Frontiers in Digital Health 10.3389/fdgth.2023.1264780

Forde-Johnston C, Butcher D, Aveyard H 2023 An integrative review exploring the impact of Electronic Health Records (EHR) on the quality of nurse–patient interactions and communication. Journal of Advanced Nursing 79:48–67 https://doi.org/10.1111/jan.15484

García-Moreno R M, Benítez-Valderrama P, Barquiel B et al 2022 Efficacy of continuous glucose monitoring on maternal and neonatal outcomes in gestational diabetes mellitus: a systematic review and meta-analysis of randomized clinical trials. Diabetic Medicine 39(1):e14703 doi: 10.1111/dme.14703 Epub 2021 Oct 13 PMID: 34564868

Gagnon J, Chartrand J, Probst S et al 2024 Content of a wound care mobile application for newly graduated nurses: an e-Delphi study. BMC Nursing 23(1):331 https://doi.org/10.1186/s12912-024-02003-x

Haydon H M, Snoswell C L, Jones C et al 2023 Digital health literacy to enhance workforce skills and clinical effectiveness: a response to 'Digital health literacy: Helpful today, dependency tomorrow? Contingency planning in a digital age'. Australasian Journal on Ageing 42(4):803–804 https://doi.org/10.1111/ajag.13257

Janes G, Chesterton L, Heaslip V et al 2024 Current nursing and midwifery contribution to leading digital health policy and practice: an integrative review. Journal of Advanced Nursing 81(1):116–139 https://doi.org/10.1111/jan.16265

Jimenez G, Spinazze P, Matchar D et al 2020 Digital health competencies for primary healthcare professionals: a scoping review. International Journal of Medical Informatics 148 10.1016/j.ijmedinf.2020.104260

Jones R, Usher K, Rice K et al 2024 The shame of sexual violence towards women in rural areas. International Journal of Mental Health Nursing 33(3):728–734 https://doi.org/10.1111/inm.13269

Jouffroy R, Jost D, Prunet B 2020 Prehospital pulse oximetry: a red flag for early detection of silent hypoxemia in COVID-19 patients. Critical Care 24:313 doi: 10.1186/s13054-020-03036-9

Kamath U, Keenan K, Somers G et al 2024 Large language models: a deep dive: bridging theory and practice. Springer Nature, Switzerland ISBN 978-3-031-65646-0.

Kilfoy A, Chu C, Krisnagopal A et al 2024 Nurse-led remote digital support for adults with chronic conditions: a systematic synthesis without meta-analysis. Journal of Clinical Nursing 00:1–22 https://doi.org/10.1111/jocn.17226

Kwasnicka D, Keller J, Perski O et al 2022 White Paper: Open Digital Health – accelerating transparent and scalable health promotion and treatment. Health Psychology Review 16(4):475–491 https://doi.org/10.1080/17437199.2022.2046482

Long H, Li S, Chen Y 2023 Digital health in chronic obstructive pulmonary disease. Chronic Diseases and Translational Medicine 9:90–103 doi:10.1002/cdt3.68

Martzoukou K, Luders E S, Mair J et al 2024 A cross-sectional study of discipline-based self-perceived digital literacy competencies of nursing students. Journal of Advanced Nursing 80:656–672 https://doi.org/10.1111/jan.15801

Moore T, Kline D, Palettas M et al 2023 Fall prevention with the Smart Socks System reduces hospital fall rates. Journal of Nursing Care Quality 38(1):55–60 https://doi.org/10.1097/NCQ.0000000000000653

Neves A L, Freise L, Laranjo L et al 2020 Impact of providing patients access to electronic health records on quality and safety of care: a systematic review and meta-analysis. British Medical Journal 29:1019–1032 10.1136/bmjqs.2019.010581

Purohit A, Smith J, Hibble A 2021 Does telemedicine reduce the carbon footprint of healthcare? A systematic review. Future Healthcare Journal 8:e85:–e91 doi: 10.7861/fhj.2020-0080

Rezaei M, Jafari-Sadeghi V, Cao D et al 2021 Key indicators of ethical challenges in digital healthcare: a combined Delphi exploration and confirmatory factor analysis approach with evidence from Khorasan province in Iran. Technological Forecasting and Social Change 167:120724.

Scott K, Hart J 2024 Digital technologies in health: implications for health professional education. Focus on Health Professional Education 25(1):i–iv https://doi.org/10.11157/fohpe.v25i1.813

Sloss E A, Jones T L 2021 Nurse cognition, decision support, and barcode medication administration: a conceptual framework for research, practice, and education. CIN: Computers, Informatics, Nursing 39(12):1041–1048 https://doi.org/10.1097/01.NCN.0000794024.07433.7f

Smith B, Magnani J W 2019 New technologies, new disparities: the intersection of electronic health and digital health literacy. International Journal of Cardiology 292:280–282 doi: 10.1016/j.ijcard.2019.05.066

Tapuria A, Porat T, Kalra D M et al 2021 Impact of patient access to their electronic health record: a systematic review. Informatics for Health and Social Care 46(2):194–206 doi: 10.1080/17538157.2021.1879810

The Lancet Digital Health 2024 Balancing AI innovation with patient safety. Lancet Digital Health 6(9):e601–e601 https://doi.org/10.1016/S2589-7500(24)00175-4

Tsagkaris C, Hoian A V, Ahmad S et al 2021 Using telemedicine for a lower carbon footprint in healthcare: a twofold tale of healing. The Journal of Climate Change and Health 1:100006–3 doi: 10.1016/j.joclim.2021.100006

Usher K, Jones R, Rice K et al 2023 Technology-facilitated sexual abuse and mental health: what mental health nurses and mental health professionals need to know. International Journal of Mental Health Nursing 32:1191–1192 https://doi.org/10.1111/inm.13178

Usher K, Williams J, Jackson D 2024 The potential of virtual healthcare technologies to reduce healthcare services carbon footprint. Frontiers in Public Health 12 https://doi.org/10.3389/fpubh.2024.1394095

van Kessel R, Wong B L H, Clemens T et al 2022 Digital health literacy as a super determinant of health: more than simply the sum of its parts. Internet Interventions 27:100500 doi: 10. 1016/j.invent.2022.100500.

Vayena E, Haeusermann T, Adjekum A et al 2018 Digital health: meeting the ethical and policy challenges. Swiss Medical Weekly 148(34):w14571–w14571 https://doi.org/10.4414/smw.2018.14571

Vijayan V, Connolly J P, Condell J et al 2021 Review of wearable devices and data collection considerations for connected health. Sensors 21:5589 10.3390/s21165589

Walker R, Usher K, Jackson D et al 2021 Addressing digital inequities in supporting the wellbeing of young Indigenous Australians in the wake of COVID-19. International Journal of Environmental Research and Public Health 22;18(4):2141 doi: 10.3390/ijerph18042141

Wannheden C, Åberg-Wennerholm M, Dahlberg M et al 2022 Digital health technologies enabling partnerships in chronic care management: scoping review. Journal of Medical Internet Research 24(8):e38980–e38980 https://doi.org/10.2196/38980

World Health Organization (WHO) 2021 Global strategy on digital health 2020-2025. WHO. Online. Available: https://www.who.int/docs/default-source/documents/gs4dhdaa2a9f352b0445bafbc79ca799dce4d.pdf

Zarif A 2022 The ethical challenges facing the widespread adoption of digital healthcare technology. Health and Technology 12(1):175–179 https://doi.org/10.1007/s12553-021-00596-w

Zhao L, Abdolkhani R, Walter R et al 2024 National survey on understanding nursing academics' perspectives on digital health education. Journal of Advanced Nursing 80:4888–4899 https://doi.org/10.1111/jan.16163

Zhou Z-H, Liu S 2020 Machine learning. Springer, Singapore ISBN: 978-981-15-1966-6

CHAPTER 15

SOCIAL JUSTICE, HEALTH DISPARITIES AND EQUITY IN NURSING

Denise Wilson, Stephen Neville and Lynore Geia

KEY WORDS

colonisation
deficit explanations
differential access
discrimination
health disparities
inequalities
inequities
intersectionality
poverty
quality of care
racism
rights
social determinants of health
social justice
victim blaming

LEARNING OBJECTIVES

After reading this chapter, readers should be able to:

- explain what health disparities are and how they are similar to or different from inequalities, disparities and inequities
- discuss how social determinants of health, such as colonisation, racism, poverty and family violence, impact access to health services and health outcomes
- explain the impact of differential access to social determinants of health, access to health services and quality of care
- discuss why listening carefully to the needs of people with health disparities is essential for quality nursing care
- explain how a social justice, equity and intersectionality framework can assist nurses in understanding and responding to the needs of people living with health disparities.

INTRODUCTION

In this chapter, we explore health disparities and the various factors influencing the quality of health services needed by people belonging to marginalised groups. We use the concepts of social justice, equity and intersectionality to explore ways to engage better with people. The focus will be primarily on Indigenous (First Nations and Māori) peoples, older people, those belonging to LGBTQI (lesbian, gay, bisexual, transgender, queer and intersex) communities, families affected by violence, and youth living in Australia and New Zealand (Aotearoa). We start with highlighting the growing body of evidence about the importance of cultural determinants of health that are linked to health benefits for Indigenous peoples (Verbunt et al 2021).

Nurses will encounter people who live with worse health status and outcomes than other people living in their communities and countries. Instead of receiving quality care to address their health disparities, those belonging to marginalised groups often encounter discriminatory behaviours and attitudes, and are negatively stereotyped when seeking health services (Komene et al 2024, Moorley et al 2020). The health disparities that people experience are often reflective of wider social inequities and a lack of access to the wider determinants of health (leading to poverty and poor housing, for example). While health disparities can impact people's access to health services, determinants of health are invariably beyond the control of nurses to make a difference. Nurses can positively influence timely access to, and engagement with, health services and the quality of care people receive. Moorley et al (2020:2450) maintain, 'Being a nurse … must mean being aware of social injustices and the systemic racism that exist in much of nursing … and having a personal and professional responsibility to challenge and help end them'.

Health disparities

Disparities, inequalities and inequities are terms commonly used in the health sector. Nurses can inadvertently perpetuate these by lacking awareness and understanding of health disparities that exist for various groups within their community (Rooddehghan et al 2019). It also increases the possibility of nurses becoming complacent and 'normalising' some people's poor health status and outcomes. Importantly, this can lead to overlooking specific health needs.

Some disparities are justifiable and expected, while others may relate to cultural expectations. For instance, inequalities such as sex-related conditions are acceptable—women are more likely to have breast cancer whereas men will have prostate cancer and women will not. In some cultures, being overweight is a sign of affluence and that the family is doing well. However, many persistent disparities and inequalities affecting groups of people in our communities are considered unfair and unjust, such as Indigenous peoples, older people, youth, those who identify as LGBTQI, or those living with family violence. These groups of people are marginalised within our health systems because the focus is on meeting the needs of the majority, often in a way that is informed by the dominant worldview and culture. The outcome of such healthcare delivery does not recognise the specific requirements of those on the 'margins'. Health inequalities occur when different population groups, like Aboriginal and Torres Strait Islanders and Māori, have persistent differences in health status and health outcomes. Not only do individuals incur great social and economic costs, but so does society. Notably, these differences are avoidable and preventable, and they are unjust and unfair, often embedded structurally within the health system and at individual and professional levels.

> It is important to recognise and remember that health is not just the absence of disease, but the existence of a totality of factors influencing our physical and mental well-being. If the underlying issue is structural, then we must address the structural factors that resulted in inequalities.
>
> (Egede et al 2024:490)

Health disparities are those differences evident in the health status and outcomes between various groups of people within a community, based on age, gender, ethnicity, race, sexual orientation or socioeconomic status. Health equity means efforts are made to eliminate the health disparities linked to social disadvantage (Egede et al 2024, Pearson et al 2020). Differences also exist in people's access to and engagement with health services, and the nature and quality of healthcare received (Wasserman et al 2019).

Not everyone has equal opportunities to access quality healthcare. Healthcare providers' discriminatory attitudes and how they approach the delivery of a person's healthcare can contribute to people feeling uncomfortable or avoiding future needed healthcare; for example, when a nurse omits or does not offer a person an aspect(s) of healthcare that others receive, or who speaks to an individual in an indifferent or offensive way (Komene et al 2024). As a consequence, those experiencing disparities and exposed to a healthcare provider who treats them in a discriminatory manner may avoid timely contact with needed health services (Komene et al 2023). Avoiding accessing healthcare services then leads to preventable and unnecessary hospitalisations or deaths. Blaming individuals does not explain why they are not proactively seeking health services in spite of their negative experiences (Windle et al 2023).

REFLECTION

Think about the people in your local community.
1. Do any one or more groups of people (e.g. belonging to distinct ethnically or socially based groups) experience health disparities and inequities in their healthcare or health outcomes?
2. How do these inequities compare with the national profile of these groups?
3. In what ways may they be treated differently when accessing health services?

FRAMING DISPARITIES WITHIN A SOCIAL JUSTICE–RIGHTS–EQUITY NEXUS

The World Health Organization (WHO) (2023) explicitly states every human being has the right to '… the highest attainable standard of physical and mental health …'. The WHO stresses the need for quality health services that avoid discrimination to be sufficiently available, accessible to everyone, ethnically and culturally acceptable, ensuring all people have human rights, and that health service providers are accountable for ensuring people's rights are respected.

Some groups of people have additional rights to health. For instance, Indigenous peoples have the United Nations (UN) Declaration on the Rights of Indigenous Peoples (UNDRIP), which was passed in 2007 although not signed by Australia and New Zealand (Aotearoa) until 2009 and 2010, respectively. In New Zealand (Aotearoa), Māori have rights afforded under Te Tiriti o Waitangi—a treaty between the government and Māori. Youth have rights under the United Nations Convention on the Rights of the Child (UNCRC). Despite these various rights existing, for those living with social and health inequities they are applied inconsistently or not observed. While there are no formal international declarations on the rights of older and LGBTQI peoples, the United Nations has highlighted the human rights challenges for both groups and promotes addressing violations (see Office of the High Commissioner for Human Rights, United Nations Human Rights website https://www.ohchr.org/en/topics).

Social justice relates to the equitable distribution of resources that enable people's optimal health and wellbeing and full participation in society (Kapiriri & Razavi 2022). Treating people equitably is underpinned by social justice; equity is the right to health and to achieving equal health outcomes. In New Zealand (Aotearoa), the Health Quality & Safety Commission (HQSC) (2019:47) states that, 'Equity recognises different people with different levels of advantage require different approaches and resources to get equitable health outcomes'. Ideally, by treating everyone fairly, using different approaches, upholding their rights and achieving equity, all groups of people should be able to reach their health potential.

Particular groups bear the burdens associated with health inequities, which are not shared by everyone. They are both avoidable and unjust (Kapiriri & Razavi 2022), but occur because of:
- variations in health status and outcomes that affect a particular group(s), consistently seen in patterns of difference in morbidity and mortality rates and higher levels of socioeconomic deprivation
- social processes (social, economic and environmental policies, for example) that privilege some groups of people over others, and
- biased and discriminatory practices leading to the unfair distribution of resources and opportunities (Edege et al 2024).

However, by nurses being sensitive to people's realities and life contexts affected by inequities, aspects of inequities are potentially modifiable. Nurses can also question dominant discourses within our society and, more specifically, within the health arenas they work within. Examples of dominant discourses are:
- 'Everyone has equal opportunities', or
- 'Everyone has equal access to healthcare services—some choose not to access them'.

Such statements overlook the challenges some groups of people face in their everyday lives, making it difficult or impossible to capitalise on opportunities or to access healthcare services. For instance, mothers affected by socioeconomic deprivation or poverty, raising their children on their own, may prioritise their money on feeding their children rather than on the costs associated with accessing health services. Also, people identifying as LGBTQI may perceive healthcare services as not readily accessible because they fear being judged or discriminated against because of their sexual orientation, and those delivering the services will not understand their needs.

REFLECTION

1. Treating everyone the same or equally does not guarantee equal outcomes or equity. Discuss with your peers why this may be so.
2. Some minority or marginalised groups aspire to having more than the same health outcomes as other population groups; that is, beyond health equity. They aspire to wellbeing as their end-goal. Discuss how wellbeing would be a loftier goal than health equity.

Social determinants of health

Social determinants of health are those factors known to protect people's health and contribute to getting the right healthcare they need. But not all people have the same access to these important

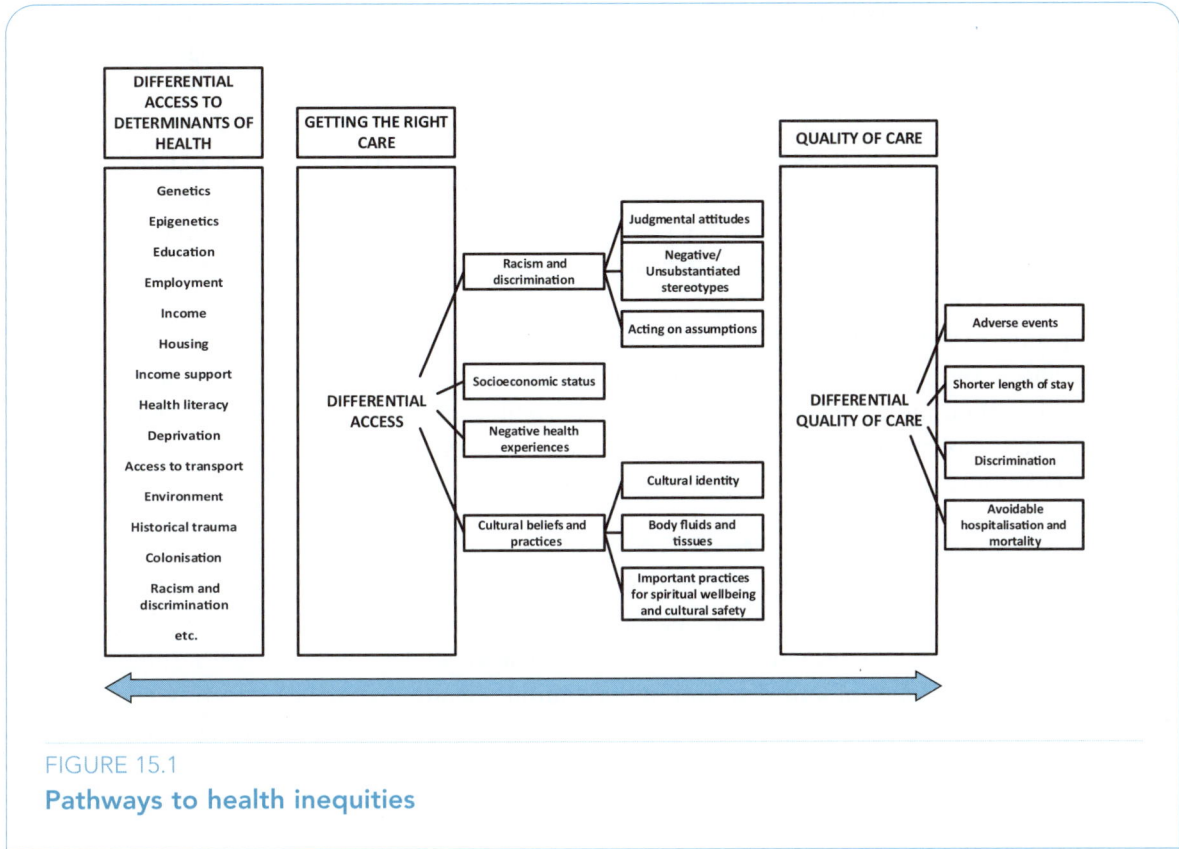

FIGURE 15.1
Pathways to health inequities

determinants of health, to healthcare services, or quality healthcare, each of which can influence health status or health outcomes. Figure 15.1 shows that health inequities can occur anywhere along a healthcare continuum. Inequities include not having necessary determinants of health (such as those listed) and experiencing differences in access to healthcare services influenced by discrimination, socioeconomic status, previous adverse health experiences or cultural beliefs and practices that differ from those of the health service. People belonging to minority groups can also experience differences in the quality of care they receive, evident in adverse events rates, and differences in length of stay in hospital from those with similar conditions (Wilson et al 2018). Having a university education, being employed, having enough money, feeling safe in your community and feeling connected to friends and family are all social determinants of health. We know those with reduced health outcomes are likely to have less education, be unemployed or employed in jobs with inadequate incomes and live in substandard housing. Furthermore, discrimination and racism severely restrict people's job and shelter opportunities and the quality of healthcare they may receive (Thurber et al 2022). Indigenous peoples' colonisation and subsequent disconnection from their traditional land, language, cultural practices and ways of life negatively impact their health—effects that persist across generations (Australian Indigenous Health*InfoNet* 2024, Cormack et al 2020).

Environment counts! Evidence shows children growing up in homes with poverty, family violence and regular exposure to discrimination have their short- and long-term health adversely impacted.

These children are more likely than those without poverty to have chronic physical and psychological health condition(s) in adulthood and die prematurely (Fanslow et al 2021b). Epigenetic research demonstrates the environments people live in can create epigenetic changes that either activate or suppress gene expression. Rogers-LaVanne et al (2023) explored the embodiment of historical trauma (sometimes referred to as 'soul wound' or intergenerational trauma) and loss (land, language and culture) was associated with DNA methylation that leads to epigenetic changes that influence how genes are expressed. They also found a positive relationship between cultural connectedness and wellbeing. The trauma associated with colonisation is likely connected with epigenetic changes (Rogers-LaVanne et al 2023).

Often people experiencing marginalisation are disregarded on more than one basis; for instance, someone who is Indigenous, a young woman and who identifies as being lesbian, may be marginalised based on their indigeneity, gender and sexual orientation. Poverty and unemployment may be additional factors compounding the total effect of being marginalised. These impact access to not only healthcare services but also the quality of healthcare.

Effects of disparities in healthcare

Intersectionality is useful to explain the multi-faceted and compounding effects of multiple forms of marginalisation (such as sexism, ableism, economic status and racism) shaping people's daily lives, and that influence their suboptimal access to necessary social determinants of health. Intersectionality can challenge our ways of knowing and understanding health disparities affecting some people (Macgregor et al 2023). The usual rhetoric that all people have equal access to healthcare implies equity exists and where it does not these people choose not to avail themselves of the opportunities afforded to them. But as we have discussed, this is far from their reality. They need compassionate and empathetic nurses who understand the challenges and barriers they face (Komene et al 2024).

Marginalisation occurs in various forms and is evident in societal inequities related to gender, race and ethnicity, age and access to necessary socioeconomic determinants of health (such as income, employment, education, reliable transport and telephones). Any form of marginalisation can negatively impact people's timely access to needed healthcare services; that is, being able to seek help before their health conditions become more acute and chronic. It is important to understand that these multiple forms of marginalisation do not present singly, but instead have compounding effects (Macgregor 2023). Furthermore, observations of differences in groups such as Indigenous peoples in access to, and quality of, healthcare resulting in a substandard quality of care include adverse events or unplanned readmission to hospital (Gatwiri et al 2021, Graham & Masters-Awatere 2020).

People's social contexts assist in shaping their health and wellbeing, yet within our wider Western-influenced societies a persistence exists in explaining health disparities regarding individuals' responsibilities and obligations. These explanations are frequently presented as false negative stereotypes that are deficit focused, negative and, as such, support victim blaming. Fundamental to reducing health inequities and promoting access to needed services and the quality of care delivered, health practitioners, like nurses, should avoid blaming individuals by using unhelpful explanations (such as negative stereotypes) or deficit accounts. Countering such references is achieved by having a critical understanding of the socioeconomic and community contexts and nature of health inequities that exist for the various groups (see Table 15.1 for examples).

TABLE 15.1
Dispelling deficit explanations

DEFICIT EXPLANATION	EVIDENCE
Deficit explanations are ways in which people belonging to particular groups have their health and social status explained	Research that shows us the realities for marginalised individuals who are in our health systems
'Poor people could eat better if they managed their money better!'	Research shows affordability of food is complex with rent and food consuming high proportions of people's weekly incomes when living in the most deprived neighbourhoods (Lewis et al 2021)
'A woman living with family violence should just leave. If this woman doesn't, she must be okay with it!'	Research highlights that women, especially Indigenous and marginalised women, are socially and systemically entrapped in their relationship by a violent partner who uses strategies, such as coercive control, manipulation, threats to their wellbeing and life (and their children's) and social isolation, and by the family violence system designed to help them. Consequently, they do not have the necessary autonomy and agency to leave (Tolmie et al 2023, Wilson et al 2019)
'[Indigenous] people spend all their money on smoking and gambling instead of feeding their kids well and correctly. They just need to get their priorities right'	Most Indigenous people reside in neighbourhoods with high deprivation (poverty), and struggle to provide the basic needs for their children daily. The introduction of tobacco was a tool colonisers used for coercive control. Poverty, trauma, stress, racism and societal marginalisation are all connected to colonisation and tobacco use (Maddox et al 2022)
'Young people are fit and healthy and do not need health services'	Contrary to this statement, young people's unmet health needs include a broad range of health and social issues, including difficulty accessing appropriate and youth-friendly services (Barbarich-Unasa 2023)
'Older people are dependent, cannot live on their own and should be cared for in residential care facilities'	While some people live in residential care, overwhelming evidence suggests 'ageing in place' or living in their home improves physical and mental health and promotes independence (Van Dijk et al 2015)
'LGBTQI people are mentally ill'	Identifying as LGBTQI is not a mental illness but mental health issues in these groups are relatively high, usually as a result of the stigma and discrimination experienced for not identifying as heterosexual (Wilson & Cariola 2020)

Responding better to those belonging to groups commonly affected by disparities

INDIGENOUS PEOPLES

Globally, Indigenous peoples experience inequities in their healthcare compared with other groups living in their respective countries, related to the ongoing effects of colonisation, discrimination and their access to necessary socioeconomic determinants of health. Social and historical circumstances make them targets for negative stereotypes and deficit explanations. The realities of their everyday lives make it difficult to access healthcare because, for example, many do not have access to reliable personal or public transport, or their experiences with healthcare providers have often been negative (Best & Fredericks 2021, Gatwiri et al 2021, Graham & Masters-Awatere 2020).

The Indigenous and First Nations peoples of both Australia (Aboriginal and Torres Strait Islanders) and New Zealand (Aotearoa) (Māori) were prosperous and healthy people before the settlement of their countries by settlers. As a consequence of Indigenous colonisation, people were systematically depopulated, disconnected from their land, cultural knowledge practices and language, and became disenfranchised socially and economically. They became minority groups within their countries. Furthermore, forcible removal of Indigenous children from their families occurred—for example, the 'stolen generation' in Australia. As a result, Indigenous peoples are affected by historical trauma, which has led to the transmission of this past trauma across the generations (Pihama et al 2020, Menzies 2019), aided by the loss of their cultural identity and connections, and their consequent assimilation. They have become socially marginalised and forced to discard their cultural ways of being in favour of new dominant cultural practices.

Indigenous and First Nations peoples of Australia and New Zealand (Aotearoa) live with notable social and health disparities compared with other people residing in their respective countries. Also, they are more likely to live with high levels of socioeconomic deprivation, develop non-communicable diseases (such as diabetes and cardiovascular disease) at younger ages, live with greater levels of ill-health and disability, and die prematurely. They are also less likely to access primary health services, instead over-represented in the avoidable hospital and mortality statistics (Australian Indigenous Health*InfoNet* 2022, Health Quality & Safety Commission 2019). While Indigenous peoples tend to be youthful populations, they are dying of diseases commonly associated with older age before they are 65 years of age. They have shorter life expectancies: male 8.8 years and female 8.1 years for Australian First Nations peoples although this increases for those living in rural and remote areas (Australian Bureau of Statistics 2023), and for Māori in New Zealand (Aotearoa) (Stats NZ 2021).

Taking a person-centred approach to practice is crucial for working with Indigenous peoples to ensure consideration of their life circumstances when planning care (Wilson et al 2018). Culture is important. Cultural identity and connection are protective factors to a certain degree; therefore, providing culturally responsive care is important for Indigenous peoples (Table 15.2). Such care provides nurses with a frame of reference to understand Indigenous peoples' worlds. In contrast to the biomedical model evident in many health services, Indigenous worldviews are holistic, relational, and spiritually and environmentally based. This multi-faceted concept of health means Indigenous peoples' spiritual wellbeing and family are of utmost importance. Establishing respectful relationships

TABLE 15.2
Culturally responsive practice

	Culturally responsive practice involves nurses being culturally competent and providing culturally safe care for the Indigenous person and his or her family. Wilson and Hickey (2015) identified three components (KAI) to culturally responsive practice
Knowledge	Identify personal, cultural values, beliefs, practices, assumptions and biases held about marginalised groups in your community and how these may impact on your practice. Critically understand the historical, socioeconomic and political influences affecting their health and wellbeing
Action	Establish respectful and non-judgmental relationships. Recognise the health (and social) needs of the person and their family. Avoid imposing your personal and professional values and beliefs on individuals and their family. Identify people's and the family's strengths and existing health-promoting behaviours and use these to inform plans of care
Integration	Include important cultural needs in an individual's care plan. Including cultural needs may require getting the assistance of a cultural advisor who understands their particular culture needs

and a partner-in-care approach is important—this should begin by saying where you are from and who you are. Recognising the significant role and obligation family plays in an Indigenous person's healthcare journey is important. Recognise the different health priorities an Indigenous person and their family might have from those of the health professional. For example, housing may be more important than the individual's health condition.

OLDER PEOPLE

The world's population is ageing, and this is particularly evident in Westernised countries. Contributing factors include decreases in global fertility and mortality rates. Other factors include advances in science and healthcare, improved standards of living, including improved nutrition and the implementation of public health measures such as the availability of clean water. In line with other Western societies, the receipt of superannuation marks the time when a person transitions from middle to old age. In New Zealand (Aotearoa), retirement age is 65 years and in Australia legislation raised the eligibility to receive superannuation incrementally to 67 years by 2023.

Santrock (2017) identifies three categories used to describe the older age group: 'young old' (those aged 65–74 years), 'old' (those aged 75–84 years) and the 'oldest old' (those aged 85 years and over). Ageing is not viewed positively in Western societies and being 65 years or over potentiates this group of people to discrimination, called ageism. Ageism is a term used to describe the negative and stereotypic bias resulting in older people's first-hand experience of society's bigoted views about being older (Burnes et al 2019). There is a significant body of research-based literature that negatively links being old to increased frailty, being dependent and not being able to live on their own, being forgetful and cognitively impaired, as well as being an economic burden on society (Ausanee & Duangjai 2019). While this may be true for some, it does not relate to all older people—Rose et al's (2023) work on ageing in place demonstrates that an older person's personal qualities and strategies, networks and community connections, home environment and accessibility of appropriate support are indicative of successful ageing in place.

Negative views on ageing are picked up by the media and translated into our everyday conversations. An example is referring to the ageing population as a 'grey tsunami'; tsunami evokes visions of death and destruction. Viewing older people in this way moves ageing from being a natural human process to positioning this group of people negatively, and old age as a burden on society. The consequences are significant regarding mental health and wellbeing. Studies reported that older participants who feel discriminated against based on how old they were had poor psychological wellbeing including stress, depression and low scores in self-rated health (Hang & Kim 2022). Hang and Kim (2022) reported that ageism was moderated by identifying with age group, nature of emotional responses, views on ageing, having a purpose in life, body esteem, and being able to adjust goals.

Negative societal attitudes to older people have also infiltrated the delivery of healthcare services to this group of individuals. Nursing research has shown that if you are older and hospitalised, especially if you are a vulnerable older adult, you may not receive active treatment or respect, could be assigned a nurse who is less experienced and could be spoken to as if you were a child (Van Wicklin 2020). As nurses have the most contact with older people in comparison with other health professional groups they are well placed to be instrumental in reducing ageism. As identified in the previous section, taking a person-centred approach to working with older people is pivotal to reducing inequities and, as a result, improving their outcomes. Person-centred care recognises the individual's uniqueness and includes the person and their family or significant other as active participants in

the care process by empowering them and providing information (Nilsen et al 2022). By taking this approach nurses can advocate for older people by:
- ensuring older people are not treated as a homogeneous group—there are generational differences between a 65- and a 90-year-old
- replacing terms like 'elderly' with 'older people' to avoid ageist connotations
- remembering that many older people remain active and live independently, while some live with dementia and frailty.

LGBTQI PEOPLE

Throughout many parts of the world, anti-discrimination laws have been passed promoting equality for same-sex attracted, gender dysphoric and intersex people. Historically this has not been the case. LGBTQI people were classified as criminals and deviant, resulting in them being imprisoned or admitted to psychiatric institutions (Taliaferro & Muehlenkamp 2017). However, despite advances in civil rights, homophobia, transphobia and not understanding what being intersexed is has remained an issue. Consequently, discrimination of these groups occurs in both subtle and overt ways.

A subtle form of discrimination is assuming everyone is heterosexual (referred to as heterosexism). For example, asking a man as part of a health screening questionnaire about his wife. Another assumption is being assigned a 'gay' label if you are not heterosexual. Such labelling does not take into account the different expressions of sexuality and gender that exist amongst LGBTQI people. More overt forms of discrimination are refusing to call a transgendered person by their preferred name, instead insisting on using their biologically assigned name or requiring transgendered people to use public restrooms by anatomy rather than identity.

Negative experiences and discrimination of these groups of individuals have been shown to result in significant social and health disparities, particularly mental health issues. When compared with the general population, people identifying as LGBTQI experience an increased risk for substance abuse, anxiety disorders, depression, self-harm and suicide (Medina-Martinez et al 2021). Also, due to negative attitudes towards LGBTQI individuals by health professionals, including nurses, these groups may be reluctant and fearful to seek healthcare. Consequently, this is a significant barrier to receiving timely, preventive, health-promoting and intervention-related health services (Sherriff et al 2019).

There are many ways nurses can be more responsive to LGBTQI people that can have a significant and positive effect on their wellbeing:
- Become knowledgeable about the diversity that exists within LGBTQI communities and the specific health and social service needs of these groups
- Be aware of the multiple ways that discrimination (subtle and overt) impacts on LGBTQI people
- Understand the social and health effects resulting from discriminatory attitudes and practices
- Have skills and attributes to engage meaningfully with LGBTQI individuals
- Be able to put aside your views and prejudices to provide a person-centred and culturally appropriate healthcare service
- Ensure the workplace is LGBTQI friendly. Friendly workplaces include making publicly visible health and social service information relating to LGBTQI communities
- Develop partnerships with LGBTQI organisations to provide support and education opportunities for staff and to refer LGBTQI people to appropriate social support agencies as required.

FAMILIES AFFECTED BY VIOLENCE

Globally, one in three women have experienced intimate partner violence and for the Indigenous and First Nations peoples of Australia and New Zealand (Aotearoa) the prevalence of violence within their families is much higher (two in three women) (Australian Institute of Health and Welfare [AIHW] 2024, Fanslow et al 2022). Family violence affects both adults and children, extending beyond intimate partners to other family members. It significantly has an impact on a person's long-term physical, psychological, spiritual and social health and wellbeing (Fanslow et al 2021a, Mellar et al 2023). Children are affected by family violence—living in homes where violence occurs has harmful effects and is considered child abuse and neglect. Family violence and child abuse and neglect are considered adverse childhood experiences, and nurses have a role in safeguarding children (Fanslow et al 2021b). Evidence indicates women and child victims of family violence often go unrecognised by health professionals and their pleas for help are disregarded (Family Violence Death Review Committee 2017). Identifying and responding to victim-survivors of family violence is critical (Box 15.1) and is addressed more fully in Chapter 16.

YOUTH

Young people who are well and healthy are vital to the health, wellbeing and productivity of our communities and respective countries. The health needs of many young people can be unmet despite facing a variety of known health needs; for instance, mental health issues (including depression and suicide), sexual health (including teen pregnancy and sexually transmitted infections), alcohol and substance use, obesity, physical activity, motor vehicle accidents and life-threatening illnesses. Sutcliffe et al (2023) reported high mental health needs in adolescents in New Zealand (Aotearoa), especially for females, Māori, Pacific and Asian young people. Indigenous youth substance misuse and binge drinking is associated with poorer health and social outcomes, especially for Māori and Rainbow youth (Ball et al 2022a, 2022b). The reasons for unmet health needs can relate to the lack of access to and quality of healthcare services (Barbarich-Unasa 2023).

BOX 15.1
How nurses can respond to those experiencing family violence

Nurses can help by:
- being genuine and having a non-judgmental and helpful manner
- becoming knowledgeable about family violence dynamics and understanding common misconceptions that are unhelpful
- understanding the time leading up to and after leaving a violent relationship is dangerous for victims and their children, with an increased risk of homicide around this time
- reviewing the language used and recording the victim's story fully and accurately
- knowing organisational policies for making a referral, and helping a victim to contact people rather than just providing a name and contact details, information leaflets or a safety plan (Wilson et al 2015).

> ### STORY
>
> Krystle is a 16-year-old Indigenous transgender student who has been exposed to persistent discrimination and racism over the last 3 years, since coming out. Krystle's parents have withdrawn support as they struggle to come to terms with the loss of their son and the transition she has undertaken. The general practitioner is concerned about Krystle's overall wellbeing and has asked you to visit her at home to determine her health needs and mental health status.
>
> #### Reflective questions
>
> Reflect on the scenario and answer the following questions. Using knowledge about the barriers and facilitators to health and wellbeing for LGBTQI students (see Crockett et al 2022) and the KAI approach to culturally responsive practice, consider the following:
>
> #### Knowledge
>
> 1. What are the assumptions and biases you hold about LGBTQI people in similar situations to Krystle?
> 2. What do you know about the realities for transgender people? What do you need to know?
> 3. What do you need to understand about Krystle's health and wellbeing needs?
>
> #### Actions
>
> 1. What things do you need to consider to establish an effective relationship with Krystle?
> 2. How would you go about engaging with Krystle?
>
> #### Integration
>
> 1. How would you go about identifying Krystle's needs as a transgender person?
> 2. Given that Krystle appears to be somewhat disconnected from her family, what things do you need to consider to strengthen her social and family connections and supports?

An Australian study found most adolescents, especially those who are socially and ethnically marginalised, have difficulties accessing healthcare, despite having health issues (Robards et al 2019). Reasons for young people not accessing health services include having confidentiality concerns, a lack of knowledge about available services, being uncomfortable disclosing a health issue, not being believed or not listened to, complicated processes to access services, or encountering discrimination and racism (Barbarich-Unasa 2023). Often young people's input and visibility in health services may be absent. For example, not including a young person in decisions made about their health and wellbeing or not participating because of perceived barriers such as staff friendliness.

Young people are not a homogeneous group—they are diverse. There is a significant difference between how a 14-year-old understands and interacts in the world compared with a 20-year-old. Therefore, co-reviewing delivery of services to young people is essential in creating youth-friendly services—importantly, creating an environment and having age-appropriate and friendly staff (Barbarich-Unasa 2023, Blignault et al 2016).

There are some things nurses can do in their practice to improve responsiveness to youth (Barbarich-Unasa 2023, Robards et al 2019):
- getting feedback from young people about what is 'youth-friendly'
- ensuring young people are involved in decision making about their health
- being clear about confidentiality and consent issues
- listening attentively and respectfully
- being flexible and using a range of approaches
- having discussions about recovery
- communicating clearly and providing meaningful information
- use of technology.

CONCLUSION

Those groups experiencing health disparities belong to marginalised groups within their communities. They face inequities in their access to and engagement with healthcare services, including the quality of care that they receive, despite health being a fundamental right of all people globally. Underpinning practice with health equity, social justice and intersectionality ensures people receive care that is fair and just, and are not subjected to deficit explanations and discriminatory attitudes and behaviours. By attending to the quality of care that they deliver, nurses can contribute to the reduction of health disparities.

REFLECTIVE QUESTIONS

Complete the following reflective exercise to determine the thoughts, biases and assumptions that you hold for each of the groups of people (Indigenous peoples, older people, those belonging to the LGBTQI community, families affected by violence, and youth). Identify where you need further development than is discussed in this chapter. Use this opportunity to be creative and note that there are no right or wrong answers.

1. What I think about [the particular group] is …
2. What I feel about [the particular group] is …
3. What I know about [the particular group] is …
4. What I need to know about [the particular group] is …

Recommended readings

Bastos J L, Harnois C E, Paradies Y C 2018 Health care barriers, racism, and intersectionality in Australia. Social Science & Medicine 199:209–218

Campbell B 2021 Social justice and sociological theory. Society 58(5):355–364

Crockett M A, Martínez V, Caviedes P 2022 Barriers and facilitators to mental health help-seeking and experiences with service use among LGBT+ university students in Chile. International Journal of Environmental Research and Public Health 19(24):16520

References

Ausanee W, Duangjai P 2019 A systematic review of factors influencing social participation of older adults. Pacific Rim International Journal of Nursing Research 23(2):131–141

Australian Bureau of Statistics 2023 Aboriginal and Torres Strait Islander life expectancy. Online. Available: https://www.abs.gov.au/statistics/people/aboriginal-and-torres-strait-islander-peoples/aboriginal-and-torres-strait-islander-life-expectancy/latest-release 7 March 2024

Australian Indigenous HealthInfoNet 2022 Overview of Aboriginal and Torres Strait Islander health status 2021. Australian Indigenous HealthInfoNet, Perth. Online. Available: https://healthinfonet.ecu.edu.au/key-resources/publications/44570 10 March 2024

Australian Indigenous HealthInfoNet 2024 Overview of Aboriginal and Torres Strait Islander health status 2023. Australian Indigenous HealthInfoNet, Perth. Online. Available: https://healthinfonet.ecu.edu.au/key-resources/publications/48279/?title=Overview+of+Aboriginal+and+Torres+Strait+Islander+health+status+2023&contentid=48279_1 10 March 2024

Australian Institute of Health & Welfare (AIHW) 2024 Aboriginal and Torres Strait Islander people. Online. Available: https://www.aihw.gov.au/family-domestic-and-sexual-violence/population-groups/aboriginal-and-torres-strait-islander-people

Ball J, Zhang J, Anderson C et al 2022a Understanding and addressing alcohol harm among Rainbow youth at secondary school. Factsheet. Alcohol Healthwatch, University of Otago & Adolescent Health Research Group, Auckland. Online. Available: https://www.youth19.ac.nz/publications 10 March 2024

Ball J, Zhang J, Roberts A et al 2022b Understanding and addressing alcohol harm among rangatahi Māori at secondary school. Factsheet. Alcohol Healthwatch, University of Otago & Adolescent Health Research Group, Auckland. Online. Available: https://www.youth19.ac.nz/publications 10 March 2024

Barbarich-Unasa T W 2023 Whakamana te reo aa ngaa rangatahi ki roto i ngaa ratonga hauora (Empowering the voices of our young people in health services). Doctoral thesis, Auckland University of Technology, New Zealand. Online. Available: https://hdl.handle.net/10292/15853

Best O, Fredericks B (eds) 2014 Yatdjuligin: Aboriginal and Torres Strait Islander nursing and midwifery care. Cambridge University Press, Port Melbourne

Blignault I, Haswell M, Jackson Pulver L 2016 The value of partnerships: lessons from a multi-site evaluation of a national social and emotional wellbeing program for Indigenous youth. Australian and New Zealand Journal of Public Health 40 Suppl 1:S53–S58

Burnes D, Sheppard C, Henderson C R et al 2019 Interventions to reduce ageism against older adults: a systematic review and meta-analysis. American Journal of Public Health 109(8):e1–e9

Cormack D, Harris R, Stanley J 2020 Māori experiences of multiple forms of discrimination: findings from Te Kupenga 2013. Kōtuitui: New Zealand Journal of Social Sciences Online 15(1):106–122

Crockett M A, Martínez V, Caviedes P 2022 Barriers and facilitators to mental health help-seeking and experiences with service use among LGBT+ university students in Chile. International Journal of Environmental Research and Public Health 19(24):16520

Egede L E, Walker R J, Williams J S 2024 Addressing structural inequalities, structural racism, and social determinants of health: a vision for the future. Journal of General Internal Medicine 39(3):487–491

Family Violence Death Review Committee 2017 Fifth data report: January 2009 to December 2015. Health Quality and Safety Commission New Zealand, Wellington

Fanslow J, Malihi Z, Hashemi L et al 2021a Change in prevalence of psychological and economic abuse, and controlling behaviours against women by an intimate partner in two cross-sectional studies in New Zealand, 2003 and 2019. BMJ Open 11(3):e044910

Fanslow J, Hashemi L, Gulliver P et al 2021b Adverse childhood experiences in New Zealand and subsequent victimization in adulthood: findings from a population-based study. Child Abuse & Neglect 117:105067

Fanslow J L, Hashemi L, Gulliver P et al 2022 Gender patterns in the use of physical violence against a violent partner: results of a cross-sectional population-based study in New Zealand. Journal of Interpersonal Violence 37(23–24):NP22890–NP22920

Gatwiri K, Rotumah D, Rix E 2021 BlackLivesMatter in healthcare: racism and implications for health inequity among Aboriginal and Torres Strait Islander peoples in Australia. International Journal of Environmental Research & Public Health 18(9):4399

Graham R, Masters-Awatere B 2020 Experiences of Māori of Aotearoa New Zealand's public health system: a systematic review of two decades of published qualitative research. Australian & New Zealand Journal of Public Health 44(3):193–200.

Hang H, Kim H 2022 Ageism and psychological well-being among older adults: a systematic review. Gerontology and Geriatric Medicine 8:23337214221087023.

Health Quality & Safety Commission (HQSC) 2019 A window on the quality of Aotearoa New Zealand health care 2019 – a view on Māori health care. HQSC. Online. Available: https://www.hqsc.govt.nz/resources/resource-library/a-window-on-the-quality-of-aotearoa-new-zealands-health-care-2019-a-view-on-maori-health-equity-2/ 10 March 2024

Kapiriri L, Razavi S D 2022 Equity, justice, and social values in priority setting: a qualitative study of resource allocation criteria for global donor organizations working in low-income countries. International Journal for Equity in Health 21(1):17

Komene E, Pene B, Gerard D et al 2024 Whakawhanaungatanga – building trust and connections: a qualitative study of Indigenous Māori patients and whānau (extended family network) hospital experiences. Journal of Advanced Nursing 80(4):1545–1558

Lewis M, McNaughton S A, Rychetnik L et al 2021 Cost and affordability of healthy, equitable and sustainable diets in low socioeconomic groups in Australia. Nutrients 13(8) https://doi.org/10.3390/nu13082900

Maddox R, Bovill M, Waa A M et al 2022 Reflections on Indigenous commercial tobacco control: 'The dolphins will always take us home'. Tobacco control 31:348–351 https://doi.org/10.1136/tobaccocontrol-2021-056571

Macgregor C, Walumbe J, Tulle E et al 2023 Intersectionality as a theoretical framework for researching health inequities in chronic pain. British Journal of Pain 17(5):479–490

Medina-Martínez J, Saus-Ortega C, Sánchez-Lorente M M et al 2021 Health inequities in LGBT people and nursing interventions to reduce them: a systematic review. International Journal of Environmental Research and Public Health 18(22):11801

Mellar B M, Hashemi L, Selak V et al 2023 Association between women's exposure to intimate partner violence and self-reported health outcomes in New Zealand. JAMA Network Open 6(3):e231311–e231311

Menzies K 2019 Understanding the Australian Aboriginal experience of collective, historical and intergenerational trauma. International Social Work 62(6):1522–1534

Moorley C, Darbyshire P, Serrant L et al 2020 Dismantling structural racism: nursing must not be caught on the wrong side of history. Journal of Advanced Nursing 76(10):2450–2453

Nilsen E R, Hollister B, Söderhamn U et al 2022 What matters to older adults? Exploring person-centred care during and after transitions between hospital and home. Journal of Clinical Nursing 31(5–6):569–581.

Pearson O, Schwartzkpff K, Dawson A et al 2020 Aboriginal community controlled health organisations address health equity through action on the social determinants of health of Aboriginal and Torres Strait Islander peoples in Australia. BMC Public Health 20(1):1859

Pihama L, Smith L, Cameron N et al 2020 He oranga ngākau: Māori approaches to trauma informed care. Te Kotahi Research Institute, Hamilton, New Zealand

Robards F, Kang M, Steinbeck K et al 2019 Health care equity and access for marginalised young people: a longitudinal qualitative study exploring health system navigation in Australia. International Journal for Equity in Health 18(1):41

Rooddehghan Z, ParsaYekta Z, Nasrabadi A N 2019 Equity in nursing care: a grounded theory study. Nursing Ethics 26(2):598–610

Rogers-LaVanne M P, Bader A C, de Flamingh A et al S 2023 Association between gene methylation and experiences of historical trauma in Alaska Native peoples. International Journal for Equity in Health 22(1):182

Rose K, Kozlowski D, Horstmanshof L 2023 Experiences of ageing in place in Australia and New Zealand: a scoping review. Journal of Community & Applied Social Psychology 33(3):623–645

Santrock J W 2017 Lifespan development. McGraw-Hill Education, New York

Sherriff N, Zeeman L, McGlynn N et al 2019 Co-producing knowledge of lesbian, gay, bisexual, trans and intersex (LGBTI) health-care inequalities via rapid reviews of grey literature in 27 EU Member States. Health Expectations 22(4):688–700

Stats NZ 2021 Growth in life expectancy slows. Online. Available: https://www.stats.govt.nz/news/growth-in-life-expectancy-slows 10 March 2024

Sutcliffe K, Ball J, Clark T C et al 2023 Rapid and unequal decline in adolescent mental health and well-being 2012–2019: findings from New Zealand cross-sectional surveys. Australian & New Zealand Journal of Psychiatry 57(2):264–282

Taliaferro L A, Muehlenkamp J J 2017 Nonsuicidal self-injury and suicidality among sexual minority youth: risk factors and protective connectedness factors. Academic Pediatrics 17(7):715–722. https://doi.org/10.1016/j.acap.2016.11.002

Thurber K A, Brinckley M-M, Jones R, et al 2022 Population-level contribution of interpersonal discrimination to psychological distress among Australian Aboriginal and Torres Strait Islander adults, and to Indigenous & non-Indigenous inequities: cross-sectional analysis of a community-controlled First Nations cohort study. The Lancet 400(10368):2084–2094

Tolmie J, Smith R, Wilson D 2023 Understanding intimate partner violence: why coercive control requires a social and systemic entrapment framework. Violence Against Women 30(1)

Van Dijk H M, Cramm J M, Van Exel J et al 2015 The ideal neighbourhood for ageing in place as perceived by frail and non-frail community-dwelling older people. Ageing & Society 35(08):1771–1795

Van Wicklin S A 2020 Ageism in nursing. Plastic Surgery Nursing 40(1):20–24

Verbunt E, Luke J, Paradies Y 2021 Cultural determinants of health for Aboriginal and Torres Strait Islander people – a narrative overview of reviews. International Journal for Equity in Health 20(1):181

Wasserman J, Palmer R C, Gomez M M et al 2019 Advancing health services research to eliminate health care disparities. American Journal of Public Health 109:S64–S69

Wilson C, Cariola L A 2020 LGBTQI+ Youth and mental health: a systematic review of qualitative research. Adolescent Research Review 5(2):187–211

Wilson D, Heaslip V, Jackson D 2018 Improving equity and cultural responsiveness with marginalised communities: understanding competing worldviews. Journal of Clinical Nursing 27(19–20):3810–3819

Wilson D, Hickey H 2015 Māori health: Māori- and whānau-centred practice. In: Wepa D (ed) Cultural safety in Aotearoa New Zealand. Cambridge University Press, Melbourne, pp 235–251

Wilson D, Mikahere-Hall A, Sherwood J et al 2019 E Tū wāhine, e tū whānau: wāhine Māori keeping safe in unsafe relationships. AUT Taupua Waiora Māori Research Centre. Online. Available: https://hdl.handle.net/10292/13068 10 March 2024

Wilson D, Smith R, Tolmie J et al 2015 Becoming better helpers: rethinking language to move beyond simplistic responses to women experiencing intimate partner violence. Policy Quarterly 11(1):26–31

Windle A, Javanparast S, Freeman T, Baum F 2023 Evaluating local primary health care actions to address health inequities: analysis of Australia's Primary Health Networks. International Journal for Equity in Health 22(1):243

World Health Organization (WHO) 2023 Human rights. Online. Available: https://www.who.int/news-room/fact-sheets/detail/human-rights-and-health 10 March 2024

CHAPTER 16

NURSING AND FAMILY VIOLENCE

Denise Wilson and Debra Jackson

KEY WORDS
child abuse and neglect
domestic violence
elder abuse
family violence
intersectionality
intimate partner violence

LEARNING OBJECTIVES

After reading this chapter, readers should be able to:

- describe family violence and how it manifests
- use social justice, equity and intersectionality to understand how family violence occurs at societal, community, family and individual levels
- discuss common misconceptions and debates related to family violence
- discuss supportive nursing practice when interacting with those affected by family violence.

INTRODUCTION

Interpersonal violence is prevalent in many families globally and more locally in Australasia. Often termed as family or domestic violence, it is 'one of the most urgent health issues of our generation and is at pandemic proportions' (Withiel et al 2022:1). Family violence is a problem that defies resolution. It affects children abused at the hands of 'trusted' people, women (and, to a lesser extent, men) killed, injured or humiliated by violent partners, or older persons mistreated by their carers. Mandela (2002) positioned it as intergenerational suffering across the life course and fostered by historical and contemporary social and economic conditions. Nurses, like other health professionals, are highly likely to encounter victim-survivors and users of family violence in their day-to-day practice. Despite Australia and New Zealand (Aotearoa) being developed countries, both have concerning family violence records.

Yet, nurses and other health professionals frequently overlook injuries inconsistent with their explanation or are unaware that those impacted by family violence are high users of health services (Withiel et al 2022). It can be difficult to talk about family violence, even in healthcare, and this is so for a range of reasons—personal discomfort, lack of time, systems-related issues, personal experiences, a lack of knowledge and preparation, misunderstandings about family violence, unvalidated assumptions, and racism and discrimination (Adams et al 2021, Rizkalla et al 2020, Spangaro et al 2016, Wilson 1997). Nurses with their own experiences of interpersonal violence can potentially identify and respond to victim-survivors better than those without experience. However, they experience higher levels of distress and may need support (Dheensa et al 2023), and they could potentially experience retraumatisation, which may have the effect of causing reluctance to respond or intervene. Withiel et al (2022) found Australian nurses' reluctance to respond to people experiencing family violence related to their confidence and lack of knowledge about family violence, something Wilson (1997) also found for nurses in New Zealand (Aotearoa). Some international literature has examined the role of nursing students in recognising and responding to intimate partner violence (IPV) and highlighted the importance of including issues around family violence in the education of undergraduate nursing students (Shaqiqi & Innab 2023).

IPV is a common form of family violence and is complex, being recently referred to as a 'wicked problem' (Jack et al 2023). Wicked problems are defined as those that are complex and resistant to usual solutions and exist in a context of volatility (Hutchinson et al 2015). Along with sexual violence, IPV is predominantly a gendered problem primarily affecting women and girls. Nevertheless, it is essential to be mindful that men, women and gender-diverse people can also be victim-survivors and/or users of violence (often referred to as perpetrators). Furthermore, nurses also interact with users of violence who often are marginalised in family violence discussions. For instance, male users of violence, especially, can also have histories of being victim-survivors of child abuse and neglect and of psychological, emotional and physical abuse (Wilson et al 2019a).

In this chapter, we explore the critical role nurses have in working with women, children and men impacted by family violence at some point in their lives. Family violence and its manifestations and misconceptions are explained regarding social justice, intersectionality and equity to assist in understanding the complexities and layers of family violence. Strategies to aid nurses in respectfully and empathically responding to and helping those impacted by abuse and violence are also presented.

Family violence—what it is and what it isn't

Family violence occurs in diverse ways and combinations, including physical, psychological, emotional, sexual, financial and spiritual (Table 16.1), which means each person's experiences are different. The term family violence is inclusive of child abuse and neglect, IPV or domestic violence, same-sex partner violence, intrafamilial violence, and abuse of older people. Family violence can occur at any time; for some people there can be points of heightened risk, such as when trying to end a relationship with a user of violence (Spearman et al 2023). For some people, abuse and violence spans their life course; for instance, being a victim as a child, a victim or perpetrator of violence as an adult, and then a victim as an older adult. Some people do not experience physical abuse or violence but face extensive psychological abuse that serves to undermine their personhood (Wilson et al 2019a). What we know is that family violence is shrouded in stigma, silence, shame and secrecy, making it difficult for people to disclose what is happening and, at times, difficult to detect.

As people age, they can become increasingly dependent on others to assist them in some aspect of their daily living—meaning older people can be at heightened vulnerability to the risk of abuse in some form. Abuse of older people occurs within the context of trusted relationships, such as those within families, with 60% of incidents of elder abuse reportedly occurring at the hands of family

TABLE 16.1
Types of violence affecting families

TYPE OF FAMILY VIOLENCE	DESCRIPTION
Family violence	Family violence is the physical, sexual, psychological and/or financial abuse or violence inflicted by one person against another person who is a family member. It is a cumulative pattern of harm over time that includes coercive control (such as manipulation, isolation, threats, imposing restrictions, surveillance and coercion), restricting a person's autonomy, agency and freedom
Abuse of older people (AOP)	Abuse of older people involves a single or repeated act or an absence of care by a person(s) where a relationship of trust results in harm or distress to an older person
Child abuse and neglect (CAN)	Child abuse and neglect, also called child maltreatment, includes physical and emotional maltreatment, sexual abuse, neglect and negligent treatment and exploitation that harms or potentially harms a child's health, development and dignity. It also includes children's exposure to IPV
Entrapment	Entrapment occurs at partner, social and systemic levels. It severely restricts a victim-survivor's capacity to resist a partner's violence or to escape the situation, making it difficult to leave or keep themselves and their children safe
Intimate partner violence (IPV)	Predominantly a gendered form of violence against women, sometimes referred to as domestic violence or partner violence
Historical trauma	A collective trauma associated with a significant historical event(s), such as colonisation, that impacts individuals, groups and communities. It can result in lifetime trauma, chronic stress, physiological and epigenetic changes, and is associated with family violence and racism
Intergenerational violence and trauma	A form of violence and trauma transmitted across generations
Intrafamilial family violence	A form of family violence that includes wider family members, such as siblings, grandparents, aunties, uncles and cousins
Sexual violence	Often referred to as sexual behaviours such as abuse, assault, harm or violation inflicted by a person(s) without a victim-survivor freely giving consent. Child sexual abuse or violence occurs to children under the age of 16
State violence	A form of violence that involves state or government agency neglect, failure to protect, abuse, abuse of power, racism and breaches of treaty agreements
Violence within Indigenous extended families (whānau)	Indigenous peoples living with family violence have additional layers of historical and contemporary complexity. It includes all forms of violence that occur against and within Indigenous families and involves the violence of colonisation, institutional racism and interpersonal violence

members (Hellwig 2023). Still, it can include people outside of family contexts, like carers and financial predators and in residential care settings (Duffy et al 2023). The harm associated with elder abuse includes physical, psychological, financial, sexual and social harms as well as neglect (World Health Organization [WHO] 2022). With ageing populations in both Australia and New Zealand (Aotearoa), the abuse of older people will increase. Elder abuse is under-reported and often not recognised for what it is (Hellwig 2023). However, the body of research is slowly growing but contains several limitations. For instance, the Australian AIFS National Elder Abuse Prevalence Study under-represented Aboriginal and Torres Strait Islander, LGBTQI and CALD populations (Qu et al 2021).

It is essential to understand that family violence is not a one-off or an isolated incident or event. It is a pattern of harm that one person (the primary aggressor) inflicts on their victim(s) over time—for some, it occurs regularly, for others episodically—often, its unpredictability reinforces the person's power over the victim-survivor. Often, this plays out as men's power over women or adults' power over children or older people. In addition to acts of abuse and violence, family violence usually involves coercive and controlling behaviours, involving manipulation, threats, isolation from family and friends, coercion to do things a person would normally not do, surveillance (including cyber-surveillance and technology like drones or phone software to monitor a partner) and stalking.

Effects of family violence

Evidence shows that health and social problems associated with living with family violence are long term, especially for children growing up amidst its destructive effects (Campbell 2002, Hashemi et al 2021). Health consequences of violence include alcohol and substance use, suicide, mental health disorders, learning difficulties, impulse control disorders, chronic pain and an array of somatic illnesses (WHO 2014a). Furthermore, the impacts of persistent violence are transmitted intergenerationally (Wilson 2016). Children growing up in adverse environments, even if they are not directly hurt or abused, are negatively impacted by the violence in their environments that results in multiple mental, physical and social health problems across their life course (Anda et al 2006, Hashemi et al 2021).

Significantly, family violence is associated with long-term physical, psychological, social, financial and spiritual consequences beyond direct exposure to violence. Family violence-related deaths are common forms of homicide in Australia and New Zealand (Aotearoa) (Boxall et al 2022, Family Violence Death Review Committee 2017). The Family Violence Death Review Committee (2022) in New Zealand (Aotearoa) recently called for a *'duty to care'*—a call to action for nurses, health professionals and others to respond more compassionately and effectively to those affected by violence in their lives.

Social justice, intersectionality and rights

The presence of violence in families' lives is a social justice issue—it is an unfair and unjust phenomenon. Importantly, it is a breach of the human right to live a dignified life free of experiences like abuse and violence (United Nations 2015). Family violence for children is a transgression of children's rights (United Nations 1990), and of Indigenous rights for Indigenous and First Nations peoples (such as Māori in New Zealand (Aotearoa) and Aboriginal and Torres Strait Islanders in Australia) (United Nations 2007). The World Health Organization (2014b) maintains a rights-based approach that includes the right to life without fear and violence, and includes self-determination and decision making, optimal quality, accessibility and acceptability of health services without discrimination, privacy and confidentiality, and access to information.

The United Nations (2015) stated that 'the inherent dignity and … equal and inalienable rights of all members of the human family is the foundation of freedom, justice and peace in the world'. Yet, for Indigenous and First Nations peoples, their disproportionate experiences of intergenerational violence and abuse are linked to ongoing historical and contemporary colonialism and their inequitable access to safety and services (Australian Institute of Health and Welfare [AIHW] 2024, Glover et al 2022, Pihama et al 2021, Wilson 2023).

Intersectionality provides a way of understanding the multiple marginalised identities and social forms of oppression that contribute to the complexities of family violence (Kelly 2011). Intersectionality refers to the compounding nature of the multidimensional positions, inequity, oppression and injustice for Indigenous and First Nations and other minoritised peoples. Kelly (2011) draws attention to a variety of oppressive influences like social structures and abusive family members. Social and health services people, including healthcare providers, require nuanced understandings of complex and multidimensional positions of inequity and oppression (for instance, race, gender, poverty, poor quality or unstable housing, unemployment, discrimination and racism, histories of colonisation) and injustices (e.g. lack of response, discrimination, unjust incarceration).

Thus, equitable outcomes for these women involve understanding the multi-faceted barriers and challenges they navigate to keep themselves and their children safe (Wilson et al 2019a).

Misconceptions of family violence

Family violence is a complex phenomenon that presents itself in many and varied ways. Nonetheless, many people rely on a variety of misconceptions to inform their understanding of what family violence is and what it is not (see Table 16.2 for examples). For instance, the minimisation of the seriousness of violence occurs with simplistic explanations like, 'it's just a domestic', or 'it just happened once', 'she should just leave', or 'they both give [punches] as good as they get', inferring the violence is a mutual endeavour. However, reliance on misconceptions to inform nursing practice means that for many, especially women and children, their plight is not recognised, perpetuating the continuance of the violence and exposing them to continued serious risk of harm and death. Tolmie et al (2024) explains the influence of how we understand family violence on practice.

> How one conceptualises intimate partner violence (IPV) influences what is seen when looking at situations involving IPV. It affects what is considered relevant or irrelevant in making sense of what is happening and the meanings derived from factors deemed 'relevant'. It also influences what one thinks is the appropriate response to IPV.
>
> (Tolmie et al 2024:1)

REFLECTION

Discuss in small groups the various factors nurses need to consider when assessing somebody who has been abused or is a victim of violence. Reflect on how each person in the group conceptualises family violence. How would the factors identified vary in presentation over the life course?

Coercive control and entrapment

Stark's (2007) seminal work on coercive control extended the understanding of IPV (sometimes called domestic violence) beyond neo-liberal and pathological conceptions of battered woman syndrome involving victim-blaming, for example, using individual women's psychological inadequacies to explain why they remain in abusive relationships.[1] Such conceptualisations position women negatively,

---

[1] For example, learned helplessness, hostage syndrome, and Stockholm Syndrome.

TABLE 16.2
Misconceptions about family violence

MISCONCEPTION	EXPLANATION
It is not an incident of family violence	Family violence is not a single or isolated event but rather is a pattern of harm inflicted by one person onto another over time that has cumulative and compounding effects. Family violence is not restricted to physical violence but also includes psychological, sexual, financial and spiritual forms of abuse and violence. It also involves coercive control (strategies include threats, control, surveillance, stalking, manipulation and social isolation)
It's not 'just a domestic'	Family or domestic violence is never just a domestic. People die as a result of violence inflicted on them by a family member, often over time, that can increase in severity and frequency. It is helpful to remember people are killed regularly in Australia and New Zealand (Aotearoa) as a result of family violence
Women cannot simply leave	Separation from a violent partner or leaving does not mean the violence stops or women and children are safe. The risk of homicide significantly increases at the time of leaving and afterwards—for some, 2 or more years after leaving. Their partner has entrapped them in the relationship. To leave and be safe women and children have to navigate potentially volatile and dangerous situations with contexts of coercion, threats and control
Family violence is not mutual acts of violence	Family violence is a gendered pattern of harm—women are significantly more likely to be seriously injured or killed. Family violence involves one person's (predominant aggressor) deliberate acts of abuse/violence (physical, psychological, sexual, financial and/or spiritual) inflicted on another person. Notably, abused people often resist to protect themselves and their children. It is more beneficial to determine who is the primary victim and who is the predominant aggressor in a relationship rather than dismissing violence as being mutually instigated
Empowerment has unintended harms	Empowerment at a time when women are at a crisis point and asking for help can be inappropriate. Empowerment requires a person to have autonomy and agency to make decisions and act on these. Its misuse shifts nurses' and other health providers' responsibilities and accountabilities. It leads to behaviours such as transactional use of safety plans, which assumes women are not doing anything about their safety and have the necessary autonomy and agency to make their own decisions
Alcohol and substance misuse is a symptom of trauma	The use of alcohol and other substances assists with coping with violent situations or helps to block out daily experiences of trauma and violence. This phenomenon often occurs when victim-survivors and users of violence are unable to secure help or support. In these situations, people affected by violence and abuse cannot be explained by partying or abusing alcohol and substances
Victims do ask for help	Contrary to popular belief, women tell or ask multiple people and agencies for help. Nurses must listen and acknowledge the seriousness of the violence they live with and show they care—that is, bring their mind AND heart to work. Women will respond to people who are kind and empathetic when they can talk about their situations—today, putting food in their children's tummies is the priority. Next week, it may be the violence. Important to note is that when women ask for help, they may have exhausted their strategies to keep themselves and their children safe
Co-occurrence of violence against women and child abuse and neglect	If women are being abused or subjected to violence, there is a reasonable likelihood that the children are also being abused and vice versa. These two forms of family violence are entangled

ignoring their resistance in the face of ongoing violence. Stark (2007) explained coercive control as how a user of violence, by preying on a victim-survivor's vulnerability and unequal status aims to:

… hurt, humiliate, intimidate, exploit, isolate and dominate their victims …

(Stark 2007:5)

Coercive control is not restricted solely to intimate or family relationships. It is designed to induce fear and uncertainty in a victim-survivor by a partner physically, psychologically, emotionally and sexually, undermining their integrity and sense of self, no matter where they are. The strategies used by an abusive partner often go unseen by outsiders. However, these strategies restrict in varying degrees a primary victim-survivor's autonomy, agency and freedom. Coercive control makes it challenging to make sense of a person's decision making. Outsiders may think, 'walk away, protect your children'. The reality is partners may have threatened children's or friends' or families' lives, or in the case of children, a sexual abuser often threatens to kill or harm a child's family members or pets. Such contexts mean victim-survivors, adults and children, often use silence, secrecy, compliance, shame and isolation as safety strategies. The power is in a person's use of coercive control and its layered and cumulative effects.

The work of Tolmie et al (2018, 2024) and Wilson et al (2019b) shifts further the understanding of family violence beyond coercive control to also examining the role of social and systemic entrapment of people in violent relationships. Social and systemic entrapment has three key dimensions:

1. A combination of intersectional inequities and state-sanctioned violence (such as ongoing colonialism in Australia and New Zealand [Aotearoa]) impinge on victim-survivors' lives and those in their support networks. Social and systemic entrapment enables a partner's coercive control and restricts access to available safety responses
2. The safety responses of community and agencies and those responsible for working with victim-survivors and their abusive partners frequently lack availability and equity, diminishing people's dignity. They are ineffective in controlling a partner's coercive control tactics
3. At an abusive partner's level, their coercive controlling behaviours restrict a victim-survivor's capacity to assert their autonomy and agency (Tolmie et al 2024).

So, on many levels, victim-survivors are pushed back when seeking help. The family violence system, which includes the health system and those who work within it, inadvertently becomes part of their entrapment. For instance, Wilson et al (2019a) reported Māori women's stories and their inability to rely on emergency assistance from the police—they received no, late or inappropriate responses and they themselves were considered to be the problem. These researchers also found that these Indigenous women participants reported significant injuries such as blunt force trauma to the head or strangulation with loss of consciousness. Yet, they reported that no-one attended to the ongoing risks associated with these life-threatening injuries.

REFLECTION

Reflect on what you 'know' and don't know about family violence.
1. How is what you 'know' different or like the information presented above?
2. Discuss with your peers how understanding family violence and its complexities can influence the development of your nursing practice.

Indigenous and First Nations peoples

Indigenous and First Nations peoples (such as Aboriginal and Torres Strait Islanders in Australia and Māori in New Zealand [Aotearoa]) experience higher rates of family violence and greater severity in injuries and homicides than others living in their respective countries. Two in three (67%) of Australian First Nations people over 15 years reported harm in the last 12 months, with family violence accounting for three in four (74%) hospitalisations (Australian Institute of Health and Welfare [AIHW] 2024). Two in three (64.1%) Māori women reported lifetime prevalence of domestic violence in comparison to just over half (54.7%) of other women living in New Zealand (Aotearoa) and experience significantly greater severity of physical violence and other forms of violence (Mellar et al 2023). Māori children are also more likely to experience maltreatment and be notified to child protection services (Rouland et al 2019). Māori women are three times and Māori children are four times as likely as non-Māori to be victims of homicide (Family Violence Death Review Committee 2017).

Understanding family violence affecting Indigenous and First Nations peoples through the lens of conventional tools and literature is limited (Klingspohn 2018, Luebke et al 2021). For instance, Wilson et al (2019a) noted biases in the framing of Māori women that focus on their deficits, driven by unvalidated negative stereotypes, without considering their strengths and actions in managing a partner's violence. Attention to the added layers of complexity associated with family violence affecting Indigenous and First Nations peoples includes the effects of colonisation, historical and contemporary colonialism, intergenerational violence and trauma, contemporary socioeconomic and political disadvantage, racism, social and systemic entrapment and inequities in social and health outcomes, generally (Tolmie et al 2024).

Culturally safe and respectful practice

How nurses respond to those affected by abuse and violence can make a difference. Nurses do not have to 'fix', but they do have a role in supporting people from all cultural and social backgrounds. Adams et al (2021) identified three 'threads' of optimal practice by nurses working in the area of family violence:

- First, validation of a person's experience by believing what they say and affirming the abuse and violence is not their fault.
- Secondly, providing respectful and non-judgmental support while remembering that it takes courage to disclose and speak about experiences of violence. These first two things signal practical safeguarding activities. It is also helpful to note that people who live in small towns and rural or remote areas do not have access to the emergency and specialist support services that those living in urban areas can access. Therefore, knowing your community and who can provide safe support is helpful.
- Lastly, be willing to be led and follow the person at their pace. Remember, victim-survivors are experts about their situation and their partner's behaviours and when they are safe or not. The time of and after leaving a violent relationship involves a heightened risk of homicide. Table 16.3 outlines the approach the WHO (2014) recommends to protect and work with victim-survivors—an approach recommended by the Australian Council of Nurses (2022).

TABLE 16.3
The WHO 'LIVES' approach to protecting victim-survivors of family violence

L	Listen	Use an empathetic and non-judgmental approach
I	Inquire	Respectfully inquire about the person's emotional, physical and social needs and concerns
V	Validate	Validate the person's experiences, showing you understand and believe what they say
E	Enhance	Act to enhance a person's safety—inquire what they are doing to keep safe and discuss a plan to keep themselves and any children safe from harm
S	Support	Help the victim-survivor by providing them with information to help them connect with the information, services and support if required

Source: Adapted from WHO 2014b

Hollingdrake et al (2022) undertook a study with women who had experienced family violence to better understand how nurses could best support women experiencing domestic and family violence. From this work these authors were able to identify 10 nursing practice recommendations as below:

1. Knowing the range of domestic violence (DV) services that are current and available locally (e.g. crisis, legal, housing) and establishing meaningful connection with DV services
2. Providing wallet-size business cards with a phone number or website for DV services, or disguising information about these services in a 'goody bag' of general health-related brochures
3. Education that enables nurses' capacity to 1) provide an effective first contact by safely initiating conversations to establish rapport; and 2) provide effective referrals to facilitate comprehensive care
4. Embodying a 'no wrong door' culture by educating health professionals about the ways healthcare services can be an effective first point of care for women experiencing domestic and family violence (i.e. this *is* in their remit)
5. Being receptive to and acting on cues from women's language and behaviours about their own safety
6. Providing trauma-informed care that is underpinned by safety
7. Providing safe, separate waiting areas for women who have disclosed an experience of domestic violence, or who are perceived to be at risk
8. Safety-netting follow-up; for example, seeking permission to contact women in 2 days to make sure referred agencies have established contact
9. Send a text message first when calling from a phone with a private number so that women are aware of who is trying to contact them
10. Prioritising women experiencing domestic and family violence for psychological health support to avoid mental health assessments (as these add a barrier for women involved in child custody negotiations), waiting lists and excess out-of-pocket payments (Hollingdrake et al 2022).

REFLECTION

Reflect on what may stop you from supporting a person presenting with signs of being a victim-survivor or seeking help and protection. What strategies would you put in place to be able to respond better?

STORY

Ruthie, a 20-year-old Indigenous woman, visits her primary healthcare practice to get her children immunised. A junior nurse, Kate, notes she is anxious and nervous—Ruthie appears uncomfortable in the healthcare setting. Her two young children, Jack, aged two, and Lizzi, aged three, accompany Ruthie, who, Kate noted, are clinging to her legs. Kate also observed that Ruthie had a bruised eye and bruising around her neck. The staff claim Ruthie always has bruising and not to worry about her, as she 'gives as good as she gets' from her partner, Marcus. They also claim that it is a miracle Ruthie bothered to bring the children in for their immunisations.

Kate decides to take Ruthie into a private room. She introduces herself and expresses concern about Ruthie's bruising, especially around her neck. Kate asks Ruthie kindly and non-judgmentally if she is safe and asks what she is doing to keep herself, Jack and Lizzi safe. Ruthie explains that Marcus is hitting her more, and she is frightened of him. Still, she can't do anything because he has threatened to kill Jack and Lizzi if Ruthie talks to anyone or attempts to leave. Ruthie shares that Lizzi's toileting has deteriorated, and she cries a lot. She says that even if she could leave, she has no money or support from her family and friends, from whom Marcus has isolated her.

Reflective questions

Using the knowledge gained from this chapter and the recommended readings, consider the following:

Knowledge

1. What assumptions and biases are informing the attitudes of the primary care staff towards Ruthie?
2. What do you know about the realities for women experiencing domestic violence? What do you need to learn?
3. What must you understand about Ruthie, Jack and Lizzi's safety, health and wellbeing needs and factors that potentially inhibit these?

Actions

1. What things did Kate do to establish an effective relationship with Ruthie?
2. How would you go about engaging with Ruthie, and why?
3. What are the strengths that Ruthie possesses?

Integration

1. How would you go about identifying Ruthie's safety needs?
2. What do you need to consider about Ruthie's connections and support?

CONCLUSION

Nurses should aim for fair, respectful and non-discriminatory practice that draws on compassionate and caring approaches, which assists in people disclosing abuse and violence. Working with people affected by family violence is a time to listen carefully, affirm the person's experience, and inquire about what the person needs to be safe. For children, it may involve following institutional policies to ensure children's safeguarding—they rely on adults to protect and keep them safe. Nurses frequently work with families and are uniquely positioned; nurses can respond to windows of opportunity to support people in protecting their safety.

Recommended readings

Hegarty K, Hindmarsh E D, Gilles M T 2000 Domestic violence in Australia: a definition, prevalence and nature of presentation in clinical practice. Medical Journal of Australia 173(7):363–367

Hellwig K 2023 Elder abuse. Home Healthcare Now 41 (6):304–308. doi: 10.1097/NHH.0000000000001196

Wilson D 2023 Violence within whānau and mahi tūkino – a litany of sound revisited. Te Pūkotahitanga – Tangata Whenua Advisory Group for the Minister of the Prevention of Family Violence and Sexual Violence. Ministry of Justice, Wellington New Zealand

Wilson D, Smith R, Tolmie J et al 2015 Becoming better helpers: rethinking language to move beyond simplistic responses to women experiencing intimate partner violence. Policy Quarterly 11(1):26–31

References

Adams C, Hooker L, Taft A 2021 Threads of practice: enhanced maternal and child health nurses working with women experiencing family violence. Global Qualitative Nursing Research 8:1–11 https://doi.org/10.1177/23333936211051703

Anda R F, Felitti V J, Bremner J D et al 2006 The enduring effects of abuse and related adverse experiences in childhood: a convergence of evidence from neurobiology and epidemiology. European Archives of Psychiatry and Clinical Neuroscience 256(3):174–186 https://doi.org/10.1007/s00406-005-0624-4

Australian College of Nurses 2022 December Position statement: nurses and violence. Online. Available: https://www.acn.edu.au/wp-content/uploads/position-statement-nurses-and-violence.pdf

Australian Institute of Health and Welfare (AIHW) 2024 Aboriginal and Torres Strait Islander people. Online. Available: https://www.aihw.gov.au/family-domestic-and-sexual-violence/population-groups/aboriginal-and-torres-strait-islander-people

Boxall H, Doherty L, Lawler S et al 2022 The "Pathways to Intimate Partner Homicide" project: key stages and events in male-perpetrated intimate partner homicide in Australia. ANROWS. Online. Available: https://www.anrows.org.au/publication/the-pathways-to-intimate-partner-homicide-project-key-stages-and-events-in-male-perpetrated-intimate-partner-homicide-in-australia/

Campbell J C 2002 Health consequences of intimate partner violence. The Lancet 359(9314):1331–1336 https://doi.org/10.1016/S0140-6736(02)08336-8

Dheensa S, McLindon E, Spencer C et al 2023 Healthcare professionals' own experiences of domestic violence and abuse: a meta-analysis of prevalence and systematic review of risk markers and consequences. Trauma Violence Abuse 24(3):1282–1299 https://doi.org/10.1177/15248380211061771

Duffy A, Connolly M, Browne F 2023 Older people's experiences of elder abuse in residential care settings: a scoping review. Journal of Advanced Nursing 00:1–14 https://doi.org/10.1111/jan.15992

Family Violence Death Review Committee 2017 Fifth annual report data: January 2009 to December 2015. HQSC https://www.hqsc.govt.nz/assets/Our-work/Mortality-review-committee/FVDRC/Publications-resources/FVDRC_2017_10_final_web.pdf

Family Violence Death Review Committee 2022 A duty to care. Me manaaki te tangata: seventh report. HQSC. Online. Available: https://www.hqsc.govt.nz/assets/Our-work/Mortality-review-committee/FVDRC/Publications-resources/Seventh-report-transcripts/FVDRC-seventh-report-web.pdf

Glover K, Gartland D, Leane C et al 2022 Development, acceptability and construct validity of the Aboriginal Women's Experiences of Partner Violence Scale (AEPVS): a co-designed, multiphase study nested within an Australian Aboriginal and Torres Strait Islander birth cohort. BMJ Open 12(8):e059576 Online. Available: https://doi.org/10.1136/bmjopen-2021-059576

Hashemi L, Fanslow J, Gulliver P et al 2021 Exploring the health burden of cumulative and specific adverse childhood experiences in New Zealand: results from a population-based study. Child Abuse and Neglect 122: 105372 https://doi.org/10.1016/j.chiabu.2021.105372

Hellwig K 2023 Elder abuse. Home Healthcare Now 41 (6):304–308 doi: 10.1097/NHH.0000000000001196

Hollingdrake O, Saadi N, Alban Cru A et al 2023 Qualitative study of the perspectives of women with lived experience of domestic and family violence on accessing healthcare. Journal of Advanced Nursing 79: 1353–1366 https://doi.org/10.1111/jan.15316

Hutchinson M, Daly J, Jackson D et al 2015 Leadership when there are no easy answers: applying leader moral courage to wicked problems. Journal of Clinical Nursing 24(21–22):3021–3023

Jack S M, Wilson D, Bradbury-Jones C 2023 Advancing nursing's response to the wicked problem of intimate partner violence. Journal of Advanced Nursing 79:e18–e20 https://doi.org/10.1111/jan.15664

Kelly U A 2011 Theories of intimate partner violence: from blaming the victim to acting against injustice. Intersectionality as an analytic framework. Advances in Nursing Science 34(3):E29–E51 https://doi.org/10.1097/ANS.0b013e3182272388

Klingspohn D M 2018 The importance of culture in addressing domestic violence for First Nation's women. Policy and Practice Reviews 9:1–7, Article 872 https://doi.org/10.3389/fpsyg.2018.00872

Luebke J, Hawkins M, Lucchesi A et al 2021 The utility of postcolonial and Indigenous feminist frameworks in guiding nursing research and practice about intimate partner violence in the lives of American Indian Women. Journal of Transcultural Nursing 32(6):639–646 https://doi.org/10.1177/1043659621992602

Mellar B, Gulliver P, Selak V et al 2023 Association between men's exposure to intimate partner violence and self-reported health outcomes in New Zealand. JAMA Network Open 6(1):e2252578–e2252578 https://doi.org/10.1001/jamanetworkopen.2022.52578

Pihama L, Cameron N, Pitman M et al 2021 Whāia te ara ora: understanding and healing the impact of historical trauma and sexual violence for Māori. Māori and Indigenous Analysis

Qu L, Kaspew R, Carson R et al 2021 National elder abuse prevalence study: final report. Australian Institute of Family Studies. Online. Available: https://aifs.gov.au/research/research-reports/national-elder-abuse-prevalence-study-final-report

Rizkalla K, Maar M, Pilon R et al 2020 Improving the response of primary care providers to rural First Nation women who experience intimate partner violence: a qualitative study. BMC Women's Health 20(1):209 https://doi.org/10.1186/s12905-020-01053-y

Rouland B, Vaithianathan R, Wilson D et al 2019 Ethnic disparities in childhood prevalence of maltreatment: evidence from a New Zealand birth cohort. American Journal of Public Health 109(9):1255–1257 https://doi.org/10.2105/ajph.2019.305163

Shaqiqi W, Innab A 2023 Attitude and preparedness of nursing students in Saudi Arabia concerning the managing of intimate partner violence. Journal of Advanced Nursing 79:1553–1563 https://doi.org/10.1111/jan.15424

Spangaro J, Herring S, Koziol-Mclain J et al 2016 'They aren't really black fellas but they are easy to talk to': factors which influence Australian Aboriginal women's decision to disclose intimate partner violence during pregnancy. Midwifery 41:79–88 https://doi.org/https://doi.org/10.1016/j.midw.2016.08.004

Spearman K J, Hardesty J L, Campbell J 2023 Post-separation abuse: a concept analysis. Journal of Advanced Nursing 79:1225–1246 https://doi.org/10.1111/jan.15310

Stark E 2007 Coercive control: how men entrap women in personal life. Oxford University Press

Tolmie J, Smith R, Short J et al 2018 Social entrapment: a realistic understanding of criminal offending of primary victims of intimate partner violence. New Zealand Law Review 2018(2):181–217

Tolmie J, Smith R, Wilson D 2024 Understanding intimate partner violence: why coercive control requires a social and systemic entrapment framework. Violence Against Women 30(1):54–74 https://doi.org/10.1177/10778012231205585

United Nations 1990 Convention on the Rights of the Child. United Nations. Online. Available: https://www.ohchr.org/en/instruments-mechanisms/instruments/convention-rights-child

United Nations 2007 United Nations Declaration on the Rights of Indigenous Peoples. United Nations. Online. Available: https://www.un.org/development/desa/indigenouspeoples/wp-content/uploads/sites/19/2018/11/UNDRIP_E_web.pdf

United Nations 2015 Universal Declaration of Human Rights. United Nations. Online. Available: https://www.un.org/en/udhrbook/

Wilson D 1997 Through the looking glass: nurses' responses to women experiencing partner abuse [Masters, Massey University]. Online. Available: http://hdl.handle.net/10179/5636

Wilson D 2016 Transforming the normalisation of intergenerational whānau (family) violence. Journal of Indigenous Wellbeing 1(2):32–43 Oline. Available: https://journalindigenouswellbeing.com/media/2017/12/84.81.Investigating-M%C4%81ori-approaches-to-trauma-informed-care.pdf

Wilson D 2023 A litany of sound revisited: violence within whānau and mahi tūkino. Te Pūkotahitanga Ministry of Justice.

Wilson D, Mikahere-Hall A, Sherwood J et al 2019a E Tū Wāhine, E Tū Whānau: Māori women keeping safe in unsafe relationships. Taupua Waiora Māori Research Centre, AUT. Online. Available: https://openrepository.aut.ac.nz/handle/10292/13068

Wilson D, Mikahere-Hall A, Sherwood J et al 2019b E Tū Wāhine, E Tū Whānau: Wāhine Māori keeping safe in unsafe relationships. AUT Taupua Waiora Māori Research Centre. Online. Available: https://openrepository.aut.ac.nz/handle/10292/13068

Withiel T D, Sheridan S, Rudd N et al 2022 Preparedness to respond to family violence: a cross-sectional study across clinical areas. SAGE Open Nursing 8:23779608221126355 https://doi.org/10.1177/23779608221126355

World Health Organization (WHO) 2014a Global status report on violence prevention 2014. WHO. Online. Available: https://www.who.int/publications/i/item/9789241564793

World Health Organization (WHO) 2014b Health care for women subjected to intimate partner violence or sexual violence: a clinical handbook. WHO. Online. Available: https://apps.who.int/iris/handle/10665/136101

World Health Organization (WHO) 2022 Tackling abuse of older people: five priorities for the UN Decade of Healthy Ageing (2021–2030). WHO. Online. Available: https://www.who.int/publications-detail-redirect/9789240052550

CHAPTER 17

RURAL AND REMOTE NURSING

Marie Hutchinson and Leah East

KEY WORDS

communities
health
healthcare
Indigenous
nursing
remote
rural

LEARNING OBJECTIVES

After reading this chapter, readers should be able to:

- identify the nature of rural communities and the major factors that influence their health status
- outline some of the challenges of providing healthcare in rural and remote locations
- describe the characteristics of rural and remote nursing and the challenges and rewards of the role
- identify the continuing challenge for nursing in addressing the health needs of rural and remote communities.

INTRODUCTION

Rural nursing is a dynamic and rewarding area of nursing practice that offers many unique professional experiences. If you have had little personal experience of living in the country, understanding how rurality shapes nursing practice and the health of these communities is a challenging task. This chapter is focused on the health of rural and remote communities, the multi-faceted nature of living in these locations and the scope of practice, challenges and rewards of rural nursing.

Rural nursing

The health of rural and remote communities, and the challenges of providing equitable and accessible healthcare in locations that are often long distances from major urban centres is an ongoing global healthcare issue (World Health Organization [WHO] 2021). Nurses have a long tradition of providing care in rural and remote locations. Nurses, midwives and Aboriginal and Torres Strait Islander Health Workers represent by far the largest group of health professionals in the rural sector (Australian Government Department of Health and Aged Care 2023). In many rural and remote communities, nurses are recognised as the backbone of healthcare and are advanced autonomous 'specialist generalists' who provide for the breadth of healthcare needs of their community, ranging from primary healthcare, mental health, maternity and child health, palliation, chronic and aged care to emergency and crisis intervention (McCullough 2022).

Distance from urban centres and population sparsity are frequently used to define the concept of rurality. These are useful concepts to initially understand the concept of remoteness. However, if you think more broadly about rurality you will come to understand that location, history, culture, economic policy, place and identity feature strongly in what it means to live in a rural or remote location. For nurses working and living in these locations, the nature of their practice is strongly influenced by all these factors, making rural nursing one of the more challenging and rewarding fields of nursing.

Introducing rural and remote populations

Approximately one-quarter of the Australian population live in rural or regional areas. Likewise, approximately 20% of New Zealanders reside in rural areas (Australian Government Department of Health and Aged Care 2023, Ministry of Health 2023). Reflecting the distance from urban centres, Australian settings are described as either being inner or outer regional, remote, or very remote areas (Australian Bureau of Statistics [ABS] 2023). Similarly, in New Zealand (Aotearoa), settings are classified into rural areas of either high, moderate or low urban influences or reliance, or highly rural/remote areas that have relative independence from employment from urban centres (Stats NZ 2020).

For the first time since 1981, coinciding with the COVID-19 pandemic, Australia's regional population grew more than the capital cities with large numbers of capital city residents migrating to the regional areas (ABS 2022). Country living became highly desirable among urban dwellers who sought a change, desiring greater space and less congestion compared with metropolitan regions, which contributes to the rich diversity of rural communities. Traditionally, rural and remote communities have been portrayed through stereotypical images of living in the sticks, farming the land and being somehow backward or inferior (Malatzky & Couch 2023). In stark contrast to these assumptions, country people do not necessarily live on a farm, and they are not inevitably rustic; instead, they live in many different places and are characterised by great diversity and innovation. The diversity of rural and remote communities can include farming, coastal and rainforest regions, communal living and tourist islands or mining towns that are characterised by their unique cultural and philosophical beliefs.

As nurses, when reflecting upon what it means to live in or come from the country, it is important to move beyond defining rural and urban in simple geographic, consumerist or material terms. Instead, it is important to give attention to understanding the subjective, deep-rooted and shared social understanding of association and identification that shape rural character and culture.

Understanding the health of rural and remote people requires that one consider the relationship between people, place and identity. Strong cultural, spiritual or generational ties can exist to the land, traditions and the people, which can shape the sense of personal and community identity. For First Nations peoples, identity is inextricably linked to community, person, land, spirituality and place, encompassing a way of being that creates complex relational bonds and reciprocal obligations (Quigley et al 2022, Ross et al 2023). These interrelated connections between culture, place and people are important for wellbeing, and having to relocate away from their place of country for healthcare can hinder wellbeing (Quigley et al 2022).

> ### REFLECTION
> Think of a rural or remote location—describe the characteristics of the people living in this community. What has shaped your impression?
> Or, if you do not have experience or knowledge of a rural or remote location, think of a film or television depiction of a rural community. How were rural people characterised? What do you think has shaped these depictions?

The tyranny of distance and population sparsity

In rural and remote contexts, the cost of delivering services is much higher compared with urban areas, and the accessibility and availability of services is lower (Australian Institute of Health and Welfare [AIHW] 2023a). As a result, resources are often spread sparsely across large areas. On average, rural and remote people are disadvantaged in their access to goods and services and may have greater exposure to risk factors that cause ill-health compared with their urban counterparts (AIHW 2023a). For these communities, the tyranny of distance is also compounded by population numbers, which in many instances may be too small to generate sufficient demand to sustain viable services. Sustainability of services is exacerbated by attracting a healthcare workforce and a decline in population as people move away in search of greater employment opportunities (Ministry of Health 2023).

Recent decades have seen significant demographic and economic change in rural and remote communities. Some communities experience the simultaneous redesign or withdrawal of services, population decline, growing unemployment and a deterioration in their living conditions as a result of, for example, climate change and natural disasters (Ministry of Health 2023). Economic and resource-driven models of service provision and urban-centric approaches to education, transport and health policy have impacted the resilience and population growth in rural and remote communities (Bec et al 2018). Cost-effectiveness and the centralisation of services have seen the redesign or loss of healthcare facilities, schools and other essential services such as banks. This change has had a profound effect on the social circumstances of people living in these communities and is said to have exacerbated economic decline and population drift (Hettihewa & Wright 2018). In contrast to this picture of decline, some rural and remote communities have experienced economic and population growth. Relocating to regional and rural communities has become attractive due to affordability, more flexible work arrangements, lifestyle and the creation of community connectiveness (Crommelin et al 2022).

These shifts in population mean that, in some communities, the distinction between rural and urban identity is no longer as clear-cut as it may have been in the past, with once rural country towns becoming large regional centres. The movement of populations in this way also amplifies the imbalance in healthcare provision, with population growth moving ahead of the capacity to provide services.

The health of rural and remote communities

People living in rural and remote communities face many challenges; in the main they experience more health disadvantage, are less healthy, experience greater illness and mortality than their city counterparts and have lower rates of GP consultation and generally higher rates of hospital admissions (AIHW 2023a). The deeply embedded economic and social disparity experienced in rural and remote communities equates to lower incomes, fewer healthcare and educational opportunities and higher rates of illness and mortality (AIHW 2023a). For conditions such as preterm birth and low birth weight, there is evidence to suggest there are significantly increased risks for both of these poorer outcomes in rural and remote areas. Babies born in remote areas are at up to twice the risk of preterm birth, with low birth weight 15% higher in very remote areas of New South Wales (Bizuayehu et al 2023). Time to diagnosis and treatment for some cancers is significantly longer for people living in rural and more remote communities (Foley et al 2023). Refer to Box 17.1 for a summary of current information related to the state of health in rural and remote populations.

For people in rural and remote regions, the limited access to healthcare services can be exacerbated by widely held attitudes to health, illness and help seeking. Research indicates that stoicism and perceived stigma are underlying factors in accessing and seeking healthcare among rural communities (Coombs et al 2022). Other research has found that access to essential healthcare services for a chronic illness is emotionally burdensome, attributed to the required travel to receive

---

BOX 17.1
The state of health in rural and remote populations

- People residing in rural and remote areas are 5.4 times more likely to experience death due to transport accidents compared with people residing in regional and city areas (AIHW 2023a)
- As remoteness increases, so does the incidence of risky behaviours, such as smoking and consuming alcohol, at levels creating risk of lifetime harm. The proportion of the population smoking tobacco daily in remote areas is twice that of people in major cities (AIHW 2023a)
- Residents of remote areas in New Zealand (Aotearoa) and Australia have fewer educational qualifications than the national average and have much lower rates of expected university completion (Sullivan et al 2018)
- In Australia, approximately 20% of Indigenous peoples live in remote or very remote areas, and on the whole their life expectancy is approximately 15 years lower compared with that of non-Indigenous people (ABS, Australian Government Department of Ageing 2023).
- Māori-Indigenous New Zealanders residing in rural areas have a lower life expectancy compared with their non-Indigenous counterparts (Crampton & Baxter 2018)

care, being away from community and family, isolation and the experienced financial hardship (Walker et al 2022) highlighting the complexity rural and remote communities experience within the context of health equity. An additional complexity rural people may face in disclosing their health concerns is that the professional may reside in their community, or alternatively, when seeking care from distant services they hold concern that cultural or behavioural differences may result in them being misunderstood. Individuals residing in rural areas, in particular men, are more likely to avoid seeking healthcare, with masculine norms predictive of more negative attitudes towards help seeking (Piatkowski et al 2023). A concerning outcome associated with these help-seeking characteristics is the elevated rates of suicide in rural and remote populations, particularly among males.

The proportion of Aboriginal, Torres Strait Islanders and Māori (First Nations) population increases with remoteness (AIHW 2023a), with their health being an important part of the fabric of rural life. Importantly, these communities typically have a younger population profile, and among young people (aged 10–24 years) there is an increased burden of chronic health problems such as mental illness, type 2 diabetes and ischaemic heart disease (Azzopardi et al 2018). The poorer health status of First Nations peoples in rural and remote communities contributes to the higher rates of morbidity and mortality (AIHW 2023b), a lower life expectancy, increased rates of low birth weight and infant mortality, and an increased risk of suicide (AIHW 2023b). A retrospective study reported the fatality rate for Aboriginal and Torres Strait Islander children admitted to the Sydney Children's Hospital was double that of non-Aboriginal children, with Aboriginal and Torres Strait Islander children under 2 years and from remote and regional communities at highest risk of excess mortality (Singer et al 2019). There is also an increased risk of developmental vulnerability, stemming from long waiting times for assessment, diagnosis and treatment, and difficulty accessing paediatric health services (Cumming 2019).

Ageing is another factor affecting rural and remote communities, with lack of access to local appropriate services being particularly problematic. Although little is known about how the experience of growing older may be different in urban and rural areas, the existing health inequity experienced by rural and remote communities is predicted to be exacerbated particularly in relation to the provision of aged care services. For example, while it is currently acknowledged that there is a shortage of aged care services in rural communities, this shortage is set to increase unless over 3000 residential healthcare places can be implemented throughout rural Australian communities (Blackberry & Morris 2023). Consideration of aged care services is warranted as many individuals may be reluctant to relocate due to healthcare needs, which can contribute to the burden of illness and potentially shorter life span experienced in rural and remote communities.

The challenge of providing health services in rural and remote locations

When regional, rural and remote locations are compared with urban centres, they often have lower levels of access to health services and the profile of the health workforce varies significantly. In general, there is a misdistribution of the health workforce between urban centres and rural and remote communities and attracting experienced healthcare professionals to these locations is a constant challenge (WHO 2021). Both Australia and New Zealand (Aotearoa) have relied extensively on overseas trained healthcare professionals to fill this void (Cosgrave et al

2019), with financial schemes and training programs continually being developed to attract healthcare professionals, including nurses, to staff regional and remote healthcare positions. Despite more than a doubling in the number of Australian-trained healthcare professionals since the 1990s, locally trained graduates are less likely to take up employment in rural communities compared with graduates from previous decades (O'Sullivan et al 2019). In response to the continuing challenge of recruitment in rural and remote communities, a number of specific models of health service have been developed—these include: Indigenous health services, which are often community-controlled organisations; multi-purpose services that provide integrated services such as aged care, medical or community services; the Royal Flying Doctor Service, which provides emergency and primary care outreach services; outreach medical and allied health services and on-call primary care services staffed by GPs and nurses. Other strategies to improve access to specialist and primary care services in outlying communities include fly-in fly-out (FIFO) services and the increased use of virtual health.

Despite innovative healthcare initiatives continuously being developed to connect healthcare to rural and remote communities, the presence of a hospital remains an important factor in the provision of health services in rural or urban communities. Yet, the closure of rural and remote hospitals continues to occur internationally, with factors such as cost and workforce issues underpinning these closures (Vaughan & Edwards 2020). As a result, the increasing use of other models of care is becoming more prominent in rural and remote communities.

The development of e-health initiatives, such as remote liaison nurses who link and support patients from remote areas to metropolitan hospitals, is an important initiative in the provision of healthcare to rural and remote communities. As IT and communication technology has evolved, digital healthcare technologies such as telehealth are being extensively employed enabling the overcoming of barriers in access to care among rural and regional communities (Butzner & Cuffee 2021). Telehealth services now deliver expert consultation in areas such as mental health, paediatrics, oncology, gerontology, palliative care, cancer care, the treatment of hepatitis C and the management of diabetes, heart failure and wounds to rural and remote communities. Telehealth ranges from computer-based support and web-based video consultation with specialist clinicians to store-and-forward diagnostics for remote interpretation. These services operate in community nursing services, hospitals, general practices and residential aged care facilities and report a high level of acceptability by patients (Orlando et al 2019). The increased use of e-health is an important strategy to address urban–rural health disparities and reduce the likelihood of patients needing to relocate for treatment. However, while virtual health and digital technologies (e-health, telehealth) are increasingly being used to connect communities to healthcare services, the effectiveness of virtual models of care is reliant on user digital literacy, preference of how care is received among individuals, infrastructure support and internet availability (Budhwani et al 2022).

The challenge of providing health services in rural and remote communities not only shapes the services available, it also has a major impact on the practice of health professionals. Imagine a serious accident over 500 km from a major health facility and 150 km to the closest town with a small hospital, and it is possible to begin to understand the challenge of providing healthcare in rural and remote contexts. In many settings, nurses will be required to respond to such an accident and, in the more isolated locations, may have little immediate support or back-up.

> **REFLECTION**
>
> Identify a rural town and conduct an internet search to identify the range of health services available to residents.
>
> Do you think that the health services provided are equitable compared to those for residents in a major urban city?
>
> Imagine you are a nurse in this community. Where might you work, what other services would be available to support you in your role and what types of telehealth services might outreach to this community?

The nature of rural and remote nursing

Rural and remote nursing is dynamic in nature and offers immense opportunity for professional and personal development. Nurses working in these locations describe their work as diverse, and the varied nature of this work provides opportunities and challenges unique from other nursing experiences (Australian Government Office of the National Rural Health Commissioner 2023). Rural and remote nurses are often somewhat embedded within the community in which they work. They establish strong relationships with community members and are frequently perceived as being a part of the community to whom they provide care (MacKay et al 2021) and for whom they care throughout the life span. The experience of nursing in a rural or remote context is often characterised by the development of deep and effective relationships in the communities that nurses serve with a sense of connection to the place and the community in which care is provided (MacKay et al 2021).

In their dual role of nurse and community member, rural and remote nurses will often personally know or have knowledge about most people in their community (Osik Szumer & Arnold 2023). This lack of anonymity, entwinement of personal and private lives and the high level of visibility create particular challenges for nursing practice. When a nurse in an urban hospital provides care, few but the immediate family of the patient know the details of the care provided. In contrast, the actions of rural nurses are more visible and known to the community. This high level of visibility can be a difficult work–life challenge for nurses who take up employment in rural and remote communities and contributes to higher levels of safety risk. Maintaining privacy and confidentiality in this context requires that nurses establish clear boundaries between their private and work life and strategies to ensure practice is in accordance with professional frameworks, codes and guidelines (Osik Szumer & Arnold 2023).

Scope of practice

Rural and remote nursing is characterised by a high degree of responsibility and autonomy, considerable flexibility and a requirement for extended or advanced skills. As broad generalists, rural and remote nurses' practice includes prevention, primary care, rehabilitation and acute interventions, and requires both clinical and cultural knowledge. In more geographically isolated areas nurses are likely to be the principal clinician on site, working at a distance from the multidisciplinary team. These nurses can experience a compression of the complexity of their role as they fulfil advanced roles, and also take on additional unplanned expectations (Australian Government Office of the National Rural Health Commissioner 2023a).

In both Australia and New Zealand (Aotearoa), the scope of practice of rural and remote nurses has been described as extended, advanced and expanded (Australian Government Office of the National Rural Health Commissioner 2023, Ross et al 2023). Furthermore, the scope of practice of nurses working in these settings varies according to the needs of the population and the range of other services available. Though scope of practice in these regions varies, rural and remote nursing encompasses both primary healthcare approaches and the provision of general nursing care, including acute and critical care, case management, health promotion initiatives and, in some instances, nurses exercise their managerial and entrepreneurial skills to forge new innovative models of care and initiatives to meet the unique needs of the communities in which they work (Ross et al 2023).

In outer regional and remote locations, additional multidisciplinary services are provided by outreach services and various forms of telecommunication support consultation. This means that nurses in these settings must establish and maintain effective working relationships with other team members who are often at a considerable distance (Crowther et al 2019, Kosteniuk et al 2019). This working relationship provides the 'cultural mentorship' that nurses require working in such a demanding environment, and helps ensure the care they provide is culturally appropriate (Liaw et al 2019).

Extended, advanced and solo nursing roles

As remoteness increases, there are a decreasing number of healthcare professionals available within communities and the scope of practice of nurses becomes more extended or advanced. For many nurses in rural and remote locations their practice extends across the scope of registered nurse practice to include the full spectrum of care, from the provision of primary healthcare to frontline emergency care (McCullough et al 2022). Working autonomously with greater responsibility for care means that nurses working in isolated rural or remote locations require not only experience, but also extensive knowledge, specialised skills and the ability to anticipate problems, negotiate safety and mobilise emergency transport systems (Smith et al 2019). Providing on-call services is also a feature of outer regional and remote locations. In these locations nurses work in partnership with doctors or, in instances where there is no doctor available, nurses are the mainstay of healthcare and on-call for the local community. Imagine providing diabetic education in the morning and by the afternoon providing frontline critical care to a patient who has been involved in a motor vehicle accident.

In a number of remote Indigenous communities, fly-in mine sites or small isolated towns, solo-nurse clinics operate to provide the only form of on-site healthcare. These nurses live and work in physically difficult circumstances, are required to undertake high levels of on-call work, have heavy workload demands and report a high level of safety risk and personal violence, particularly at single nurse posts or during callouts (Wright et al 2021). Nurses working in these settings are often unable to take leave and are on 24-hour call for long periods of time (McCullough et al 2022). High staff turnover resulting from these pressures increases the workload for remaining nurses and is associated with poorer health outcomes for Aboriginal people living in remote communities (Zhao et al 2019). These issues have been of longstanding concern to remote area nurses, with a growing consensus that solo-nurse services should be abandoned in favour of teams of nurses with suitable qualifications and experience to undertake this role.

In New Zealand (Aotearoa), there has been a significant increase in the rural postgraduate-qualified primary healthcare nursing workforce with healthcare reforms positioning nurses at the foreground of primary healthcare delivery in rural communities (Ross et al 2023). In Australia, while there is a large rural and remote nursing workforce, the nurse practitioner role has developed strongly around specialised areas of clinical practice, with 70% of these advanced practice nurses working in metropolitan areas, rather than in underserviced rural and remote communities (Rossiter et al 2023). Even though university courses and government initiatives have been introduced to support the rural nursing workforce, and some nurses working in remote communities have expanded their knowledge and undertaken postgraduate qualifications, research suggests that many are still ill-equipped and poorly prepared for the demands of extended and advanced practice roles (McCullough et al 2022).

To meet the demands of underserviced healthcare needs in the community, remote nurses fulfil advanced practice roles far wider than that of the nurse practitioner, often with minimal formal preparation for the role and outside of the legislated boundaries of registered nurse practice (MacLeod et al 2019). A continued criticism of Australian rural health policy has been an almost exclusive policy focus on medical workforce supply issues. While it is important to acknowledge the importance of doctors, any solution to the critical problems faced by rural and remote communities must also address nursing workforce issues.

> ### REFLECTION
> What do you think the differences would be in working in a remote community such as Coober Pedy in Australia or the Gisborne region of New Zealand (Aotearoa) as either a registered nurse or an undergraduate nurse compared with working in a large metropolitan referral hospital in a capital city?
> Have you or would you consider undertaking a clinical placement in a remote community? Why or why not?

The challenge of sustaining the rural and remote workforce

Although rural and remote area nurses have greater autonomy and can work to their full scope of practice, a downside of the role is that this group of nurses are more likely to experience high levels of occupational stress. The demands of working in rural and remote settings are said to be compounded by workload and scope of practice, poor resources and violence and safety concerns (McKay et al 2021). In the face of these challenges, rural and remote area nurses can experience considerable role stress (McKay et al 2021) with additional pressures stemming from unrealistic expectations of communities and health services that cannot be met (McKay et al 2021).

One study among rural and remote nurses highlighted the difficulties and the contention between scope of practice and sustaining life in addition to the accountability felt by nurses working remotely. The increase in responsibility resulting in a decline of services has increased the demand on nurses, which is also exacerbated by the ongoing challenge of providing care for emergency presentations for which they may not feel skilled or have the experience to manage (Whiteing et al 2021). Rural and remote nursing is characterised by many challenges that increase the likelihood of experiencing psychological distress, which has continued to be recognised for at least the last two decades (Whiteing et al 2021). Interventions such as greater professional development, review of scope of practice and generally greater support may in part assist the emotional demands experienced by rural and remote nurses (Whiteing et al 2021). For nurses working in rural and remote communities the support and mentorship of colleagues and managers is also a crucial factor in retention (McKay et al 2021).

Recruiting and retaining a health workforce is a significant issue across Australia and New Zealand (Aotearoa). In response, educational providers have developed a range of undergraduate clinical placement initiatives to expose students to practices in rural and remote settings. In addition to a rural background or previous rural living, factors known to increase interest in a rural health career include rural placement programs that provide unique clinical experiences and influence more positive views about future work in such areas (Crossley et al 2023). Research following the longitudinal trajectory of undergraduate students into their postgraduate years suggests that these placements provide students with preparation and support, a rural or remote health experience, and exposure to rural lifestyles and socialisation (Crossley et al 2023). However, living and studying in rural communities can create particular challenges for students and preceptors. Preceptors may struggle to make themselves available to students and educating metropolitan academics is important to ensure they select students who will maximise the opportunities presented (Walsh et al 2023), while students report that a sense of isolation can increase stress (Crossley et al 2023).

In rural areas, new graduates have the added challenge of transitioning to work roles that demand a broader knowledge base and range of generalist skills. Crossley et al (2023) highlight the importance of providing additional support for graduates to ensure they successfully transition to practice in the rural workforce. These types of support programs provide increased opportunities for learning, as well as additional guidance as graduates adapt to the unique aspects of the rural nurse's role and responsibilities (Crossley 2023). A number of initiatives are also in place to attract graduates to rural areas. However, these are largely, but not exclusively, targeted towards medical graduates. These initiatives include salary incentives to work in areas of greatest need, bonded scholarships and a range of non-financial incentives for graduates.

STORY

Providing telehealth to three very remote communities

Gangan, Yilpara and Wandawuy are three very remote communities in the Northern Territory. These small communities are 200 km (on unsealed roads) from the nearest larger town, and 750 km from Darwin. The health clinics in these communities are staffed by Aboriginal Health Practitioners (AHP), with weekly nursing visits and a periodic general practitioner. In these remote communities the whole family is involved in decision making, with relevant family members needing to be present during important healthcare consultations to allow for family decision making.

During a weekly visit the nurse talks with a community member about them needing to travel to Darwin for further investigation and urgent treatment of a tumour. Understanding the need for whole-family decision making, the nurse liaises with the AHP who arranges a telehealth consultation with important family members across a number of different communities. This telehealth consultation allowed the whole family to be involved in the consultation with the treating surgeon and a decision made about treatment.

Given the distances and difficulty with travel between these communities, prior to the advent of telehealth it may have taken many weeks for this type of family conversation and decision making to occur. This delay would have risked a poorer outcome and potentially an inoperable tumour. Telehealth allowed group decision making that respected culture, with conversations in the patient's preferred language. This facilitated a timelier decision and reduced the burden of travel.

Each week nurses, GPs and AHPs in these communities use telehealth for a wide range of consultations, and when emergencies arise, the accurate assessment of the need for emergency retrieval. This real-time remote assessment has been a game changer in these remote communities, allowing for earlier detection and treatment. Expanding these types of telehealth services requires improved access to broadband in remote communities.

Reflective questions

1 Critically reflect upon this situation and consider the possible impact of missed or delayed care for people living in rural and remote communities. How might telehealth reduce these risks?
2 Imagine you are the nurse at the remote nursing station in this scenario. What additional skills would you need for this type of telehealth consultation? Think about the type of equipment (such as an audio stethoscope) that you might need in this telehealth clinic.

(Clair et al 2019)

The circumstances described in the telehealth care story above demonstrate how technology is transforming the provision of healthcare in rural and remote locations. Supporting early cancer treatment is a national priority, particularly in rural and remote communities where rates of cancer and poorer cancer outcomes are higher. The inability to support community or extended family decisions for Aboriginal and Torres Strait Islander people living in remote communities may impact health trajectories and risk increased trauma related to travel (Clair et al 2019). Aboriginal and community-controlled health organisations have been very effective in improving health outcomes in their communities, and there have been calls to increase training for Aboriginal Health Workers (Dossetor et al 2023). Combined with initiatives such as telehealth, there is the potential to significantly address barriers to healthcare experienced by rural and remote communities. Nurses are at the forefront of leading many of the telehealth initiatives in regional, rural and remote communities. This technology will continue to influence how nurses undertake assessment, and create additional challenges with regard to consent, patient education, confidentiality and record keeping.

CONCLUSION

Nursing has a long-established tradition of providing healthcare in rural and remote locations, often in the face of great adversity. The determinants of health for people living in rural and remote locations are poorer than for their urban counterparts. This disadvantage arises from a complex interplay of geographic, economic, social and policy factors. This disadvantage impacts not only on the people living in these communities and seeking healthcare, but also on the healthcare workers who support these communities. In recognising these challenges, educational programs and government support and incentives are continually being implemented to foster growth, safety and improved working conditions among rural and remote nurses and to facilitate optimal care for people residing in rural and remote communities. Despite these challenges, rural and remote nursing is a highly rewarding career that offers unique and rich experiences that can be both professionally and personally fulfilling.

REFLECTIVE QUESTIONS

1. Consider the health status of rural and remote Australia or New Zealand (Aotearoa). What are the major health issues? Identify strategies to improve this situation. How might nurses implement or incorporate these strategies in their practice?
2. Working in a rural setting means nurses often work autonomously with few immediate supports. What type of supports could be introduced to assist rural and remote nurses and reduce burnout?
3. Reflecting back on your undergraduate preparation, what additional skills would you need to work in a rural and remote location? What type of education do you think would prepare you for the role of a beginning rural or remote area nurse?

Recommended readings

Australian Institute of Health and Welfare 2023 Rural and remote health, Canberra. Online. Available: https://www.aihw.gov.au/reports/rural-remote-australians/rural-and-remote-health 22 November 2023

Ministry of Health 2023 Rural Health Strategy. Wellington: Ministry of Health

References

Australian Bureau of Statistics (ABS) (July 2021–June 2026) (ABS) 2023 Remoteness areas. Online. Available: https://www.abs.gov.au/statistics/standards/australian-statistical-geography-standard-asgs-edition-3/jul2021-jun2026/remoteness-structure/remoteness-areas#cite-window1

Australian Bureau of Statistics (ABS) 2022 Gangan, Yilpara and Wandawuy, ABS. Online. Available: https://www.abs.gov.au/media-centre/media-releases/more-growth-regions-during-pandemic 9 January 2024

Australian Government Department of Health and Aged Care 2023 Summary statistics, remoteness area. Online. Available: https://hwd.health.gov.au/resources/data/summary-remote.html 27 November 2023

Australian Government Office of the National Rural Health Commissioner 2023 The National Rural and Remote Nursing Generalist Framework 2023–2027. Online. Available: https://www.health.gov.au/sites/default/files/2023-03/the-national-rural-and-remote-nursing-generalist-framework-2023-2027.pdf

Australian Institute of Health and Welfare (AIHW) 2023a Rural and remote health, Canberra. Online. Available: https://www.aihw.gov.au/reports/rural-remote-australians/rural-and-remote-health 22 November 2023

Australian Institute of Health and Welfare (AIHW) 2023b Aboriginal and Torres Strait Islander Health Performance Framework: summary report July 2023. Online. Available: https://www.indigenoushpf.gov.au/ 28 November 2023

Azzopardi P S, Sawyer S M, Carlin J B et al 2018 Health and wellbeing of Indigenous adolescents in Australia: a systematic synthesis of population data. The Lancet 391(10122):766–782

Bec A, Moyle B, Moyle C L 2018 Resilient and sustainable communities. Sustainability 10(12):4810

Bizuayehu H M, Harris M L, Chojenta C et al 2023 Maternal residential area effects on preterm birth, low birth weight and caesarean section in Australia: a systematic review. Midwifery 123:103704 doi: 10.1016/j.midw.2023.103704. Epub 2023 May 3. PMID: 37196576.

Blackberry I, Morris N 2023 The impact of population ageing on rural aged care needs in Australia: identifying projected gaps in service provision by 2032. Geriatrics (Basel) 27;8(3):47 doi: 10.3390/geriatrics8030047. PMID: 37218827; PMCID: PMC10204523

Budhwani S, Fujioka J, Thomas-Jacques T et al 2022 Challenges and strategies for promoting health equity in virtual care: findings and policy directions from a scoping review of reviews. Journal of the American Medical Informatics Association 29(5):990–999 doi: 10.1093/jamia/ocac022. PMID: 35187571; PMCID: PMC9006706.

Butzner M, Cuffee Y 2021 Telehealth interventions and outcomes across rural communities in the United States: narrative review. Journal of Medical Internet Research 23(8):e29575

Clair M S, Murtagh D P, Kelly J et al 2019 Telehealth a game changer: closing the gap in remote Aboriginal communities. Medical Journal of Australia 210: S36–S37 https://doi.org/10.5694/mja2.50036

Coombs N C, Campbell D G, Caringi J 2022 A qualitative study of rural healthcare providers' views of social, cultural, and programmatic barriers to healthcare access. BMC Health Service Research 22:438 https://doi.org/10.1186/s12913-022-07829-2

Cosgrave C, Malatzky C, Gillespie J 2019 Social determinants of rural health workforce retention: a scoping review. International Journal of Environmental Research and Public Health 16(3):314

Crampton P, Baxter J 2018 Rural matters. New Zealand Medical Journal 131(1485):6–7

Crommelin L, Denham T, Troy L et al 2022 Understanding the lived experience and benefits of regional cities, AHURI Final Report No. 377. Australian Housing and Urban Research Institute Limited, Melbourne. Online. Available: https://www.ahuri.edu.au/ research/final-reports/377, doi: 10.18408/ahuri7126301

Crossley C, Collett M, Thompson S C 2023 Tracks to postgraduate rural practice: longitudinal qualitative follow-up of nursing students who undertook a rural placement in Western Australia. International Journal of Environmental Research and Public Health 20:5113 https://doi.org/10.3390/ijerph20065113

Crowther S, Deery R, Daellenbach R et al 2019 Joys and challenges of relationships in Scotland and New Zealand rural midwifery: a multicentre study. Women and Birth 32(1):39–49

Cumming T 2019 Lived experiences of seeking support for rural and remote children with developmental challenges. White Paper. Charles Sturt University. Online. Available: https://www.royalfarwest.org.au/wp-content/uploads/2019/02/Lived_Experiences_-White_-Paper_T_Cumming_CSU.pdf

Dossetor P J, Freeman J M, Thorburn K et al 2023 Health services for Aboriginal and Torres Strait Islander children in remote Australia: a scoping review. PLOS Global Public Health 3(2):e0001140 doi: 10.1371/journal.pgph.0001140

Foley J, Wishart L R, Ward E C et al 2023 Exploring the impact of remoteness on people with head and neck cancer: utilisation of a state-wide dataset. Australian Journal of Rural Health 31(4):726–743

Hettihewa S, Wright C S 2018 Nature and importance of small business in regional Australia, with a contrast to studies of urban small businesses. Australasian Journal of Regional Studies 24(1):96

Kosteniuk J, Stewart N J, Wilson E C et al 2019 Communication tools and sources of education and information: a national survey of rural and remote nurses. Journal of the Medical Library Association 107(4):538–554

Liaw S T, Wade V, Furler J S et al 2019 Cultural respect in general practice: a cluster randomised controlled trial. Medical Journal of Australia 210(6):263–268

McCullough K, Bayes S, Whitehead L et al 2022 Nursing in a different world: remote area nursing as a specialist–generalist practice area. Australian Journal of Rural Health 2022; 30:570–581 doi:10.1111/ajr.12899

MacKay S C, Smith A, Kyle R G et al 2021 What influences nurses' decisions to work in rural and remote settings? A systematic review and meta-synthesis of qualitative research. Rural and Remote Health 21:6335 https://doi.org/10.22605/RRH6335

MacLeod M, Stewart N, Kosteniuk J 2019 Rural and remote registered nurses' perceptions of working beyond their legislated scope of practice. Nursing Leadership 32(1):20–29

Malatzky C A R, Couch D L 2023 The power in rural place stigma. Bioethical Inquiry 20:237–248 https://doi.org/10.1007/s11673-023-10260-9

Ministry of Health 2023 Rural health strategy. Ministry of Health, Wellington

Osik Szumer R, Arnold M 2023 The ethics of overlapping relationships in rural and remote heathcare. A narrative review. Journal of Bioethical Inquiry 20:181–190

O'Sullivan B, Russell D J, McGrail M R et al 2019 Reviewing reliance on overseas-trained doctors in rural Australia and planning for self-sufficiency: applying 10 years MABEL evidence. Human Resources for Health 17(1):8

Piatkowski T, Sabrus D, Keane C 2023 The relationship between masculinity and help-seeking among Australian men living in non-urban areas. The Journal of Men's Studies 32(2):199–218 https://doi.org/10.1177/10608265231207997

Quigley R et al 2022 Aging well for Indigenous peoples: a scoping review. Frontiers in Public Health 10

Ross J, Crawley J, Parmee R 2023 The rural way: rural nurses' contribution to new models of care, reducing health disparities – stories from practice. Rural Health – Investment, Research and Implications. IntechOpen. Online. Available: http://dx.doi.org/10.5772/intechopen.109768

Rossiter R, Phillips R, Blanchard D et al 2023 Exploring nurse practitioner practice in Australian rural primary health care settings: a scoping review. Australian Journal of Rural Health 31(4):617–630 doi: 10.1111/ajr.13010. Epub 2023 Jun 23. PMID: 37350494

Singer R, Zwi K, Menzies R 2019 Predictors of in-hospital mortality in Aboriginal children admitted to a tertiary paediatric hospital. International Journal of Environmental Research and Public Health 16(11):1893

Smith T, McNeil K, Mitchell R et al 2019 A study of macro-, meso- and micro-barriers and enablers affecting extended scopes of practice: the case of rural nurse practitioners in Australia. BMC Nursing 18(1):14

Stats NZ 2020 Urban accessibility – methodology and classification. Online. Available: www.stats.govt.nz

Sullivan K, McConney A, Perry L B 2018 A comparison of rural educational disadvantage in Australia, Canada, and New Zealand using OECD's PISA. SAGE Open 8(4) https://doi.org/10.1177/2158244018805791

Vaughan L, Edwards N 2020 The problems of smaller, rural and remote hospitals: separating facts from fiction. Future Healthcare Journal 7(1):38–45 doi: 10.7861/fhj.2019-0066. PMID: 32104764; PMCID: PMC7032574

Walker R C, Hay C, Walker C et al 2022 Exploring rural and remote patients experiences of health services for kidney disease in Aetearoa New Zealand: an in-depth interview study. Nephology 27(5):421–429

Walsh S M, Versace V L, Thompson S C et al 2023 Supporting nursing and allied health student placements in rural and remote Australia: a narrative review of publications by university departments of rural health. Medical Journal of Australia 219 Suppl 3:S14–S19 doi: 10.5694/mja2.52032. Erratum in: Medical Journal of Australia 2023 Sep 18;219(6):256. PMID: 37544003

Whiteing N, Barr J, Rossi D M 2021 The practice of rural and remote nurses in Australia: a case study. Journal of Clinical Nursing Online. Available: https://doi.org/10.1111/jocn.16002

World Health Organization (WHO) 2021 WHO guideline on health workforce development, attraction, recruitment and retention in rural and remote areas. Online. Available: https://iris.who.int/bitstream/handle/10665/341139/9789240024229-eng.pdf

Wright L K, Jatrana S, Lindsay D 2021 Workforce safety in the remote health sector of Australia: a scoping review. BMJ Open 11(8):e051345 doi: 10.1136/bmjopen-2021-051345. PMID: 34452968; PMCID: PMC8404439

Zhao Y, Russell D J, Guthridge S et al 2019 Costs and effects of higher turnover of nurses and Aboriginal health practitioners and higher use of short-term nurses in remote Australian primary care services: an observational cohort study. BMJ Open 9(2):e023906

CHAPTER 18

PRIMARY HEALTHCARE AND NURSING

Elizabeth Halcomb

KEY WORDS
community health
health literacy
health promotion
nursing in the community
nursing roles
primary healthcare

LEARNING OBJECTIVES
After reading this chapter, readers should be able to:
- explain the concepts of primary healthcare and the social determinants of health
- identify how nurses contribute to healthcare in the community
- discuss a range of roles for nurses in community settings.

INTRODUCTION

The nursing profession is so much more diverse than the nursing care provided in hospital settings. While nursing in a hospital is vital to manage acute conditions or exacerbations and provide proactive healthcare, nursing in the community is critical to keep people well and out of the hospital. One of the most dynamic aspects of nursing is how nursing roles continue to evolve to meet the changing needs of individuals, their families and communities. As the population ages and the prevalence of chronic conditions continues to grow, so too does the need for healthcare in the community. This chapter introduces the concept of primary healthcare and highlights the important and diverse roles of nurses working in the community.

Primary healthcare

Nursing in the community is based on the principles of primary healthcare (PHC). PHC considers the needs and circumstances of individual people, their families and communities in a whole-of-society approach to health (Halcomb & Ashley 2023). Nurses recognise that health is created and shaped in the social, cultural and physical environments of people's lives, which can enhance or inhibit health and wellbeing. In providing care, PHC professionals seek to overcome social disadvantage and address the social determinants of health. There are some differences in the definition of PHC between contexts and the definition has evolved. Since the 1978 Declaration of Alma-Ata the definition of PHC has been revised to place greater emphasis on individual needs and circumstances, as well as care across the life span and the physical, mental and social domains. At the Astana conference, the World Health Organization and United Nations Children's Fund (2018) released its revised definition, stating that: 'PHC is a whole-of-society approach to health that aims at ensuring the highest possible level of health and wellbeing and their equitable distribution by focusing on people's needs and as early as possible along the continuum from health promotion and disease prevention to treatment, rehabilitation and palliative care, and as close as feasible to people's everyday environment' (viii).

Nurses practising within a PHC framework take on an enabling role, working with individuals, families and communities to build capacity and empower them to take control of their health and wellbeing. PHC nurses seek to promote equal access to health services, address the social determinants of health, and emphasise health promotion and prevention. A common thread running through these principles is an attitude of inclusiveness, which means being sensitive to individual differences and personal choices, including cultural differences, individual identities and/or social preferences for religion or lifestyles.

The World Health Organization (WHO) (2018) has identified three key components of PHC; namely, integrated health services, multi-sectoral policies and actions and empowered people and communities. Integrated health services refers to the provision of health services that are responsive to people's needs and preferences at both an individual (primary care) and community (population health) level (World Health Organization and United Nations Children's Fund 2018). Multi-sectoral policies and actions refers to the policies and actions of non-health sectors that influence community health and wellbeing. For example, policies about education, employment, urban planning and transport have a significant influence on the availability of resources within a local community. Additionally, policies that affect childcare, disability support, migration, rights of same-sex partners or retirement age also create inequalities that have a negative impact on health. Finally, the third component of PHC involves health professionals working with individuals and communities to empower them to plan and implement community support for health and wellness. In this process the community plays a key role in identifying and setting healthcare priorities (Behera et al 2022).

You have a university assignment to complete, which involves learning more about healthcare in your local community.

> **Reflective questions**
>
> Reflect on the scenario and answer the following questions:
> 1. What opportunities are there for community members to inform or shape health services?
> 2. What is an example of how multisectoral policy impacts on the health of the community?
> 3. What kinds of services are provided by nurses in your community?

Nursing roles in the community

Nursing in the community is diverse and can involve working with a range of groups in various settings (Guzys & Halcomb 2024). Community-based nursing roles include opportunities for all designations of nurse from assistants in nursing, enrolled and registered nurses to nurse practitioners. Additionally, roles can be highly specialised (e.g. breast care nurse, drug and alcohol nurse) or more of a generalist role (e.g. general practice nurse, school nurse). A key feature of all community-based roles is the emphasis on health promotion and preventive care. That is, working to keep the health and wellbeing of people, their families and communities as good as it can be. Many community-based nursing roles offer nurses the opportunity to be relatively independent in the planning and delivery of care and to work closely with multidisciplinary health and other professionals to improve health and wellness. This does not mean that there are not employer expectations, practice boundaries or challenges in being somewhat professionally isolated, but in many situations, the nurse can make relatively autonomous decisions about client needs, planning assessments, management strategies and workflow. Many nurses find this type of practice motivating and embrace the chance to make a difference to people's health and wellbeing.

It is an exciting time to be working as a nurse in the community setting. As the community is ageing and the health needs of the population are changing, the importance of keeping people well in the community is increasingly recognised. More and more governments are recognising the importance of nurses and investing in building and developing the nursing workforce in the community (Australian Government Department of Health 2022, Nursing Council of New Zealand 2019). However, to optimise the impact of nurses on the health and wellbeing of people living in the community it is vital that nurses in the community are supported and enabled to work to the extent of their practice scope within the context of the multidisciplinary and inter-sectoral team (Stephen et al 2023).

It is impossible to list all the possibilities for nurses working in the community as there is an ever-growing range of career opportunities. Some key areas where nurses work in the community include community nursing, residential aged care facilities, schools, general practices, occupational health settings, correctional facilities, public health units, specialist services (e.g. breast cancer care, stomal therapy, mental health) and health services for vulnerable groups, such as refugee health, homeless outreach, LGBTQI+, sexual health and drug and alcohol services (Guzys & Halcomb 2024). While all community-based roles share commonalities, each role involves specific types of nursing care that is delivered in a somewhat unique context to a particular community group. This diversity offers rich career opportunities for nurses to build expertise in a diverse range of practice areas. Such diversity allows the nurse to find an area of clinical practice that they find interesting, stimulating and engaging.

Finding an area of practice that fits with the individual nurse's interests and personal characteristics is vital in supporting job satisfaction, workforce retention and high-quality clinical practice.

SCHOOL HEALTH NURSES

School nurses deliver nursing care in a range of educational contexts including both day only and boarding schools (Australian Nursing and Midwifery Federation 2019). As Australia does not have a formal national school health service, nurses are employed by individual schools or jurisdictions (Moyes et al 2023). In Australia, school nursing continues to evolve; the development of the Australian School Nurses' Practice Standards was a major step towards recognition of the importance of the role (Australian Nursing and Midwifery Federation 2019). In New Zealand's (Aotearoa's), public health nursing teams and secondary school nurses provide school health services.

School nurses provide support for the physical and mental health needs of students, families and the school community (Jones et al 2020, McCluskey et al 2019). The school nursing role differs depending on the age of the students, demographics and social determinants of the school community and specific local health needs (Jones et al 2020). However, the role primarily addresses healthcare needs, provides health assessment, screening and referrals, as well as health promotion and education and creation of a safe environment (Halcomb & Chalmers 2024). School nurses address healthcare needs by supporting students with known health conditions, such as diabetes, epilepsy or severe allergies, and managing acute illness, injury or social, emotional or mental health concerns (Halcomb & Chalmers 2024). This also includes ensuring that teachers are educated to respond to potential health emergencies and liaising with services to advocate for students' needs (Sanford et al 2020).

The nature of health assessments and screening is related to students' age. Primary school nurses usually focus on developmental, behavioural and sensory assessment and screening. However, high school nurses likely have a greater emphasis on general health checks, gender issues and sexual health concerns and mental health assessment. During these assessments, nurses must consider the impact of issues such as family dysfunction, poor social support, financial concerns, abuse and bullying on student health and wellbeing.

All aspects of the school nurse role incorporate age-appropriate health education and promotion (Australian Nursing and Midwifery Federation 2019, WHO 2021). In primary schools, young children often need health education on preventing disease by improving hand hygiene and appropriate techniques for coughing, body issues such as body image and puberty, and healthy living issues such as good food choices and physical activity. In high schools, health issues often become more complex and include eating disorders, sexual and gender issues, chronic conditions, mental health challenges, vaping/smoking and substance abuse. A range of social and environmental issues will exacerbate these health issues, such as poverty, homelessness, violence, family breakdown and bullying (Australian Child Rights Taskforce 2018, Blakemore 2019). To improve health outcomes, the school nurse must identify students affected by these factors and support them to access appropriate services.

The school environment must be safe for all. Firstly, this relates to physical safety. The school nurse may contribute to environmental assessments to identify and minimise physical risk, as well as exploring factors such as canteen foods to facilitate making healthy choices. Secondly, it is important that schools address risks such as violence, bullying and marginalisation of vulnerable groups that can lead to negative mental health impacts. However, school bullying is not new; social media has changed the dynamic and nature of such behaviour as well as its health impacts (Jadambaa et al 2019). Beyond bullying, safe environments are those that are welcoming and conducive to learning for all, including those from priority groups, such as racial groups, LGBTQI and those with special needs (Halcomb & Chalmers 2024). The school nurse can be a trusted person that people can come to and disclose feelings and safety concerns.

GENERAL PRACTICE NURSES

While nurses have worked in general practice for many decades in countries like New Zealand (Aotearoa) and the United Kingdom, the Australian general practice nurse workforce has only really developed in the last 20 years (Halcomb et al 2021). In response to positive government policy and funding for nursing roles, an increasing number of Australian general practices have employed nurses. However, the need to strengthen primary care services in response to the ageing population and rise in the prevalence of chronic conditions has prompted shifts in the general practice workforce internationally (Australian Government Department of Health 2022, Heywood & Laurence 2018). Building a more multidisciplinary team-based general practice workforce increases the access to services within the community to promote lifestyle risk reduction (e.g. quit smoking, reduce body weight, increase activity), enhance self-literacy and promote self-management. The nursing role in general practice may complement the services of the general practitioner, extend the scope of clinical services available or the nurse may substitute for the general practitioner in providing some aspects of care, releasing them to undertake more complex tasks (Thompson & Halcomb 2024).

A key difference for general practice nurses (GPNs) compared to other nursing roles is the business structure of general practice. While there are some differences in the health system model between Australia and New Zealand (Aotearoa) there are also broad similarities. In both health systems, hospitals are part of government-funded health services. However, most general practices are either small businesses, which are usually owned by doctors, or a part of larger corporate chains (Australian Government Department of Health 2022, General Practice New Zealand 2024). This has implications for the way in which nurses work, as within small business practices they are often the employees of their general practitioner peer (McInnes et al 2017), and they are working in a smaller organisation that is a business rather than a pure service. As such, GPN roles often have a strong focus on activities that generate remuneration from Medicare reimbursement or other funding schemes. Additionally, balancing the dual relationship of peer and employer with general practitioners can create some unique challenges (McInnes et al 2017).

Despite this, nurses working in general practice provide a diverse range of services depending on the needs of the specific practice population, preferences of the multidisciplinary team, the nature of the business and locally available services (Thompson & Halcomb 2024). Such services include physical and mental health assessment, acute symptom management, chronic disease education and support, preventive activities such as screening and immunisation and practice population activities such as recalls for blood pressure checks or pap smears. The general practice nurse has a key role in working with general practitioners and consumers to ensure that care needs are met and that access to appropriate services is available.

An evolving body of research has shown that GPN-led services are both feasible and effective in improving health outcomes in chronic conditions, such as hypertension, pulmonary disease, diabetes and cardiovascular disease (Aranburu-Imatz et al 2022, Crowe et al 2019, Li et al 2020, Stephen et al 2022, 2023). In these studies, nurses have been integral in identifying at-risk people, undertaking health assessments, co-developing action plans/goal setting for behaviour change in conjunction with patients and providing guidance on strategies to support self-management (Stephen et al 2022). Registered nurses working in general practice have been shown to be effective in promoting patient satisfaction, improving quality of life, enhancing self-efficacy and modifying health behaviours (Lukewich et al 2022).

Internationally, much work is being undertaken to generate evidence to support multidisciplinary models of general practice care and promote strategies to achieve truly team-based care. This is a great opportunity for nurses to work in a close-knit team context where they have significant relational continuity with patients across the life span.

OCCUPATIONAL HEALTH NURSES

Occupational health nurses (OHNs) can work in any workplaces, from offices and factories to mines and construction sites. Their role incorporates activities such as workplace surveillance and risk assessment, health education and promotion, case finding and management of occupational diseases, treating ill or injured workers, ensuring compliance with workplace health and safety policies and research (Gok Metin & Yildiz 2023, Gonzalez-Caballero 2024). In recent years, there has been a shift in focus beyond worker safety and work-related injury and health problems, to also encompass broader health issues that affect workers (Abe & Nishikido 2023, Jain et al 2021, Jimenez-Merida et al 2021). However, they often have a varied scope of practice depending on the nurses' skills and experience, as well as the needs of the specific workplace (Onyeador et al 2023).

OHNs work in partnership with workers, managers and employers to maintain healthy and safe working practices and a healthy and safe work environment (Gonzalez-Caballero 2024, Harriss 2020). Surveillance is a major part of ensuring environmental safety, aimed at identifying workplace risks (Gok Metin & Yildiz 2023). This requires in-depth knowledge of work structures, processes and products, to design injury and illness prevention strategies. Surveillance and monitoring in the workplace often involves ergonomic assessments to provide information on the fit between the worker and the environment. Ergonomic risks can include boredom, glare, repetitive motion, poor workstation–worker fit, lifting heavy loads or tasks that require the worker to assume an abnormal position. Physical hazards can include such things as extremes of temperature, noise, radiation or poor lighting. Biological hazards include exposures to chemical or biological agents. Psychosocial hazards are those that produce inordinate stress, such as shiftwork, or negative interpersonal relationships on the job, such as bullying and incivility. As with other nursing roles, careful documentation is a pivotal part of the OHN role, particularly when disputes arise over differences in expectations by employers and employees, or when it becomes necessary to demonstrate the measurable value, or return on investment of their services to the organisation (Mastroianni 2018). Given the potential sensitivity of situations where the nurse participates in lobbying for safe working conditions, which may be costly to the employer, nurses need high-level communication skills, in-depth understanding of interpersonal and industrial relations, and familiarity with professional and government standards and legislation (Gonzalez-Caballero 2024, Harriss 2020).

The OHN needs to maintain high-level skills in first-aid procedures, crisis intervention and trauma management, including threats from workplace violence. Some OHN undertake health intervention programs to engage workers while they are recovering from illness or injury. They may also provide intervention for those with substance abuse problems, smoking cessation, workplace health and fitness programs or pain management, especially for those with chronic conditions (Abe & Nishikido 2023, Jimenez-Merida et al 2021, Sok et al 2019). Successful implementation of rehabilitation or health promotion programs relies on a primary healthcare approach, empowering workers to self-manage, helping them overcome any injuries or disabling conditions without discrimination, ensuring equal opportunity, access to support and inclusion in decision making. These activities require an extensive referral network, including knowledge of workers' general practitioners for timely referrals, which creates an impetus to liaise with other community-based nurses.

CORRECTIONAL NURSES

Correctional nurses work in a range of settings, including correctional facilities, forensic hospitals, courts and police cells (American Nurses Association 2021, Kinghorn et al 2024). The roles and required skills will vary across these settings. Those who work in police cells and courts likely have a role focused on assessment and specialist advice on health issues. However, those in correctional centres or forensic hospitals likely have a more 'traditional' PHC nursing role delivering direct patient care. This may involve the provision of specialist services, such as forensic mental healthcare, or more general health assessment, chronic condition management and general health education and promotion (Kinghorn et al 2024). Additionally, correctional nurses may be faced with being the first responder to significant acute injuries sustained through violence or suicide attempts (Woods & Peternelj-Taylor 2022). While the role may be similar to other PHC nursing roles, the environmental context is very different. Correctional nurses must balance the patients' health needs against the safety and security of those incarcerated or in custody and the security and health of staff (Kinghorn et al 2023). This can be challenging to nurses as they have to reconcile the conflicts between maintaining security and providing person-centred care (Bouchaud et al 2018, Gorman et al 2018, Sasso et al 2018).

In Australia, 32% of the prison population identifies as being Aboriginal or Torres Strait Islander people (ABS 2022) and in New Zealand (Aotearoa) some 52.8% of those in prisons are Māori (Ara Poutama Aotearoa Department of Corrections 2023). This creates a need for culturally sensitive support to address health and social issues. People in prisons often experience significant disadvantage in terms of economic, environmental, social and lifestyle factors (Ismail et al 2021). As a result, they often have much higher rates of mental illness, chronic conditions, acquired brain injury and substance misuse than the general population (AIHW 2023, McLeod et al 2020). Additionally, those in prison frequently under-utilise primary and preventive healthcare in the community and may have their first recent interaction with health services during incarceration (Borschmann et al 2020). This represents an opportunity for nurses to improve the health and wellbeing of incarcerated people by identifying health issues and implementing appropriate care (Besney et al 2018, Bouchaud et al 2018, Lafferty et al 2018). Addressing the social determinants of health and returning people to the general community in better health than when they were incarcerated has benefits for the individual, their families and the community (Gould & Brent 2020).

> **REFLECTION**
>
> What might it be like to be a nurse working in the community? What would be some of the good parts of the job? What might some negatives of this kind of work be?
> Is there a particular role within the community that interests you?

CONCLUSION

Nurses can make a positive difference to health and wellbeing in many different community-based settings. Practising in the community offers diverse opportunities to work with a range of community groups that have varying needs and challenges. By taking a PHC approach to care, nurses working in the community are a key component of integrated health services that seek to empower people and communities to optimise their health and wellbeing. The embedded nature of nursing in the community and the degree of autonomy of practice makes them some of the most rewarding roles in nursing.

REFLECTIVE QUESTIONS

1. What clinical skills do you think are most important in community-based nursing? How are these skills similar and different to those needed in a hospital setting?
2. What general skills are required for nurses to work across different community-based settings?
3. What are the advantages and disadvantages of working in a community-based nursing role?

Recommended readings

Guzys D, Halcomb E J 2024 An introduction to community and primary health care, 4th edn. Cambridge University Press, Melbourne

World Health Organization (WHO) and United Nations Children's Fund 2018 A vision for primary health care in the 21st century: towards universal health coverage and the Sustainable Development Goals. (Vol. Licence: CC BY-NC-SA 3.0 IGO.) WHO, Geneva

References

Abe H, Nishikido N 2023 Effectiveness of a support program for balancing treatment and work in small and medium-sized enterprises promoted by occupational health nurses using a web meeting system: a cluster randomized controlled trial. Journal of Occupational Health 65(1): e12407

American Nurses Association 2021 Correctional nursing: Scope and standards of practice, 3rd edn. American Nurses Association

Ara Poutama Aotearoa Department of Corrections 2023 Prison facts and statistics - March 2023. Online. Available: https://www.corrections.govt.nz/resources/statistics/quarterly_prison_statistics/prison_stats_march_2023 10 June 2024

Aranburu-Imatz A, López-Carrasco JD, Moreno-Luque A, et al 2022 Nurse-led interventions in chronic obstructive pulmonary disease patients: a systematic review and meta-analysis. International Journal of Environmental Research and Public Health 19(15): 9101

Australian Bureau of Statistics (ABS) 2022 Prisoners in Australia. Online. Available: https://www.abs.gov.au/statistics/people/crime-and-justice/prisoners-australia/latest-release 10 June 2024

Australian Child Rights Taskforce 2018 The Children's Report: Australia's NGO coalition report to the United Nations Committee on the Rights of the Child. Online. Available: https:// www.unicef.org.au/Upload/UNICEF/Media/Documents/Child-RightsTaskforce-NGO-Coalition-Report-For-UNCRC-LR-Spreads.pdf

Australian Government Department of Health 2022 Future focused primary health care: Australia's Primary Health Care 10 Year Plan 2022-2032. Online. Available: https://www.health.gov.au/resources/publications/australias-primary-health-care-10-year-plan-2022-2032

Australian Institute of Health and Welfare (AIHW) 2023 The health of people in Australia's prisons 2022 Online: Available: https://www.aihw.gov.au/getmedia/e2245d01-07d1-4b8d-81b3-60d14fbf007f/aihw-phe-33-health-of-people-in-australias-prisons-2022.pdf?v520231108163318&inline5true 18 February 2024

Australian Nursing and Midwifery Federation (ANMF) 2019 National School Nursing Standards for Practice: Registered Nurse. ANMF Federal Office, Melbourne

Behera BK, Prasad R, Shyambhavee 2022 Primary health-care goal and principles. Healthcare Strategies and Planning for Social Inclusion and Development 221–39

Besney JD, Angel C, Pyne D, et al 2018 Addressing women's unmet health care needs in a Canadian remand center: catalyst for improved health? Journal of Correctional Health Care 24(3): 276–294

Blakemore SJ 2019 Adolescence and mental health. Lancet 393(10185):2030–2031

Borschmann R, Janca E, Carter A, et al 2020 The health of adolescents in detention: a global scoping review. The Lancet Public Health 5(2):e114-e126

Bouchaud MT, Brooks M, Swan BA 2018 A retrospective analysis of nursing students' clinical experience in an all-male maximum security prison. Nurse Educator 43(4):210–214

Crowe M, Jones V, Stone M.-A, et al 2019 The clinical effectiveness of nursing models of diabetes care: a synthesis of the evidence. International Journal of Nursing Studies 93:119–128

General Practice New Zealand 2024 Securing sustainable general practice in Aotearoa. Online. Available: https://www.nzdoctor.co.nz/sites/default/files/2024-01/Sustainable%20general%20practice%20in%20Aotearoa%20New%20Zealand%202024%20GPNZ.pdf

Gok Metin Z, Yildiz AN 2023 Update on occupational health nursing through 21st century requirements: a three-round Delphi study. Nurse Education Today 120:105657

Gonzalez-Caballero J 2024 Occupational health nursing: realities and challenges. International Nursing Review

Gorman G, Singer RM, Christmas E, et al 2018 In a spirit of restoration: a phenomenology of nursing practice and the criminal justice system. Advances in Nursing Science 41(2):105–117

Gould L, Brent J 2020 Handbook on American prisons. Taylor and Francis

Guzys D, Halcomb EJ 2024 An introduction to community and primary health care, 4th edn. Cambridge University Press

Halcomb E, Ashley C 2023 Primary health care. In: Liamputtong P (ed) Handbook of Social Sciences and Global Public Health. Springer, Cham

Halcomb E, Bird S, McInnes S, et al 2021 Exploring job satisfaction and turnover intentions among general practice nurses in an Australian primary health network. Journal of Nursing Management 29(5): 943–952.

Halcomb EJ, Chalmers L 2024 School nursing. In: D Guzys, E J Halcomb (eds) An introduction to community and primary health Care, 4th edn. Cambridge University Press

Harriss A 2020 Name of the game – is it time for OH to change its name? Occupational Health & Wellbeing 72(4):26–30

Heywood T, Laurence C 2018 An overview of the general practice nurse workforce in Australia, 2012–15. Australian Journal of Primary Health 24(3):227–232

Ismail N, Lazaris A, O'Moore É, et al 2021 Leaving no one behind in prison: improving the health of people in prison as a key contributor to meeting the Sustainable Development Goals 2030. BMJ Global Health 6(3):e004252

Jadambaa A, Thomas HJ, Scott JG, et al 2019 Prevalence of traditional bullying and cyberbullying among children and adolescents in Australia: a systematic review and meta-analysis. Australian New Zealand Journal of Psychiatry 53(9): 878–888

Jain A, Hassard J, Leka S, et al 2021 the role of occupational health services in psychosocial risk management and the promotion of mental health and well-being at Work. International Journal of Environmental Research in Public Health 18(7):3632

Jimenez-Merida MR, Romero-Saldana M, Molina-Luque R, Molina-Recio G, Meneses-Monroy A, De Diego-Cordero R Vaquero-Abellan M 2021 Women-centred workplace health promotion interventions: a systematic review. International Nursing Review 68(1):90–98

Jones D, Randall S, White D, et al 2020 Embedding public health advocacy into the role of school-based nurses: addressing the health inequities confronted by vulnerable Australian children and adolescent populations. Australian Journal of Primary Health 27:67–70

Kinghorn G, Bosworth R, Halcomb EJ 2024 Correctional nursing. In: Guzys D, Halcomb E J, (eds) An introduction to community and primary health care, 4th edn. Cambridge University Press

Kinghorn G, Froggatt T, Thomas S, Halcomb E 2023 The experience of nurses moving into forensic mental health employment: a qualitative study. International Journal of Mental Health Nursing 32(2): 524–533

Lafferty L, Chambers GM, Guthrie J, et al 2018 Measuring social capital in the prison setting: lessons learned from the inmate social capital questionnaire. Journal of Correctional Health Care 24(4):407–417

Li C, Liu Y, Xue D, et al 2020 Effects of nurse-led interventions on early detection of cancer: a systematic review and meta-analysis. International Journal of Nursing Studies 110:103684

Lukewich J, Martin-Misener R, Norful AA, et al 2022 Effectiveness of registered nurses on patient outcomes in primary care: a systematic review. BMC Health Services Research 22(1):1–34

Mastroianni K 2018 AAOHN Member opinions on demonstrating value: a closer look at the findings. Workplace Health Safety 66(5):241–251

McCluskey A, Kendall G, Burns S 2019 Students', parents' and teachers' views about the resources required by school nurses in Perth, Western Australia. Journal of Research in Nursing 24(7):515–526

McInnes S, Peters K, Bonney A, et al 2017 The influence of funding models on collaboration in Australian general practice. Australian Journal of Primary Health 23(1):31–36

McLeod KE, Butler A, Young JT, et al 2020 Global prison health care governance and health equity: a critical lack of evidence. American Journal of Public Health 110(3):303–308

Moyes A, McGough S, Wynaden D 2023 Hidden and unacknowledged: the mental health and psychosocial interventions delivered by school nurses in Western Australia. International Journal of Mental Health Nursing 33(2):463-47

Nursing Council of New Zealand 2019 The New Zealand Nursing Workforce: a profile of Nurse Practitioners, Registered Nurses and Enrolled Nurses 2018–2019

Onyeador CC, Umberger RA, Robb M 2023 Scope of practice for occupational health nurses: a concept analysis based on Walker and Avant methods. Nursing Forum 2023:1-7

Sanford C, Saurman E, Dennis S, Lyle D 2020 'We're definitely that link': the role of school-based primary health care registered nurses in a rural community. Australian Journal of Primary Health 27:76–82

Sasso L, Delogu B, Carrozzino R, et al 2018 Ethical issues of prison nursing: a qualitative study in Northern Italy. Nursing Ethics 25(3):393-409

Sok SR, Kim OS, Park MH 2019 Effects of obesity management program provided by occupational health nurse in worksite. Western Journal of Nursing Research 41(5):728–742

Stephen C, Halcomb E, Fernandez R, et al 2022 Nurse-led interventions to manage hypertension in general practice: a systematic review and meta analysis. Journal of Advanced Nursing 78(5): 1281–1293

Stephen C, Halcomb E, Zwar N, et al 2023 Impact of a general practice nurse intervention to improve blood pressure control: the ImPress study. Australian Journal of General Practice 52(12):875–881

Thompson C, Halcomb EJ 2024 Nursing in general practice. In: Guzys D, Halcomb E J (eds) An introduction to community and primary health care, 4th edn. Cambridge University Press

Woods P, Peternelj-Taylor C 2022 Correctional nursing in Canada's prairie provinces: roles, responsibilities, and learning needs. Canadian Journal of Nursing Research 54(1):59–71

World Health Organization (WHO) 2021 WHO guideline on school health services: web annex B: brief exploratory review of school health services globally: methodology and select findings. WHO, Geneva

World Health Organization and United Nations Children's Fund 2018 A vision for primary health care in the 21st century: towards universal health coverage and the Sustainable Development Goals. World Health Organization and the United Nations Children's Fund (UNICEF), Geneva

CHAPTER 19

SIMULATION LEARNING IN NURSING

Kerry Reid-Searl, Melanie Barlow, Danny Sidwell and Colleen Ryan

KEY WORDS
extracurricular simulation
fidelity
modalities of simulation
simulation
simulated clinical environment

LEARNING OBJECTIVES
After reading this chapter, it is hoped that readers will:

- gain an appreciation of what simulation can offer in your journey as a nursing student
- develop an understanding of the different types of simulation
- gain an understanding of how you can maximise your learning in simulation.

INTRODUCTION

Welcome to this chapter on simulation. Simulation can best be described as the creation of learning opportunities intended to replicate reality, which in the context of nursing, means real-world clinical experiences. Said another way, simulations, and the scenarios created, are designed to help prepare you for your clinical placement. Through simulation, you can practise clinical skills, and apply clinical reasoning and decision making, which helps bridge the gap between theory and practice. Because simulations occur in a setting away from 'real patients' you can practise hands-on experience where it is okay to make mistakes, learn from your mistakes and refine your skills without consequences to real patients. As a result of participating in simulations, you also have opportunities for feedback, and to practise self-reflection. In this chapter, we will discuss aspects of simulation pertinent to you as a student.

Where simulation-based learning occurs

Simulation-based learning can occur in a variety of contexts, including the classroom, online or in a clinical simulation laboratory. When simulations are within a clinical simulation laboratory, students may feel confronted due to the reality of equipment surrounding them, the simulations occurring and being surrounded by peers whom they may be expected to work with or even perform in front of. For some students, the simulations may trigger their emotions, and simulation-based assessments may create feelings of anxiety or concern. Later in this chapter there is information on physical and emotional safety in simulation. However, to help alleviate some of the potential anxiety, it is important to make yourself familiar with the settings and equipment and being prepared for your class. Participating in briefing and debriefing is very important; so too is having a voice to speak up if you have concerns. You should consider the clinical simulation laboratories as a place where you apply knowledge, practising what you have learned from the theory. This means that you come to the clinical simulation laboratory having completed pre-readings or online material. It is hoped that after you have read this chapter, the importance of preparation in simulation will make sense.

Bridging theory and practice

As a nursing student you will spend much time learning theoretical content, in lectures, workshops, tutorials and through self-directed learning. This theoretical learning will be both vast and varied and will cover a range of topics from nursing ethics to anatomy. Not only will this new learning make you a knowledgeable nurse, but it will help you talk like a nurse, think like a nurse and apply clinical reasoning like a nurse. Theory alone, however, will not be able to help you act and 'do' like a nurse. As is described by Kolb (1984:38), 'learning is the process whereby knowledge is created through the transformation of experience'. Put simply, to be able to truly become a nurse you must experience being a nurse. As you can imagine, experiencing how to perform like a nurse can be rather daunting without the ability to practise, hence the need for simulation.

> But hold on. Surely if I watch a video on how to administer an intramuscular injection, I will have enough knowledge on how to do it on a patient? I've learned the various muscle groups, how to measure for the perfect injection site, I know how to hold the skin while I inject and how quickly to inject. So do I really need to practise within a simulated environment?

The above is great information and the theory learned is very important to underpin what is being performed; however, there remains a small gap in understanding. What is unable to be understood through theory alone is how the syringe will feel in your hand, how you may prefer to hold the syringe, and how much force is needed for the needle to pierce the skin and enter the muscle. It is, however, possible to fill in these gaps in theoretical knowledge through hands-on practice and simulation.

The bonus of simulated practice is the increased confidence you will develop in your knowledge and skills, as well as an increase in competence that demonstrates your proficiency in performing a task (Bromley 2019). More importantly, however, is that through simulation and competency building you will start your journey in becoming a capable nurse; with capability described by Stephenson and Yorke (2013:3) as '… an integration of knowledge, skills, personal qualities and understanding used appropriately and effectively—not just in familiar and highly focused specialist contexts but in response to new and changing circumstances'. Therefore, through simulation you will develop your competence and ability to perform a task, but through ongoing practice you will be able to develop the ability to apply this skill in new and unknown clinical environments, thus becoming a capable nurse. Let's consider Emma's story to understand how she built competence which later developed her capability.

> **STORY**
>
> ### The value of simulation: Emma's story
>
> As a nursing student, Emma had always been diligent in her studies, but it wasn't until she started to really prepare for simulations in her assigned courses and attend extracurricular simulations that she began to understand the practical application of her knowledge. Little did she know that these simulation experiences would play a pivotal role in shaping her confidence and competence during a significant event on her clinical placement.
>
> One of the activities that Emma's lecturers had created in the simulated learning environment at her university was an up-to-date resuscitation trolley with information clearly available about each item. Emma's lecturers had advised all students about the importance of being aware of where emergency equipment is located and had spoken on many occasions about their role in basic life support (BLS) and how they may be asked to seek the trolley in the event of a real-life patient collapse or cardiac arrest.
>
> Emma made it her business to really get to know the contents of the trolley. She then commenced a unit of study that involved a simulation involving a deteriorating patient and, ultimately, a cardiac arrest. During the simulation Emma was quick to put together the bag valve mask and inserted an oral adjunct airway. Emma's lecturers commented on her performance.
>
> It was only a week later that Emma commenced her placement in a surgical ward. Emma was in a four-bed ward when one of the patients experienced a cardiac arrest. While the registered nurses (RNs) were present and escalated care, it was Emma who retrieved the resuscitation trolley and quickly assembled the bag valve mask, connected it to the oxygen and managed the patient's airway. After the experience, the RNs commended Emma on her performance. Emma reflected on the experience. She felt that the continual practice in the simulated learning environments at university facilitated both her confidence and competence. Emma realised just how much her participation in simulations had prepared her for moments like these. She understood now that the simulated scenarios, while artificial in nature, had equipped her with the knowledge and confidence needed to navigate an unknown real-world clinical challenge. They had not only bridged the gap between theory and practice but had also shaped her into the confident and capable nurse she was becoming—one simulation at a time.

You will return to Emma's story again in this chapter. Now it is time to learn more about the functional aspects of simulated learning, such as the different kinds or modalities that may be used at your university.

Types of simulation in nursing education

The simulations you will experience in your studies may all be very different. The following descriptions of the more common types might help you prepare for simulations by understanding the kind of simulation your teachers are using. The teachers will choose the simulations depending on the kind of skill or the intent of the learning session.

Augmented Reality (AR) is an interactive experience that combines the real world and computer-generated content. As seen in Figure 19.1, the Virtuali-Tee is embedded with links that when used with a smartphone app help you to learn about anatomy and physiology.

Sometimes goggles are used with AR to enhance the experience. Periodically students may experience cyber sickness, including dizziness, nausea or vertigo. Should this occur, the student should remove the goggles and let your facilitator know. There are many kinds of goggles (Fig. 19.2).

Mask-Ed™ is a modality of simulation where the experienced and trained teacher adorns themself in a silicone mask and other silicone products to transform into another person or character. The educator becomes disguised, and the newly created person/character has a back story/history that enables them to become a person with knowledge and experience and they pass on their wisdom to students (Reid-Searl 2020). For example, the teacher taking an undergraduate nursing class could transform into an older person who is a retired nurse (Fig. 19.3). As students care for the retired nurse (the hidden teacher) they pass on valuable information to

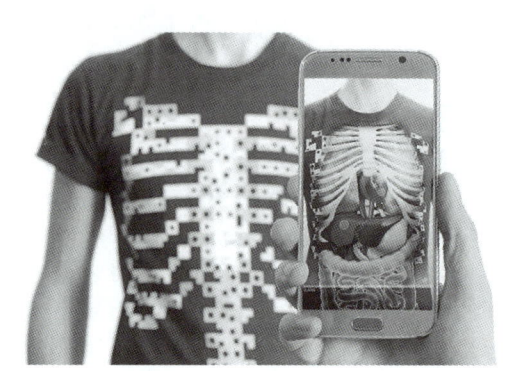

FIGURE 19.1
Virtuli T
Source: https://www.curiscope.com/

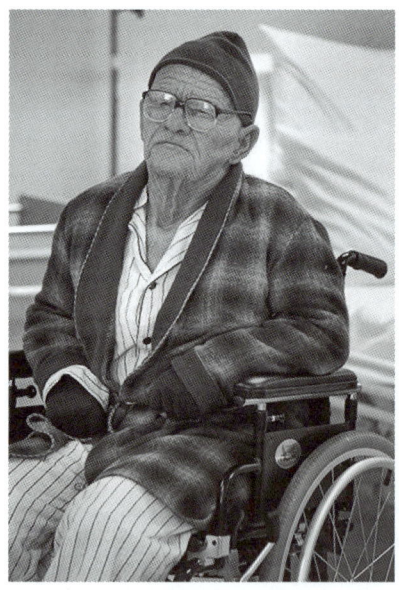

FIGURE 19.3
Image of Professor Kerry Reid-Searl adorned with a mask to become the character Cyril Smith
Courtesy: CQUniversity

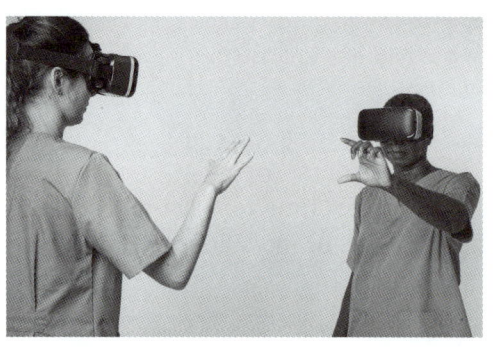

FIGURE 19.2
Goggles used with AR to enhance the experience
Source: Shutterstock/Rawpixel.com

the student because they have an abundance of knowledge to share. In this modality of simulation, students may find it confronting to see the teacher transform into another person. This is a reason why participation in both the briefing and debriefing is important.

Manikin simulations (Fig. 19.4) use full body size manikins made of plastic or fibreglass that allow you to perform invasive procedures such as chest compressions or administer intravenous, subcutaneous or intramuscular medications. You can listen to the manikin's breathing and much more.

Part-task trainer simulations (Fig. 19.5) use parts of the body, such as an arm, to allow you to practise specific skills such as cannulation, venipuncture, or a chest to practise managing an intercostal catheter.

Role play is simply playing the role of another person and in nursing simulations this could mean a person is assigned to play the role of a patient, a doctor or a relative, for example. As a student you might have to be a patient while another student plays the part of the nurse. You might have to ask the nurse specific questions from the script given to you. This means your colleagues are practising the content and then you get to feel what it is like to be a patient. As the patient you may have to give your colleagues feedback. See the section on feedback in this chapter to learn more. If you participate in role play it is important to consider the three Ds. These include 1) don a prop so that you are no longer yourself; 2) do not play yourself, stick to the role and script; 3) doff the prop as you de-role and debrief.

Serious games or virtual games are simulations designed for more than just entertainment. Serious games have an explicit and carefully thought-out educational purpose. Real-world events are used, and you will be expected to solve a problem to meet the learning objectives. Escape room simulations are another example of serious games.

Try this free online escape room not related to nursing. It is a Hogwarts experience that will

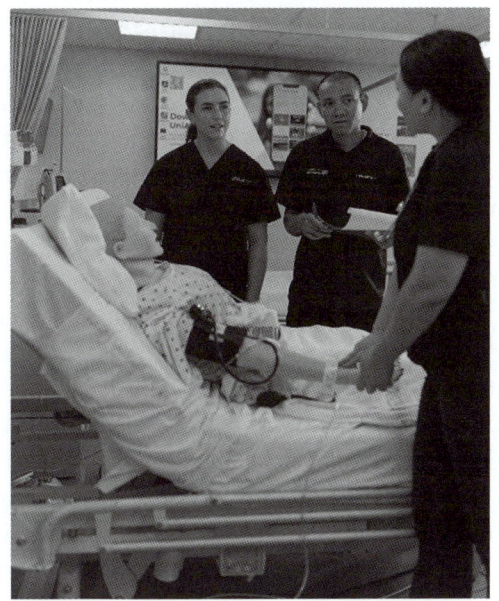

FIGURE 19.4
Manikin simulations

Source: With kind permission from University of Tasmania/OiStudios.

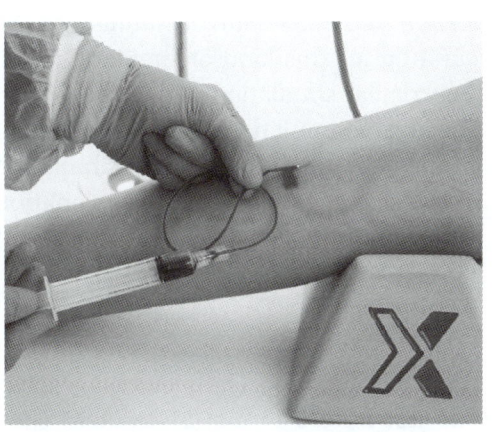

FIGURE 19.5
Part-task trainer simulations

Source: www.medical-x.com

take you about 10–15 minutes to escape. All the tips to work out the clues are included in links except for one where you will have to look up a map of America: https://docs.google.com/forms/d/e/1FAIpQLSflNxNM0jzbZJjUqOcXkwhGTfii4CM_CA3kCxImbY8c3AABEA/viewform_ (created by Sydney Krawiec, Youth Services Librarian at Peters Township Public Library in McMurray, PA, US).

Simulated patient is a trained actor or a person with lived experience of a medical condition or a healthcare experience. Simulated patients are used in role plays and act as the patient for you to interact with. These patients can be used to provide sudden deterioration and other unpredictable events for you to learn to manage. In some scenarios the simulated patient will also give you feedback on your performance.

Virtual simulation (VS) is a scenario that you will access on your laptop, phone or computer screen that requires you to participate in the scenario by doing something, usually with your computer mouse. Some advanced forms of these simulations will include speech and voice recognition, artificial intelligence to provide you with feedback and much more. Watch this space as these simulations continue to develop using the newest technology.

Virtual reality (VR). These simulations are also on your computer or laptop but project you into a 3D world. This is another simulation where you may wear goggles.

Virtual reality simulation (VRS). Simulations that use a variety of immersive, highly visual, 3D characteristics to replicate real-life situations and/or healthcare procedures. VRS is distinguished from computer-based simulation in that it generally incorporates physical or other interfaces, such as a computer keyboard, a mouse, speech and voice recognition, motion sensors, or haptic devices.

Objective Structured Clinical Examinations (OSCE) or **Objective Structured Clinical Assessments (OSCA)** are what are known as high stakes simulations. This is because you will be required to participate in these simulations to assess your knowledge and for you to show how you apply your knowledge and skills to certain situations. The kind of simulation (part-task trainer, manikin etc.) used in an OSCE/OSCA will depend on the skills for which you are being assessed. You will need to prepare yourself for your OSCE/OSCA by managing your anxiety and learning how to perform in these assessment simulations. Your lecturers will normally give you lots of practice and preparation for this kind of simulation. Sometimes this may be in your own time (see section on extracurricular simulation in this chapter).

There is a simulation dictionary (https://www.ssih.org/dictionary) if you want to learn more about the definitions and types of simulation used.

As we have mentioned in the explanation of an OSCE/OSCA, sometimes the simulations will be extra to your unit of study. Read more about extracurricular simulations now.

Participation in extracurricular simulation

Extracurricular simulations are not practice simulations; rather, they are carefully designed simulations on specific topics complementary to your study program. They are not compulsory and generally do not have a formal assessment component. These simulations can be nursing specific or on some occasions can involve students and staff from another discipline. This becomes a great way to have interprofessional collaboration. You may be asking why you should bother to attend extracurricular simulations when you have the competing demands of tutorials, lectures, assignments, simulated learning requirements with units/subjects, OSCEs and professional experience placements. Furthermore, you may also have to balance family and work, so finding time to attend extra learning opportunities is daunting.

However, when you do participate in extracurricular simulations, there are myriad benefits, some of which are included below.

IMMERSION IN REALISTIC SCENARIOS

These simulations provide you with a chance to immerse yourself in realistic scenarios that may not be covered in your standard curriculum. They can expose you to a broader range of patient situations, each presenting its own set of challenges and learning opportunities. By stepping into these scenarios, you gain practical experience that can help bridge the gap between theory and real-world practice.

DEVELOPMENT OF CLINICAL REASONING SKILLS

Extracurricular simulations, like most simulations, are designed to mimic real-world situations. They occur in a relatively controlled environment and can provide you with basic to complex scenarios. They give you an opportunity to develop your clinical reasoning skills and at times make decisions about practice when under pressure; however, you can experiment with different approaches, analyse the consequences of your actions, and learn from successes and mistakes. This learning helps with the clinical judgment skills you will require as a competent registered nurse.

AN OPPORTUNITY TO PRACTISE WITHOUT ASSESSMENT

Most extracurricular simulations do not have a formal assessment. This means you can focus on learning and improving your skills without the stress of assessment. The extracurricular simulations can, however, present as an opportunity for you to gain some feedback from peers or the facilitator with regard to your performance. This becomes an opportunity to reflect and identify areas that you did well in and those where you can practise improving.

WORKING WITH OTHER DISCIPLINES

Extracurricular simulations can provide you with an opportunity to work with peers from other healthcare disciplines. This is a great opportunity to gain an understanding of their roles, and they gain an insight into yours. You can practise interprofessional communication, which is central to patient safety. Simulations involving other disciplines give you an opportunity to really apply communication frameworks such as ISBAR. Most of all you can gain an understanding of collaborative practice and in doing so gain confidence in delegating tasks and coordinating care. This experience can serve you well in future clinical practice.

PERSONAL AND PROFESSIONAL GROWTH

Extracurricular simulations contribute to your personal and professional growth. They challenge you to step out of your comfort zones, adapt to unfamiliar situations, and develop the resilience needed in your role as a registered nurse. These simulations can foster a sense of confidence and self-assurance that will serve you well throughout your career.

> **STORY**
>
> **Simulation: the challenge of speaking up; Lucy's story**
>
> As a final year undergraduate student, Lucy was undertaking her last clinical placement in a busy medical ward. Lucy was on a late shift and under the supervision of registered nurse Ben. Lucy's preceptor was sick for the shift and Ben was assigned to Lucy. However, Ben expressed to Lucy at the commencement of the shift that he really was too busy for a student and hoped that she would be able to keep up to his pace. It was 4 p.m. and several patients were due for their medications. Lucy indicated that she would like to prepare the medication for one of her assigned patients. The patient required two oral medications, one being a restricted medication requiring a two-nurse check. Lucy gathered the patient's medication chart and proceeded to go to the medication preparation area. Lucy requested that Ben be present. Ben agreed and together they checked the medications against the medication order. Ben hurried Lucy in the process, which made Lucy feel anxious.
>
> Lucy and Ben left the medication preparation area and proceeded towards the patient's bed. At this point Ben signed the medication chart and indicated to Lucy that he needed to get on with other medications and she was fine to proceed to the patient and administer the medications herself. Ben suggested to Lucy that she was on her final placement, so she had best get ready for the real world of practice. Lucy was reluctant to speak up and therefore did not ask Ben to come with her to the patient to provide direct supervision (as she had been taught). Anxious and hesitant, Lucy knew that her actions were wrong but proceeded to give the patient the medication without Ben.
>
> Lucy shared the experience with her preceptor the next day, knowing that she had breached safe practice. While the preceptor and Lucy managed the situation, upon reflection Lucy understood that patient safety had been compromised and she spoke about guilt, the fear of doing something wrong and yet the need to feel accepted by Ben. Lucy did not want to 'rock the boat' by speaking up and requesting that Ben provide direct supervision. Lucy had heard about her friends attending an extracurricular simulation and how the simulation focused on medication administration and the challenging situations that students could find themselves in. Her friends shared examples of how they were taught to speak up when they felt patient safety was compromised. At the time Lucy said she had so many other commitments and didn't have time to attend. Lucy felt that if she had participated in the simulation it may have helped her to respond to Ben using communication skills that could have resulted in Ben providing the safe level of supervision necessary.

Thinking about the two different stories from Lucy and Emma we hope you might be thinking more about engaging with simulation. To begin your preparation for learning through simulation the next section introduces some benefits and challenges for you to consider.

Benefits and challenges of participating in simulation

Now you know about the different kinds of simulation that you might be asked to participate in we would like you to think back on a time when you did experience a simulation.

REFLECTION

Think about a recent simulation you participated in. This could be a role play, a manikin simulation, an OSCE/OSCA or even an escape room like the Hogwarts one provided in the section on escape rooms in this chapter. If you have never participated in a simulated experience perhaps you have been in an IMAX theatre or watched a 2D or 3D film? These experiences are simulations. Or you could spend some time doing the Hogwarts escape room introduced earlier.

What we would like you to do is list 3–5 points of what you thought was good about your simulation experience—what did you learn, was it enjoyable and so on.

Now list 3–5 challenges you may have experienced. This could be things like: you felt unprepared; you didn't know what to expect; you wanted more time to get the answers right and so on.

Keep your list as we will ask that you reflect on it at the end of this next section on the benefits and challenges for students learning with simulation.

BENEFITS OF SIMULATION

Availability. If you have access (within timetable requirements) to the simulation rooms where you are studying you may find that the equipment or scenario is already set up for you to practise your skills. This is a great benefit of simulation for you to develop competence and confidence.

Adaptability occurs when the simulations are designed to target your specific skills and knowledge deficits. Why not ask your lecturers if you can use the equipment when it suits you? This way you can **practise the skills and knowledge** you need to develop.

Simulations can be arranged so you **develop skills** to manage critical and stressful situations, for example a **deteriorating patient**. It is not always likely that you will care for different kinds of deteriorating patients (e.g. cardiac, respiratory, aggressive, trauma) during your clinical placements; however, you still need to learn these skills. Simulation scenarios are excellent for **allowing you to practise caring, critical thinking and clinical reasoning for many kinds of patients**.

Sometimes caring for high acuity (very ill) patients places the patient and yourself at risk because you may not have the knowledge or are not yet confident in performing skills. Simulation **allows you to make mistakes without harming real patients, staff or yourself**. Think about learning how to give an injection or insert a nasogastric tube. It is **safer** for you to practise on a manikin than a real patient.

Simulations allow you to **practise deliberately** by concentrating on specific skills and also give you the opportunity for **repeated practice**.

Feedback is a key benefit of simulation and once you have received feedback then you can repeat the skill to master it. This leads to another benefit of simulation that is **gaining confidence and competence**.

CHALLENGES OF SIMULATION

Students will sometimes comment that the simulations **are not real** or are not as real as a real-life situation or what you might experience in the clinical setting.

Similar to this complaint is that the patient scripts or the **scenarios may be stereotypical and therefore cultural considerations** and specifics of patients, such as the patient experiencing a mental health crisis, are not always portrayed **accurately**.

Problems with technology not working is a common complaint.

Access to the internet can also make computer simulations and virtual simulations challenging.

Some students have found that the debrief or the reflective conversations are not always helpful to their learning. Sometimes this is because we don't understand the reason for the reflective conversation, or we don't understand how to reflect. There is a section on reflection in this chapter to help you develop your reflective skills and understanding.

Remember, everyone has to learn new skills and sometimes your teachers may be new to simulation so this could be a challenge. This means at times you may not feel comfortable during the simulation. This chapter provides a whole section for you to think about how you can feel safe and prepare yourself for the simulation.

Table 19.1 shows there are many more benefits than challenges for learning with simulation.

REFLECTION

These two papers are about students' experiences of debriefs that might help you prepare for your next simulation-based learning experience:

Fey M K, Scrandis D, Daniels A, Haut C 2014 Learning through debriefing: students' perspectives. Clinical Simulation in Nursing 10(5): e249–e256 https://doi.org/10.1016/j.ecns.2013.12.009

Ryan C, Delport S, Channell P, et al 2021 Nursing and paramedicine student and academic perceptions of the two phase debrief model: a thematic analysis. Nurse Education in Practice 51: 103001–103001 https://doi.org/10.1016/j.nepr.2021.103001

TABLE 19.1
Benefits and challenges identified in virtual simulation

BENEFITS	CHALLENGES
Knowledge	Technology
Repeated and deliberate practice	Design flaws
Engaging	Unrealistic
Reduces theory–practice gap	Staff need training
Patient-centred	Being an avatar is hard
Student-centred	Development costs
Consistent learning	Difficult navigating virtual worlds
Communication	Minimal debriefing
Realistic	
Teamwork	
Confidence	
Satisfying	
Accessible	

Source: Cant et al 2023

> ## REFLECTION
>
> ### An introduction to reflection
>
> If you haven't learned how to reflect or why we need to, we introduce the concept later in this chapter. Have a go at this very simple reflective exercise first.
>
> Return to the list of benefits and challenges you made at the start of this section. Now think about the new things you have learned from reading this section.
>
> Reflect on your list and the new points you read about and add to your list several points that could improve your experience and the experience of your nursing friends in simulated learning.
>
> This kind of reflection helps you to think about and identify what you could do differently to improve your practice. You can do this simple reflection every time you perform a skill or learn something new either in simulated or the real practice.

Now you have read about the kinds of simulation available and the benefits and challenges to you of learning with simulation, the next section explains more ways to gain the most out of simulation.

Tips to gain the most out of simulation

Your teachers are responsible for creating the essential content for your learning. How you personally engage with that learning will influence the level of knowledge, skills and understanding you will achieve. So how can you personally get the most out of your simulation-based activities, so you feel ready for clinical placement or your practical assessments? Here are some tips!

1. Read the information given to you. Your teachers put considerable thought into how to set you up for success in the simulation laboratory. The suggested or required pre-reading and activities give you the foundational knowledge required for the session. This is, in fact, part of your pre-briefing. Having this knowledge before you step into the simulation laboratory allows you to spend more time practising, getting feedback and clarifying any concerns. If this isn't done, then many students waste the first half of the session trying to figure out what they are meant to do and miss the opportunity to practise. **Tip number 1:** preparation enhances practice

2. Your teachers think carefully about how the simulation activity is designed. Although the patient may not be real, for example your patient may be a manikin or a peer, the skill you are practising is real, and the conversations you may have with your fellow team members in the simulation are real. If you can, as much as possible, treat the simulated patient as real, then you will find it easier to engage in the activity and the more learning you can achieve (Rudolph et al 2014). For example, you are practising inserting an indwelling urinary catheter on a female pelvis part-task trainer. If you engage with that part-task trainer as if there is a woman attached to the pelvis, you can not only practise the physical skill, but also your therapeutic communication, treating the whole person. You will find that the fact you are only practising on a piece of plastic will be become less obvious and you will begin to feel both cognitively and emotionally

that you are putting a catheter in a real patient. Rehearsing a skill while having to think about the person as a whole and managing your own emotions is fundamentally replicating what it is like in real practice. The more you can practise this in the simulation laboratory, not just the skill, but learning self and patient management strategies, the easier it will be in real practice and the better practitioner you will be. **Tip number 2:** engage as much as you can that the patient/environment/team is real

3. It's all in the attitude. Look, we all have bad days, but approaching your time in simulation with a positive attitude will help to advance your learning. This may seem hard when you are struggling to master a skill, you receive some difficult feedback, or you are making mistakes. The simulation laboratory, though, is the place to make mistakes (outside of formal assessment)! Making mistakes and receiving constructive feedback to understand what went wrong is a powerful learning tool. So, to help you be kind to yourself, give yourself the Basic Assumption© (Clark & Fey 2020, Rudolph 2022). That is, you are intelligent, capable, care about doing your best and you are there as you want to improve. Giving yourself and others the Basic Assumption allows you to hold yourself in high regard, while also maintaining a high standard of practice. **Tip number 3:** give yourself and your peers (even your teachers!) the Basic Assumption

4. You will hear a lot that simulation is the place to make mistakes, and it is absolutely correct. In simulation you can practise without hurting or harming a patient. Simulation, though, is also the place to learn from success! You will do many things successfully when practising in the simulation laboratory. Sometimes you may not understand how you came to be successful. Receiving feedback on your success and exploring how you got there is fantastic learning. If you know how you were successful, then you know how to repeat it in the future. **Tip number 4:** remember to learn from success as well as from your mistakes.

Feedback, self-reflection and reflective conversations

THE IMPORTANCE OF FEEDBACK

Feedback comes in many forms. It can be obvious, such as a grade on your paper, or it can be very subtle, such as your teacher in the classroom agreeing with your point made. In simulation, feedback is usually delivered in varying ways, such as direct feedback from your peers or teacher on your actions when you are practising a skill. It could be in the form of successful completion of a patient care episode in VR, or it is often in reflective conversations (often referred to as a debrief) where a facilitator helps you to reflect upon your own and/or your team's performance. This is to understand what went well, what did not go to plan and most importantly, why. You may not know at first why, but through facilitated reflection, you can begin to work through your thinking (cognitive processes), your behavioural responses (attitudes, communication strategies and approaches to situations) and your technical skills. Elite athletes and musicians achieve their success by not just practising, but by deliberately practising **with** coaching and feedback (Ericsson 2006). They regularly self-assess their own performance, for example watch video recordings of their performances, alongside actively seeking feedback from their coach (teacher) and mentors. In the simulation laboratory, you can do this too. Many simulation laboratories have audio-visual systems for the purpose of rewatching performance, and through the facilitated coaching and reflective conversations (debriefs). Simulation, in fact, is the ideal environment to give and receive feedback. You have opportunities to work independently, with peers and with your facilitator/coach. Best thing of all, you can practise and make mistakes, learn, and get feedback, try again and no patients get hurt! Bloxham and Campbell (2010) suggest you might even like to use prompts with your teachers or peers in seeking feedback:

- What are the strengths of my performance?
- What are the weak points of this performance?
- What I would like your feedback on is …

When you are out on clinical placement, take a moment to watch a great nurse in action. They can in the moment be doing a care or intervention and then pause, reflect, and then change their approach if something isn't working. This is because they can reflect in action. Your learning in the simulation laboratory will help you learn how to reflect **on** your actions. If you keep practising reflecting on your actions, and actively seeking feedback, you will then be able to start reflecting **in** action (Schön 2017). That means, like that great nurse, you can reflect while 'doing'. You have a heightened level of self-awareness, making you a safer practitioner.

Giving respectful, helpful and constructive feedback is a vital skill. The simulation laboratory is an ideal environment to learn how to give feedback to others; in particular, to your peers. One day soon you will be a qualified nurse and will have a student working with and learning from you. As their preceptor, you will want them to do well and be safe; this means you will need to be effective at giving feedback. Simulation laboratories provide amazing opportunities to learn so much more than technical skills!

RECEIVING FEEDBACK

A key to success is not just receiving feedback, but how you receive the feedback provided. Receiving feedback can be hard, particularly when it does not align with your own self-assessment of your performance. To be effective in receiving feedback, you need to be able to manage your emotions, be able to listen to understand the message, and to get curious enough to clarify and seek further understanding (Barlow et al 2023). This is easier to do when you are in a learning environment where you feel safe to try a new skill and make mistakes, to question and to seek further clarification if you do not understand the feedback provided. This is where pre-briefing (mentioned earlier) is so important as it helps to establish your understanding on how to engage during the activities, how to question and how to get feedback.

Effective reception of feedback requires the ability to listen. Listening is a participatory activity, meaning it requires your attention and effort. Listening involves both hearing and understanding of what is being said. Often, we receive feedback that may not align with our own evaluations or may even challenge perceptions we have of ourselves or a situation. This can be difficult, and it is easy to get defensive. When we jump into defending our position without trying to understand the other person's perspective, we are fundamentally *listening to respond*. When we listen to respond, we are not taking the time to understand what is actually being said to us, and as a result we may judge the message or the person's intent incorrectly. This does not mean you have to agree with all the feedback you are given, but taking the time to listen to understand the feedback, getting curious about what the other person means and seeking clarification is what is called *listening to learn* (Carnegie 2018). If you can manage your emotions, hold the belief that feedback is helpful to enhance your performance and position yourself to be willing to seek further clarification, you will find your learning will be enhanced and, in turn, you will start actively seeking more feedback in the future. This is an amazing continual cycle of self-improvement. If you want to understand more about how to effectively receive feedback, check out these resources (Barlow et al 2023, Stone & Heen 2015).

Learning to self-reflect: participating in a reflective conversation

We introduced you to a simple reflective conversation earlier in this chapter. Reflection is a large concept that we do not expect you to master from this chapter. Learning to reflect will help you improve your competence, confidence and capabilities for skills performance, critical thinking, problem solving and even empower you to be the nurse you want to be. You can start to learn to reflect by thinking about and answering these guiding self-reflective questions (Colomer et al 2013):

1. What are my emotions in response to the situation?
2. What knowledge did I have that helped me in the situation related to (this identifies your strengths):
    a. my emotions
    b. my actions
    c. my attitude?
3. Do I need to improve my (this identifies your areas for improvement):
    a. oral communication skills
    b. self-reflective learning skills
    c. knowledge and practical skills
    d. attitude
    e. emotions, stress and anxiety
    f. something else meaningful to you?
4. What does my learning plan for this situation look like?
5. Who will help me enact my learning plan?
6. How do I like to learn—self-directed, lecture, video, simulation, on my own, in a group, what else?
7. What difficulties am I currently having learning?
8. What is working for me and what isn't?

During your studies you may also be introduced to any number of these reflection approaches. To learn how to reflect you could start by using a different approach each time until you develop your own or choose one that works for you.

▸ Read: Gibbs Reflective Cycle (https://www.ed.ac.uk/reflection/reflectors-toolkit/reflecting-on-experience/gibbs-reflective-cycle)

▸ Watch: Gibbs Reflective Cycle (https://youtu.be/Rp-gaV-uSIo?si=a6TiY2VAxAScjXH6) (3 minutes with practice examples)

▸ Read: 5 Rs of Reflecting: Reporting, Responding, Relating, Reasoning, Reconstructing (https://crowjack.com/blog/strategy/reflection-models/5r-framework-of-reflection)

- Read: Johns Model of Reflection (https://www.toolshero.com/personal-development/johns-model-of-reflection/)
- Watch: Kolbs experiential cycle (https://youtu.be/Rp-gaV-uSIo?si=a6TiY2VAxAScjXH6) (1 min 47)

ADDITIONAL LEARNING

There are many different models your teachers can use when facilitating the simulation activity and associated debrief/reflective conversation. Here are two resources you might want to look at to deepen your understanding of simulation and reflective conversations (debriefing):

1. The PEARLS debriefing model: explains how a simulation debrief can be structured to enhance safe reflective practice
   - Eppich W, Cheng A 2015 Promoting Excellence and Reflective Learning in Simulation (PEARLS): development and rationale for a blended approach to healthcare simulation debriefing. Simulation in Healthcare 10(2):106–115. Read more here: PEARLS Debriefing Tool – Debrief2Learn (https://debrief2learn.org/pearls-debriefing-tool/)
2. The Debriefing Assessment for Simulation in Healthcare (DASH). This resource helps to assess a debriefer's performance, whether it is self-reflection (instructor version), student feedback to the debriefer on their experience being in the debrief, or debriefing expert feedback to debriefer (rater):
   - Handbook: DASH Rater's Handbook (https://harvardmedsim.org/resources/dash-raters-handbook-en/)
   - Student version of the DASH: DASH© Score Sheet Student Version (https://harvardmedsim.org/resources/dash-score-sheet-student-version-long-form/)
   - Colomer J, Pallisera M, Fullana J, et al 2013 Reflective learning in higher education: a comparative analysis. Procedia – Social and Behavioral Sciences 93(C):364–370 https://doi.org/10.1016/j.sbspro.2013.09.204.

REFLECTION

Think of a time when you were practising a skill with a peer, and they did something you deemed was incorrect. This could be in the simulation laboratory, clinical context or, if you are just starting your study, in your part-time job. Examples might be they made an error in following the asepsis protocol or forgot to check allergies before administering a medication.
- What did you say?
- What did you not say? Why didn't you say it?
- What do you think may be the future impact of you not providing feedback to your peer?

Think of a time when you received feedback from your teacher. Hold that thought …

Now think of a time when you received feedback from a peer. Ask yourself:
- How did you react receiving feedback from a peer as opposed to your teacher/lecturer?
- Did it feel different receiving feedback from a peer as opposed to your teacher/lecturer? If so, how and why?
- Did you evaluate or perceive the feedback differently depending on who gave you the feedback?
- What did you do with the feedback they provided?

Safe learning environment

PHYSICAL SAFETY

In Australia between 2021 and 2022, 15.3% (76,100) of healthcare and social assistance staff (including nurses) were injured or suffered illness as part of their job (Australian Bureau of Statistics [ABS] 2023). This number is sadly higher than other industries that are considered 'dangerous', such as mining at 1.7% (8300) and construction at 11.4% (56,600) (ABS 2023). It is no surprise then that safety is an important consideration when thinking of nursing practice, real or simulated.

Simulations are designed as much as possible to replicate the real clinical world, or at the very least a small part of it. While this helps create an authentic practice environment it does present some risks if we are not careful and mindful of what we are doing. Manual handling, the use of sharps and environmental hazards are all things that can pose a problem if we are not vigilant. How do we try and avoid these risks? Safety checks should be something that everyone does before any simulation; these may be a formal process requested by your teacher, or something that you do individually. These safety checks will not only mitigate any current risks but will also get you into the practice of performing safety checks at the start of your clinical shift. But what should be included?

- Is the environment free of clutter?
- Are the bed brakes on?
- Are the beds at the right height?
- Is all the equipment (IV pumps, hoist, ECG machine etc.) working?
- Is there enough hand gel and/or soap?
- Is there enough PPE?
- Are the sharps bin not full?

Additionally in Australia there are approximately 180,000 healthcare-associated infections (HCAI) annually, accounting for around 2 million hospital bed days and 7000 deaths (Australian Council on Healthcare Standards [ACHS] 2023). This is alarming, but how does that affect you in simulation? Well, what we practise is what we remember and take into the clinicalsetting. You might think that wearing a watch or having painted nails won't do any harm in simulation and maybe you're right. But what happens if practising with a watch and painted nails reinforces that practice when you work clinically? Do you really want to be the reason that a patient suffers from an HCAI because of something you took to them on the band of your watch?

EMOTIONAL SAFETY

As we have previously discussed, simulation and the various activities that you will be involved in are a great way for you to practise and sharpen your nursing skills before performing them on a real-life patient. Of course, this will ultimately help improve the safety of the patients that you will care for, as you can practise a skill for the very first time with no fear of risk to a patient. Ultimately this provides you with the opportunity to learn new things with no negative consequence if things do not go according to plan; although, when things go well in simulation you will be able to grow confidence in your own ability.

Learning anything new can, however, be difficult and stressful. Combining this difficulty with having to demonstrate new knowledge and skills in a simulation lab for others to see can soon lead to becoming overwhelmed and feeling uncomfortable and fearful of doing the wrong thing. The good news is most of the other students in the room are feeling the same way; however, knowing this is unlikely to add to your own confidence and make you feel ready to engage in the lesson. So how can we help ourselves and the others around us feel more comfortable during simulation and gain the most out of the lesson?

The most important thing to remember is that no-one is perfect the first time they try something. Mistakes will happen and will often be the most useful thing to help us learn and get better. If we didn't need to practise and improve, we wouldn't need simulation. Walk into any large hospital and you will find nurses of all experience levels taking part in simulations, from cannulation to resuscitation. If an experienced nurse needs to improve through simulation, then you should feel comfortable about having to do the same thing. Be kind to yourself and understand that you do not have to be perfect, but rather you need to be willing to improve. If something goes wrong, rather than think 'I can't believe I did that', think 'what will I do better next time?' While this may seem like a simple thing, by role modelling this behaviour and thought process, others around you will start to feel more comfortable and join in with your way of thinking.

Remember, however, that while you need to create a safe space for you and others around you, it is equally important to challenge yourself. It can sometimes be easy to shy away from something that scares us, although this can mean that we might miss out from valuable experience and learning. Being involved in simulation role play is something that can be fearful for many students. Not everyone likes to talk in public and most of us do not want to appear silly in front of others. Because of this fear we might decide to say no and sit and watch others. The trouble is, nursing is full of scary things the first time we need to do them, such as the first time having to give an intramuscular injection or the first time providing chest compressions. Being able to deal with and work through that fear can be just as important as the nursing care you are providing. Don't let fear be the reason you miss out on valuable learning; rather, let fear be the reason you want to learn.

REFLECTION

Picture yourself in a simulation lab practising a skill for the first time. You don't really know the student you are partnered with very well, but it is clear they are nervous and a little anxious. You want them to feel comfortable and be okay with just having a try but you don't know what to say.

1. What have you learned with others in the past (driving, public speaking etc.) when you have felt uncomfortable, anxious or stressed?
2. Did someone say or do something that made you feel better? Could you use this with your simulation partner?
3. Did someone say or do something that was unhelpful and made you feel worse? What was this and how will you avoid the same mistake?
4. If you are the person feeling anxious, what could you say to your partner to let them know?

Moving forward with simulation as part of your learning journey

It is now time to bring all the content of this chapter together. Making a plan for how to prepare yourself for the next time you are going to engage with simulation is a good way to do this.

Using your notes from the reflection activities and from Emma and Lucy's stories will help you make your plan. Here are some key questions to guide the content of your plan.

Spend some time now making a few notes to answer the following points:

1. Start by thinking about the kind of simulation you will be participating in
2. List the challenges and benefits of this kind of simulation that you know and that are relevant to you and how you will engage and learn
3. Dot point how will you manage the challenges and really learn from benefits you have identified.

> **TIP**
>
> Revisit the chapter sections and your notes, particularly on preparing to engage with simulation, giving and receiving simulation feedback, reflection, physical and emotional safety, and Emma and Lucy's stories.

To keep benefiting from simulation at your university:

1. Consider how you could access the simulation lab or extracurricular simulations
2. Think about making a time management plan so you can attend more simulations. Think about all the things you have to do, such as work, study, life, family
3. Get together with other nursing colleagues and share your plan
4. Perhaps you can help your nursing friends make their own plan.

See Lucy's plan (Box 19.1) as an example:

I heard that there was going to be an extracurricular simulation day at my university, and I really want to attend. One of the scenarios is role play about a student needing to manage their RN supervisor on clinical practice when giving medications. The other scenario is a manikin-based OSCE to manage anaphylaxis. Now realising simulation could really help me, I made a plan. I'd like to share with you so that we can all learn more from simulation.

BOX 19.1
Lucy's plan: the simulation is role play and the other is manikin OSCE

CHALLENGES THAT MIGHT AFFECT ME

- The role play might be challenging because I might have to act as the patient, or the student—I don't like being the centre of attention
- What if no-one wants to act? Will I be brave enough to put my hand up?
- In the manikin one—what will I have to do and learn?
- What if the technology goes wrong?
- How will I know how to use the manikin?
- What if the teachers are too direct when they give feedback? I'm not feeling that confident right now

BOX 19.1
Lucy's plan: the simulation is role play and the other is manikin OSCE—cont'd

BENEFITS FOR ME
- I'll get to practise speaking up to the RN in the role play so I know how to do it when on clinical placement
- I might learn some communication phrases that help me manage RNs like Ben in future placements
- I'll get to manage the anaphylaxis situation
- I'll learn heaps of skills using the manikin, giving medication, IV medication administration and management, IV fluids administration and management, patient communication, escalating a deteriorating patient, taking observations in a stressful situation ... that's what's important to me
- I'll get to understand about the manikins
- I might feel more confident and capable at the end, especially if I get to act in the role play as the student nurse
- If I play the role of the patient, I can better understand their perspective when someone is caring for me

HOW I WILL MANAGE THE CHALLENGES
- Get there early and see if I can have access to the manikin
- Trust that the lecturers will give us an orientation to the manikin, and we can have a play first—I've heard they are good at doing that anyway
- Believe that other students will be the same as me—nervous and not very used to working with manikins and not wanting to be the centre of attention
- I'll be very positive about the whole experience; after all, nothing can go wrong (I can't hurt the patient) and this isn't an assessment
- I'm going to practise my self-reflection so that I can do that every time I do something in the role play or the manikin simulation
- I'm going to try and speak up when I don't know something
- To keep myself and my colleagues safe I'll do the safety check

Now being anxious and stressed is a big thing for me. I don't like speaking up. But I know I need to develop my confidence:

- I will practise some breathing techniques like breathing slowly and trying to calm myself before I get into the simulation
- If I get anxious, I will ask the lecturers if I can have some time out
- I will let my lecturers and nursing friends know that I get anxious
- I know the more I practise managing my anxiety or nerves in the simulation lab, the more I will know what works for me and what doesn't. This will make it easier to manage my nerves when I'm out on placement

Continued

> **BOX 19.1**
> **Lucy's plan: the simulation is role play and the other is manikin OSCE—cont'd**
>
> TO MAXIMISE MY LEARNING FROM THE SIMULATION I WILL …
>
> - Read all the material sent to me about the simulations
> - Complete the required pre-learning activities so I have the required knowledge and therefore I can spend my time practising and applying that knowledge
> - Be on time
> - Think about anaphylaxis and what it is and how to manage it
> - Understand I don't know everything—I am learning
> - Be open to receiving (and giving) feedback
> - Have my self-reflection model in my mind
> - Participate in the reflective conversations in the debrief
> - Take responsibility for my own emotional health and the actions I decide to implement (even if they are not quite right)
> - Turn up with an attitude to learn and improve

Now, making time for this simulation and other simulations is always going to be a bit tricky. I have work, family, study, exercise, just like everyone else. This simulation is actually all day on a Wednesday 0900–1700. I normally have no lectures and work half a day on Wednesdays. I also study and go to football training at 4.30 p.m. I need to work. I'm sort of up to date with my study and I don't need to go to footy training every week. Here is my plan:

1. I've emailed the teacher on the flyer and asked if I can attend from 12 noon or the afternoon only. They said yes! So, looks like I'm going to my first extracurricular simulation
2. I've organised to go with some other nursing friends. We are all meeting at 11.30 a.m. and going in one car. We are all going to make sure we all go—no backing out
3. We all have made a plan like this, and we are going to email our plans to each other so we can help each other get the most out of this.

I think that in the future I will be able to plan like this and fit in more simulations and access the simulation labs when they are open so that I can keep developing my confidence, competence and capability using simulation.

CONCLUSION

This chapter has introduced fundamental components of simulation. You will now have an idea of the different kinds of simulations that are available. You have learned about the benefits and challenges of learning with simulation. We hope you have read about the many ways you can obtain the most from simulated learning. Key to simulation learning is getting involved and working with your peers and lecturers to learn from the experience. Self-reflection is very important, as is participating in the reflective conversations in the debrief—when the simulation is all pulled together for your learning. We hope you now have a plan for how you will engage with simulation and prepare yourself for simulated learning at your university or education centre.

Simulation is so important for developing your confidence, competence and capabilities so you can be the nurse you want to be and contribute to shaping the next generation of nursing students.

References

Australian Bureau of Statistics 2023 6324.0 Work-related injuries, 2021–22: Table 4. Occupation and Industry of job where work-related injury occurred, 2021-22 [Data table]. Online. Available: https://www.abs.gov.au/statistics/labour/earnings-and-working-conditions/work-related-injuries/latest-release

Australian Council of Healthcare Standards 2023 Australasian clinical indicator report: 2015–2022, 24th edn. Online. Available: https://www.achs.org.au/news/acir2015-22

Barlow M, Watson B, Morse K et al 2023 React, reframe and engage. Establishing a receiver mindset for more effective safety negotiations. Journal of Health Organization and Management https://doi.org/10.1108/JHOM-06-2023-0171

Bloxham S, Campbell L 2010 Generating dialogue in assessment feedback: exploring the use of interactive cover sheets. Assessment & Evaluation in Higher Education 35(3):291–300 https://doi.org/10.1080/02602931003650045

Bromley P 2019 A paradigm shift from competence to capability in neonatal nursing. Journal of Neonatal Nursing 25(6):268–271 https://doi.org/10.1016/j.jnn.2019.04.003

Cant R, Ryan C, Kelly M 2023 Use and effectiveness of virtual simulations in nursing student education. CIN: Computers, Informatics, Nursing 41(1):31–38 doi: 10.1097/CIN.0000000000000932.

Carnegie D 2018. Listen!: the art of effective communication. G&D Media

Clark C, Fey M 2020 Fostering civility in learning conversations: introducing the PAAIL communication strategy. Nurse Educator 45(3):139–143 https://doi.org/https://doi.org/10.1097/NNE.0000000000000731

Colomer J, Pallisera M., Fullana J et al 2013 Reflective learning in higher education: a comparative analysis. Procedia - Social and Behavioral Sciences, 93, 364–370 https://doi.org/10.1016/j.sbspro.2013.09.204

Eppich W, Cheng A 2015 Promoting Excellence and Reflective Learning in Simulation (PEARLS): development and rationale for a blended approach to health care simulation debriefing. Simulation in Healthcare 10(2):106–115

Ericsson K A 2006 The influence of experience and deliberate practice on the development of superior expert performance. The Cambridge Handbook of Expertise and Expert Performance 38(685–705):2–2.

Kolb D 1984 Experiential learning: experience as the source of learning and development. Prentice Hall

Reid-Searl K 2020 Mask-Ed (KRS Simulation) an approach to deliver intimate care for neophyte nursing students: the creator's experience. British Journal of Nursing 29(12):S8–S10.

Rudolph J 2022 What's Up with the Basic Assumption™? Center for Medical Simulation. Online. Available: https://harvardmedsim.org/blog/whats-up-with-the-basic-assumption/ 3 January 2022

Rudolph J W, Raemer D B, Simon R 2014 Establishing a safe container for learning in simulation: the role of the presimulation briefing. Simulation in Healthcare 9(6):339–349 https://doi.org/10.1097/sih.0000000000000047

Schön D A 2017 The reflective practitioner: how professionals think in action. Routledge https://doi.org/10.4324/9781315237473

Stephenson J, Yorke M 2013 Capability and quality in higher education. Routledge

Stone D, Heen S 2015 Thanks for the feedback: the science and art of receiving feedback well. Penguin

Virtual Reality Oasis 2019 Beginners guide to virtual reality – which headset should you buy? Available at https://www.youtube.com/watch?v=T0taTtOgqd8 24 September 2024

CHAPTER 20

PREPARING FOR AND MAKING MEANING OF CLINICAL PLACEMENT

Lynda Hughes and Sandra Johnston

KEY WORDS
accountability
clinical judgment
clinical decision making
clinical learning
curriculum
feedback
information literacy
lifelong learning
theory–practice gap
transition
reflective practice

LEARNING OBJECTIVES
After reading this chapter, readers should be able to:
- value both clinical and theoretical knowledge in nursing and appreciate the need to integrate clinical and theoretical knowledge for lifelong learning and professional development
- identify personal attributes and strategies that maximise the acquisition of clinical and theoretical knowledge.

INTRODUCTION

This chapter is designed to encourage nurses to view learning as a continuum of development and lifelong learning that has the unifying goal of achieving and maintaining competence within the complexities of contemporary practice. The chapter explores the process of connecting theoretical and clinical knowledge for safe and effective nursing practice through clinical judgment. The importance of both the 'classroom' and clinical setting for learning is discussed.

The interconnection of theoretical knowledge and clinical knowledge is explored in the broader context of ways of knowing as well as the sociopolitical context of nursing practice. It is suggested that although connecting clinical and theoretical knowledge has been argued to be difficult for students, the development of a set of abilities for learning is essential for effective practice and career development in nursing. An exploration of the elements of reflective practice, self-assessment, engaging with feedback and information literacy outlines the approaches to development of key requirements of the professional registered nurse. As the transition from student to graduate can be a particularly challenging period, the importance of having developed a range of strategies that assist in integrating clinical and theoretical knowledge during transition is emphasised.

Connecting clinical and theoretical learning

Nursing is a discipline that integrates both theoretical and practical components to ensure that safe evidence-based care is provided. The capacity to respond appropriately and effectively in nursing practice is dependent upon the extent to which one connects the clinical and theoretical knowledge to make sense of situations. Such sense-making requires clinical judgment. 'Clinical judgement is a reflective and reasoning process that draws upon all available data, is informed by an extensive knowledge base and results in the formation of a clinical conclusion' (Connor et al 2023). By this definition, clinical judgment is more than clinical reasoning, critical thinking or clinical decision making. It is the collective process drawing on all these skills and processes to 'make sense' of a clinical situation. This requires both theoretical knowledge and clinical knowledge.

The Nursing and Midwifery Board of Australia (NMBA) identify in their Decision-Making Framework that clinical judgments and decisions must be contextually appropriate (NMBA 2022). Therefore, there is a need for learners to be able to transfer concepts between the learning cultures typical of classrooms (i.e. theoretical knowledge) and apply these to a variety of clinical contexts (i.e. clinical knowledge). Furthermore, there is a need for graduates to continue to develop the skills of integrating and applying theoretical and clinical knowledge as they transition to practice. In her often-cited classical work about the development of registered nurses, Benner (1984) has identified that the ability to integrate theory knowledge to practice to the point of being able to generalise is essential to the development from novice (first year of nursing education) to the advanced beginner (new graduates) to more advanced levels of nurse-mastery (Benner 2021).

Being a nurse requires the ability to actively respond with nursing interventions, to think about the clinical judgments made and the consequences of action taken and to develop a capacity to articulate that thinking to others. It moves beyond theoretical and clinical knowledge and ensures registered nurses underpin their nursing actions with ethical competence; reflecting caring, empathy and trust which are all vital to nursing today (Vabo et al 2022). These elements contribute to the development of the nurse and demonstrate the different knowledge required in modern nursing. There are five ways of knowing in nursing: empirical (how things work and sensory knowledge); personal (awareness of self and others); aesthetic (unique meaning and intent on nursing situations); moral/ethical (nature of right and wrong); and emancipatory (issues of social justice) (Chinn et al 2021). By integrating these ways of knowing, nurses as health professionals demonstrate the knowledge-intensive capabilities necessary to provide expert and reflective nursing practice (Chinn et al 2021).

Student nurses must be able to recognise the connections between clinical and theoretical knowledge of nursing within a broader framework of learning that integrates his or her experience and enables the outcomes of education to be applied in order to practise safe, effective and reflective nursing.

As nurses progress through their education, the nurse develops awareness that the range of factors beyond their knowledge and the immediate client care situation impact upon nursing. Examining the political, economic, technological and sociocultural (PETS) factors that have an impact on care is necessary to ensure wholistic and patient-centred care is provided. When nurses seek to enhance their knowledge, they should reflect upon the extent to which these factors shape themselves and what informs the context of care. Having a political understanding of influences in healthcare broadly enables nurses to challenge the status quo in terms of inequalities and injustice in healthcare (Chinn et al 2021). Understanding economic influences enables nurses to discern market workforce issues and the public versus private healthcare sectors. Understanding of digital health is vital to effectively function in healthcare services of today and in providing safe, effective and sustainable healthcare to our patients (World Health Organization 2020). Sociocultural influences can be evident both individually as well as in the larger community. Figure 20.1 provides an example of the application of

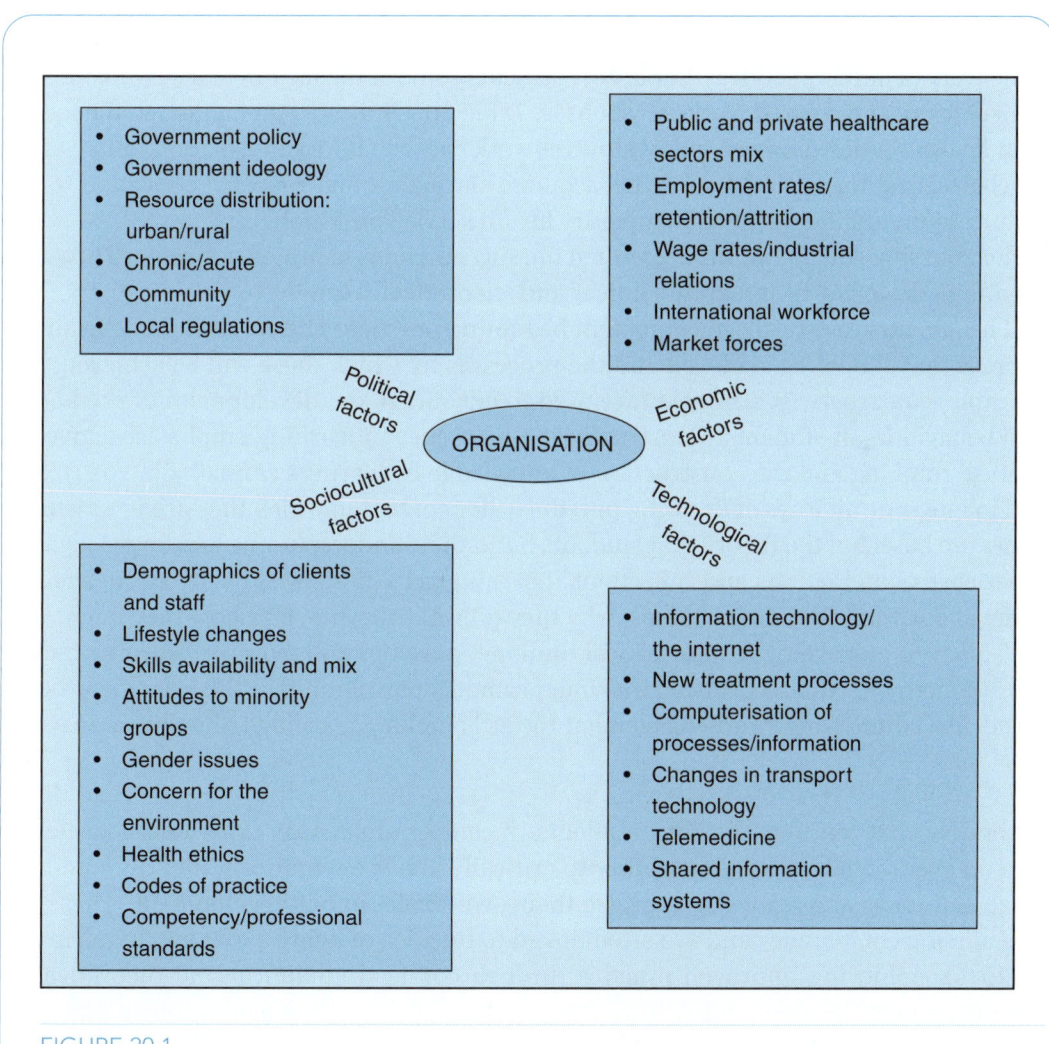

FIGURE 20.1

Application of the PETS framework to explore professional change in nursing

TABLE 20.1
Worker responses to a changing health service

HEALTH SERVICE CHALLENGES	HEALTH WORKER RESPONSE
Technology: clinical and information systems interface Fragmented patient experience Changing health patterns: chronicity and consumerism Changing workforce: unaligned skill mix and case mix Inappropriate structures and processes Changing professional roles and functions Rigidity in professional frameworks and knowledge bases	Procedurally competent, information-fluent personnel Contributors to systems review Effective managers of consumer expectations, competing value systems and tensions in resource allocation Coordinators of throughput and care processes Participants in networked organisation and healthcare teams Personnel who focus on consumer needs and outcomes rather than profession-specific outcomes

PETS to delivery of nursing services. Table 20.1 presents some of the factors that shape contemporary healthcare delivery and desired worker responses. Table 20.1 indicates that although the factors that impact on health service delivery and healthcare work can be viewed in isolation, nurses require a range of clinical and theoretical knowledge acquired through a multi-faceted education to respond meaningfully to the challenges in contemporary health service provision.

In formal nursing education, the accredited nursing curriculum provides structure to a student's learning and is designed to integrate clinical and theoretical learning to develop the knowledge, skills and behaviours that result in competent beginning practice. The curriculum determines both the outcomes that should be achieved and the processes by which these will be achieved. In classroom learning, constructivist strategies are used to encourage the development of the knowledge, skills and behaviours of students. Constructivist approaches to learning emphasise active engagement, critical thinking and the construction of knowledge by learners (Abualhaija 2019). Students also need to integrate all ways of knowing into the wider context in which they are practising. These approaches are based on the theory that students build their understanding and knowledge through their experiences, interactions and reflections. Learning activities should actively engage students in thinking about what they do as nurses, why they do what they do, and how they might do it differently. This type of learning fosters critical thinking, develops collaborative learning techniques, supports autonomy in clinical decision making, promotes partnership in the learning process, and builds students' commitment and engagement towards lifelong learning (Abualhaija 2019).

Developing knowledge

It is imperative that learners, be they students, recent graduates or experienced professionals, capitalise on events that foster their ability to critically analyse situations, identify underpinning knowledge and ideas and critically appraise their own professional development. These abilities underpin nursing competency and are often linked to the idea of being a lifelong, inquiring learner (NMBA 2016). Achieving improved practice through connecting clinical and theoretical knowledge requires active development of the process skills of lifelong learning, including reflective practice, acceptance of the outcomes of self-assessment and effective use of learning resources, including peers and people with qualifications and experiences such as clinical facilitators and nurses in the workplace.

REFLECTIVE PRACTICE FOR LIFELONG LEARNING

Classroom learning activities provide a relatively safe environment to explore what we know, what we do and who we are as nurses, so that we are more prepared for professional practice situations. Clinical learning activities provide the opportunity both to test out what has been learned in practice and to confront new situations to further learning. To be lifelong learners in relation to nursing practice, there is a need to become reflective practitioners. Following a review of theoretical concepts around reflective practice a working definition of reflection is: 'a careful examination and bringing together of ideas to create new insights through ongoing cycles of expression and re/evaluation' (Marshall 2019:411).

That means students need to reflect on what they do as nurses, how they respond as nurses and individuals and what they would do again in a similar situation. The skills of reflective practice unite theoretical and clinical knowledge, allow for consideration of the affective aspects of nursing experience and provide opportunity to explore how the learner as a reflective practitioner felt about the experience. Such an approach is particularly useful in nursing, as it acknowledges human and emotional, as well as intellectual, domains of decision making and encourages self-regulation and autonomy in learning.

As students develop the skills, knowledge and professional behaviours throughout their nursing program, it is important that students take the opportunity to critically evaluate the nursing practice they observe and to create and consider alternatives to this practice. The imagination of possibilities can only occur when nurses think about nursing. In other words, each of us has a professional responsibility to make a conscious decision to think about our own practice and link both our clinical and theoretical knowledge to clearly establish the relationship between our theoretical understandings, judgment and action taking.

Thinking about nursing needs to both direct and emerge from practice. Through the active process of inquiry, students work with, connect and form the ideas that shape their practice as nurses. The intent here is not to give the impression that nurses should only 'think about' nursing. The goal of nursing programs is to develop a graduate who can apply concepts to practice, manage complex nursing situations and accept accountability for practice. To make effective decisions, nurses require the ability to analyse situations and respond appropriately. How nurses interpret and analyse situations depends upon how they think about them. As their thinking about nursing develops, the meaning given to situations changes and learning occurs. This learning is then taken with us to the next situation and new meanings and experiential knowledge are created. This is more formally contextualised in the NMBA's Registered Nurse Standards for Practice (2016). Captured within the first standard for practice: Thinks critically and analyses nursing practice, the Standards for Practice clearly outline that the registered nurse: 'develops practice through reflection on experiences, knowledge, actions, feelings and beliefs to identify how these shape practice' (NMBA 2019:3). The ability to critically examine and appraise personal performance and be accountable for our own actions is essential to learning and professional career development.

Feedback for lifelong learning

Reflective learning requires the ability to conduct a realistic self-assessment. Self-assessment can be viewed as the assessment of one's own abilities, processes and products to improve one's own

overall practice (Andrade 2019). Essentially, self-assessment is a feedback tool on one's own practice. Self-assessment is a process by which people can:
- confirm outcomes of previous experience
- identify areas of strength
- identify areas for development
- remotivate and energise
- help predict and identify personal potential, and
- acknowledge performance against existing standards.

Self-assessment consists of assessing accomplishments and performance to make an informed judgment about strengths and limitations to identify areas for improvement. It is a mechanism which students use to evaluate and improve learning (Yan & Carless 2022). The ability to self-assess and be a reflective practitioner can in part be determined by a person's mindset. Popularised by psychologist Carol Dweck, the growth mindset represents beliefs individuals hold about their abilities, talents, intelligence and potential for growth (Yeager & Dweck 2020). A growth mindset enables students to thrive through challenges and continue to improve over time through effort, learning and persistence. People with a growth mindset embrace challenges as opportunities to learn and see mistakes as part of the learning process (Yeager & Dweck 2020). A student's mindset can influence the outcomes of reflective practice, so it is essential that students understand their own mindset through a systematic approach to self-assessment. Self-assessment is an ongoing process that can be informed by, but is not limited to, the formalised feedback sessions that occur among learners and educators. To ensure a proactive role in self-assessment students need to seek and use feedback from those stakeholders around them (Yan & Carless 2022). Figure 20.2 outlines the interplay between self-assessment and feedback.

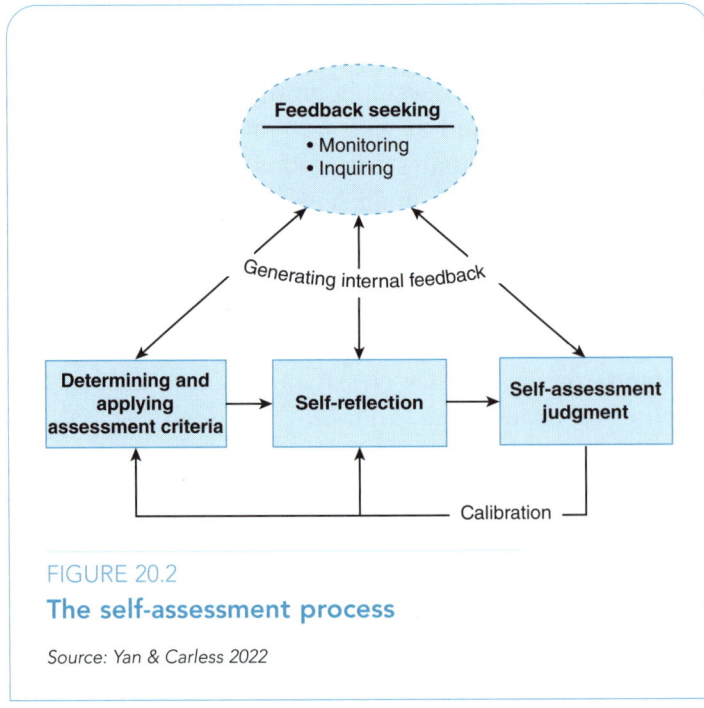

FIGURE 20.2
The self-assessment process

Source: Yan & Carless 2022

> **REFLECTION**
> - Consider your own mindset. How do you rate your own mindset?
> - Do you see yourself as capable of significant growth or see your intelligence as unchanging—you were never the smart one?
> - Do you avoid challenges and see them as potential threats or do you embrace them?
> - Do you persist when encountering difficulties in your learning?
> - Do you seek out critical feedback from targeted sources or do you see feedback as a list of faults and personal attacks?
> - Do you hide or ignore mistakes or see them as high potential for learning?
> - Do you turn down help and support or seek it out?
> - How have you responded to feedback in the past?

Feedback is an essential part of the learning process and contributes to patient safety. Feedback reinforces good practices and motivates the learner towards positive learning outcomes. Students who adopt an active role in feedback conversations have better performance outcomes (Ossenberg et al 2023). However, students often remain dissatisfied with their feedback experiences (Nobel et al 2020). All too often, feedback can be perceived or experienced as reactive and punitive, rather than as a respectful and meaningful vehicle for development through identifying one's own and others' strengths. Feedback involves both openness and vulnerability and it should be authentic, active, meaningful and constructive for nurses as well as those they work with such as clients and peers. Clinical facilitators, academic staff, clinical staff, peers and consumers can provide such feedback contributing to overall understanding of the student's current performance (Hughes 2019). Such critique needs to be managed carefully to maintain perspective and avoid negative responses (Nobel et al 2020). Developing feedback literacy in students is key to mitigating negative responses through learner agency and reflective practice. Feedback literacy development constitutes the following features: seeking information on learning performance, processing feedback information and acting upon feedback information (Malecka et al 2022). These elements, along with developing an understanding of one's growth mindset, enables students to fully engage with learning opportunities.

Connecting clinical and theoretical knowledge in clinical settings

Clinical learning experiences provide the opportunity to integrate classroom theory in 'real-life' practice situations. To be able to provide the care required, nursing students must be able to make deep connections between theoretical knowledge and patient care and effectively transfer theoretical knowledge to address specific patient care situations (Carless-Kane & Nowell 2023). This is not always easy as the complexities of the clinical learning environment can place additional challenges on learning transfer for nursing students (Carless-Kane & Nowell 2023). The clinical environment is characterised by change, rapid advancements in technology and organisational factors. Students are often rotated through a variety of settings in different healthcare settings and the support and supervision in the learning environment may vary (Panda et al 2021). Unlike well-structured theory classes where there is time for concepts to be discussed and 'unpacked', unplanned events often occur in clinical settings. In clinical environments, there is a 'busy-ness', which poses difficulties for students in that connections previously formed between theory and practice may not be immediately recognisable during direct patient care situations. Reflection is a powerful pedagogical approach to stimulate linking classroom theory to practice (Ekelin et al 2021). During clinical placement, opportunities for reflection may occur in the format of a reflective discussion or 'debriefing'. Debriefing is a directed, intentional conversation to discuss actions and thought processes involved in a particular situation (such as the theory that underpins the clinical decision), encourage reflection to foster clinical judgment, decision making and critical thinking (Littlewood & Szyld 2015). Clinical supervisors may lead debriefing sessions, for example, at the end of the week, where students can discuss patient-related topics, observations of behaviours and clinical practices and consider their actions and actions of others in a meaningful way. Debriefing may also occur after critical incidents, including the death of a patient, a violent patient episode and cardiopulmonary resuscitation (CPR) efforts (Toews et al 2021). Practice during clinical placement may be good, challenging and even confronting, but reflection on practice will assist in exploring, questioning and learning from these experiences.

To assist students in making the theory–practice connections, simulation is increasingly being used as an adjunct to clinical placement in nursing education. Simulation has been incorporated into nursing education to such an extent that in some countries, such as the UK and US, it has even been used as a replacement for clinical placement hours (Roberts et al 2019). Whereas the opportunities to practise application of skills and knowledge in the clinical area vary, simulation can provide complex and dynamic clinical and professional situations that can be replicated for all students in a controlled environment. Simulation has been reported to increase students' confidence, learning satisfaction, knowledge and skills, and critical thinking (El Hussein & Cuncannon 2022). Simulation can also enhance teamwork and situation awareness, supporting the enhancement of clinical reasoning (Theobald et al 2021). The clinical scenario is undoubtably an important component of simulation, but debriefing is considered a critical component in learning from the simulated experience (Johnston et al 2019). During debriefing, the simulation facilitator guides a reflection on the actions that occurred during the simulation and encourages learners to discuss and explore the critical elements of experience to gain understanding and insight, thereby promoting the linkage of theory and practice (International Nursing Association for Clinical Simulation and Learning [INACSL] Standards Committee 2021).

REFLECTION

- Reflect on the last simulation you were involved in. What new knowledge, skills or attitudes did you acquire?
- Even though the simulation context may be different to your current clinical placement, how can you apply this knowledge to your clinical practice?
- Reflect on the feedback you received during your last simulation experience. What were the strengths and weaknesses of your performance? How can you use this feedback to improve your clinical practice?

While clinical educators, lecturers and unit staff share in structuring the clinical experience (whether it be real world or simulated), students are also accountable for their own learning. Similar to other country regulatory requirements, the Australian Registered Nurse Standards for Practice (NMBA 2016) embeds concepts of responsibility and accountability in its framework, through reference to critical thinking, reflective practice and a lifelong learning approach to continuing educational development. Being accountable for one's own learning during clinical placement can be demonstrated by taking the initiative to learn. Students who show initiative are well regarded by members of the healthcare team as this is seen as a sign of willingness to learn and potentially leads to being provided with additional learning opportunities (McTier et al 2023). Taking initiative to enhance the learning experience must be balanced with providing safe, quality patient care. This can be achieved by nursing students articulating their scope of practice and learning objectives to the nursing staff they work with (Cusack et al 2020). Clinicians are often uncertain about what students want or have to achieve while on placement and often question student scope of practice; therefore, students must understand their scope of practice and the clinical activities they are permitted to do so that they can be appropriately supported by supervising staff and achieve their learning goals in clinical practice.

REFLECTION

In preparation for clinical placement, reflect on your previous placement and identify what went well and what are areas for further development. Use the NMBA Standards of Practice (2016) to guide your thinking.

NMBA STANDARDS OF PRACTICE	HOW DID I DEMONSTRATE LEARNING?	HOW CAN I DEVELOP FURTHER IN THIS AREA?
Thinks critically and analyses practice		
Engages in therapeutic and professional relationships		
Maintains the capability for practice		
Compressively conducts assessments		
Develops a plan for nursing practice		
Provides safe, appropriate and responsive quality nursing practice		
Evaluates outcomes to inform nursing practice		

- Write three goals for placement based on the identified areas for further development
- Access your scope of practice document appropriate to your university and year of enrolment. How do your learning goals align with your scope of practice?
- Plan how you will discuss your learning goals and scope of practice with staff you work with during clinical placement.

Connecting clinical and theoretical knowledge to transition to practice

In Australia, the NMBA (2016) provides a set of professional standards that nurses must meet to practise in Australia. The professional standards define the practice and behaviour of nurses and include codes of conduct, standards for practice and codes of ethics. To be eligible for registration, students are required to demonstrate they have met these standards by providing safe and effective practice during clinical placement throughout their undergraduate education. Despite having met the required standards for registration, the phrase 'theory–practice gap' is often used in nursing literature in relation to newly graduated nurses. This has been described as 'the gap between the theoretical knowledge and the practical application of nursing, most often expressed as a negative entity with adverse consequences' (Greenway et al 2019). This theory–practice gap is a metaphorical void; that is, experienced yet not easily measurable or quantifiable. This term has persisted in nursing education and generally has negative connotations. A new graduate is a beginning practitioner, but they are often expected to be competent in many areas of nursing. These unrealistic expectations may cause stress and a sense of inadequacy (Charette et al 2023). Rather than perceiving the theory–practice gap as negative, it may be useful to reframe this in a manner that can facilitate change. The new graduate who consciously strives to be curious and to question and use those critical thinking, reflective skills developed during undergraduate education is well placed to become a lifelong learner able to respond to the challenges in any clinical environment (Barbagallo 2019).

The transition period of the first year of practice as a new graduate has been of great interest in nursing literature. The term 'reality shock' was first termed by Kramer (1975) and has since been used to describe the experiences of new graduates when they perceive they are not work ready for their role as registered nurse when they first enter the clinical environment (Masso et al 2022). Characteristics of work readiness include problem-solving skills including the ability to manage daily tasks and workplace challenges; clinical expertise such as psychomotor, clinical assessment and communication skills; and professional capabilities such as collaboration, teamwork and organisational knowledge (Baumann et al 2019, Mirza et al 2019). Practice readiness therefore relies not only on knowledge and skills but also on the ability to relate to others and an awareness of organisational dynamics. While some knowledge and skills have been developed during undergraduate education, other attributes that are workplace related are likely to be developed through experience and workplace exposure and may also be out of an individual's control.

It is important that the healthcare organisation provides support for new graduates. Many healthcare organisations provide a transition program. A well-structured graduate support program aligned with a new graduate's progressive development can provide the support required and positively impact satisfaction with employment, retention in the workforce and practice competence (Charette et al 2023). The strategies that have been found to be beneficial to new graduates as part of a successful transition program include orientation to the wider healthcare organisation and socialisation to the specific ward, systems and processes; regular constructive feedback on performance, which enhances confidence and capability; and dedicated support people who can facilitate learning (Rogers et al 2021). The feeling of being supported has been found to be a factor that has helped new graduates develop confidence and competence (Charette et al 2023).

> **REFLECTION**
> 1 Clinical skills are considered important in the transition to new graduate. Reflect on the clinical skills taught during your nursing course. What skills have you consolidated and what skills require further consolidation?
> 2 In the clinical environment, who can assist you with meeting your needs particularly when confronted by novel or challenging situations?
> 3 What are the strengths you take as a learner and a student of nursing to future practice?

Connecting clinical and theoretical knowledge in 'classroom' learning

Substantial reference has already been made to the nature of reciprocity between clinical and theoretical knowledge and the importance of focused learning experiences related to nursing in either classroom or clinical settings. Through the design of the nursing curriculum, classroom learning provides opportunities to identify and apply theoretical knowledge, explore options and alternatives, justify thinking and learn from examples drawn from practice. It also gives students opportunities to develop the scholarly approaches necessary for contemporary nursing practice.

Contemporary nursing practice requires nurses to be enablers of practice change, but to create change, the skill of information literacy is required (Cantwell et al 2021, Fetter et al 2023). Information literacy is described as the skill to discover, understand and use information (Association of College and Research Libraries 2015). There has been an exponential increase in the amount and complexity of information available to nursing students and healthcare practitioners, therefore efforts to structure nursing practice around the efficient and effective use of healthcare information have been strongly endorsed (NMBA 2016). The application of evidence-based practice (EBP) requires that nurses have the skills to find information, evaluate the quality and apply relevant research findings to practice (Fetter et al 2023). Nursing organisations and professional bodies reflect this emphasis; for example, within its standards for RNs, the NMBA asserts that to improve current practice, nurses must be able to participate in the review of guidelines based on research, and to identify and disseminate any changes in practice in the clinical area (NMBA 2016). Problem solving, decision making, and research are ongoing needs in the healthcare environment. Therefore, the relevance of information literacy can be framed within not only undergraduate nursing education, but also as part of lifelong learning (Cantwell et al 2021).

In the classroom, the collaboration between nurse educators and health/nursing liaison librarians to scaffold information and literacy concepts throughout the course has been demonstrated to be an effective strategy in providing students with a baseline understanding of information literacy (Mahmoud & Withorn 2023). Health liaison librarians have dedicated expertise, which can provide assistance with concepts such as developing clinical questions, identifying scholarly databases; using key words and Boolean searching; and applying limiters to retrieve more relevant and focused results (Sabey & Biddle 2021). Developing knowledge on information literacy prior to entering the workplace can assist with engaging in EBP as a new graduate (Fetter et al 2023).

The contemporary healthcare environment is characterised by rapid technological advances (Brown et al 2020) and working within healthcare requires sound digital capabilities. Digital literacy is described as having the capability needed for living, learning and working in a digital environment (Pearce 2017). Evidence has shown that nurses with skills relating to digital literacy are better able to use their skills in a variety of ways and embrace and use technology at the bedside, potentially increasing the quality of patient care, improving communication between healthcare workers and decreasing clinical errors (Brown et al 2020, Shin et al 2018). The development of digital literacy facilitates engagement with effective decision making, problem solving and research (Terry et al 2019). Technological advances are in constant development in healthcare, therefore maintenance of digital literacy in order to engage with effective decision making, problem solving and research is a professional obligation (Nes et al 2021). The importance of digital literacy is recognised by professional nursing bodies such as the Australian Nursing and Midwifery Federation who have developed the National Nursing and Midwifery Digital Health Capability Framework (Australian Digital Health Agency 2020). This framework can be used by organisations to introduce and adopt technology and innovation but can also be used by individuals. As part of a lifelong learning approach, new graduates can use the framework to assess their own capability across a range of digital health specific domains, and to identify learning and developmental needs or inform personal and professional development plans relevant to their current or future workplace or role.

REFLECTIVE QUESTIONS

Reflect on your current digital skills and identify areas for improvement:
1. What resources are available to help you improve your digital skills?
2. How can you incorporate these resources into your learning?
3. How can you use digital tools to improve patient care? What are some examples of digital tools that can be used to improve patient care?

CONCLUSION

While there is increasing emphasis on the development of cognitive abilities in nursing, this should not lead to what has been labelled as a theory–practice gap. Practical and theoretical nursing knowledge are inevitably and infinitely intertwined. Nursing practice and nursing education have increasingly recognised the need to integrate thinking and doing to create informed action. Students should view their learning to become nurses as occurring in two distinct yet interdependent contexts: the classroom and the clinical setting. Furthermore, they should use their experiences as students to develop foundational knowledge and skills for effective, confident and competent transition to employment.

The past few decades have provided evidence that there is a paradigm shift in education, which now views learning as the construction of meaning in context rather than what to learn and how to do things. Nurse education is about the ability—indeed flexibility—to examine situations, deconstruct them from a number of perspectives and reconstruct them around core concepts essential to nursing practice. When students engage in reflective practice in a manner that enacts individual agency, they are able to reinforce self-worth, retain confidence and self-esteem and expand knowledge and skills.

Contemporary nursing practice demands that clinicians question and justify decisions in context, and emphasise the ability to think about nursing, as well as the ability to perform nursing actions to best manage nursing situations. The challenge for students is to develop an integrated approach to practice, which values thoughtful, highly skilled and efficient action, and to continue with lifelong learning and professional development.

Recommended readings

Australian Digital Health Agency 2020 National Nursing and Midwifery Digital Health Capability Framework. Australian Government, Sydney

Barbagallo M S 2019 Completing reflective practice post undergraduate nursing clinical placements: a literature review. Teaching and Learning in Nursing 14(3):160–165

Benner P 2019 Skill acquisition and clinical judgement in nursing practice: towards expertise and practical wisdom. In: Higgs J (eds) Practice wisdom, volume 3. Brill Sense, The Netherlands, Leiden, pp 225–240

References

Abualhaija N 2019 Using constructivism and student-centered learning approaches in nursing education. International Journal of Nursing and Health Care Research 5(7):1–6

Andrade H L 2019 A critical review of research on student self-assessment. In: Frontiers in Education (Vol. 4, p. 87). Frontiers Media SA

Association of College & Research Libraries. Framework for information literacy for higher education. 2015. Online. Available: www.ala.org/acrl/standards/ ilframework 12 February 2023

Australian Digital Health Agency 2020 National Nursing and Midwifery Digital Health Capability Framework. Australian Government, Sydney, NSW

Barbagallo M S 2019 Completing reflective practice post undergraduate nursing clinical placements: a literature review. Teaching and Learning in Nursing 14(3):160–165

Baumann A, Crea-Arsenio M, Hunsberger M et al 2019 Work readiness, transition, and integration: the challenge of specialty practice. Journal of Advanced Nursing 75(4):823–833

Benner P 2021 Novice to mastery. Teaching and learning for adult skill acquisition: applying the Dreyfus and Dreyfus Model in different fields. Online. Available: https://educatingnurses.com/from-novice-to-mastery-ii-the-dreyfus-and-dreyfus-model-of-skill-acquisition-in-nursing-practice/

Benner P 1984 From novice to expert: excellence and power in clinical nursing practice. Addison Wesley, Menlo Park, California

Brown J, Morgan A, Mason J et al 2020 Student nurses' digital literacy levels: lessons for curricula. CIN: Computers, Informatics, Nursing 38(9):451–458

Carless-Kane S, Nowell L 2023 Nursing students learning transfer from classroom to clinical practice: an integrative review. Nurse Education in Practice 103731

Cantwell L P, McGowan B S, Planchon Wolf J et al 2021 Building a bridge: a review of information literacy in nursing education. Journal of Nursing Education 60(8):431–436

Charette M, McKenna L, McGillion A et al 2023 Effectiveness of transition programs on new graduate nurses' clinical competence, job satisfaction and perceptions of support: a mixed-methods study. Journal of Clinical Nursing 32(7–8):1354–1369

Chinn P L, Kramer M K, Sitzman K 2021 Knowledge development in nursing ebook: theory and process. Elsevier Health Sciences, New York

Connor J, Flenady T, Massey D, Dwyer T 2023 Clinical judgement in nursing – an evolutionary concept analysis. Journal of Clinical Nursing 32(13–14):3328–3340

Cusack L, Thornton K, Drioli-Phillips P G et al 2020 Are nurses recognised, prepared and supported to teach nursing students: mixed methods study. Nurse Education Today 90:104434

Ekelin M, Kvist L J, Thies-Lagergren L et al 2021 Clinical supervisors' experiences of midwifery students' reflective writing: a process for mutual professional growth. Reflective Practice 22(1):101–114

El Hussein M T, Cuncannon A 2022 Nursing students' transfer of learning from simulated clinical experiences into clinical practice: a scoping review. Nurse Education Today 116:105449

Fetter K A, Wilford B, Brodie J et al 2023 Integrating information literacy into nursing education. Nursing 53(9):17–19

Greenway K, Butt G, Walthall H 2019 What is a theory-practice gap? An exploration of the concept. Nurse Education in Practice 34:1–6

Hughes L J 2019 Australian assessors' experiences of grading nursing student performances in clinical courses when that performance is not a clear pass or fail. Doctoral dissertation

International Nursing Association for Clinical Simulation and Learning (INACSL) Standards Committee, Decker S, Alinier G et al 2021 Healthcare Simulation Standards of Best Practice™ The Debriefing Process. Clinical Simulation in Nursing 58:27–32 https://doi.org/10.1016/j.ecns.2021.08.011

Johnston S, Nash R, Coyer F 2019 An evaluation of simulation debriefings on student nurses' perceptions of clinical reasoning and learning transfer: a mixed methods study. International Journal of Nursing Education Scholarship 16(1):20180045

Kramer M 1975 Reality shock: why nurses leave nursing. American Journal of Nursing 75(5):891

Littlewood K E, Szyld D 2015 Debriefing. In: Palaganas J C, Maxworthy J C, Epps C A (eds) Defining excellence in simulation programs. Wolters Kluwer, Philadelphia, pp 558–571

McTier L, Phillips N M, Duke M 2023 Factors influencing nursing student learning during clinical placements: a modified Delphi Study. Journal of Nursing Education 62(6):333–341

Mahmoud S, Withorn T 2023 Faculty-librarian collaboration to enhance information literacy skills in an online nursing course. Nursing Education Perspectives 10–1097

Malecka B, Boud D, Carless D 2022 Eliciting, processing and enacting feedback: mechanisms for embedding student feedback literacy within the curriculum. Teaching in Higher Education 27(7):908–922

Marshall T 2019 The concept of reflection: a systematic review and thematic synthesis across professional contexts. Reflective Practice 20(3):396–415

Masso M, Sim J, Halcomb E et al 2022 Practice readiness of new graduate nurses and factors influencing practice readiness: a scoping review of reviews. International Journal of Nursing Studies 129:104208

Mirza N, Manankil-Rankin L, Prentice D et al 2019 Practice readiness of new nursing graduates: a concept analysis. Nurse Education in Practice 37:68–74

Nes A A G, Steindal S A, Larsen M H et al 2021 Technological literacy in nursing education: a scoping review. Journal of Professional Nursing 37(2):320–334

Noble C, Billett S, Armit L et al 2020 "It's yours to take": generating learner feedback literacy in the workplace. Advances in Health Sciences Education 25:55–74

Nursing and Midwifery Board of Australia (NMBA) 2016 Registered nurse standards for practice. Online. Available: http://www.nursingmidwiferyboard.gov.au/News/2016-02-01-revised-standards.aspx

Nursing and Midwifery Board of Australia (NMBA) 2022 Decision-making framework for nursing and midwifery. Online. Available: https://www.nursingmidwiferyboard.gov.au/Codes-Guidelines-Statements/Frameworks.aspx

Ossenberg C, Mitchell M, Burmeister E et al 2023 Measuring changes in nursing students' workplace performance following feedback encounters: a quasi-experimental study. Nurse Education Today 121:105683

Panda S, Dash M, John J et al 2021 Challenges faced by student nurses and midwives in clinical learning environment – a systematic review and meta-synthesis. Nurse Education Today 101:104875

Pearce, L 2017 Digital literacy. Nursing Standard 31(48):18

Roberts E, Kaak V, Rolley J 2019 Simulation to replace clinical hours in nursing: a meta-narrative review. Clinical Simulation in Nursing 37:5–13

Rogers S, Redley B, Rawson H 2021 Developing work readiness in graduate nurses undertaking transition to practice programs: an integrative review. Nurse Education Today 105:105034

Sabey A, Biddle M 2021 Building capacity among health care librarians to teach evidence-based practice—an evaluation. Journal of the Medical Library Association: JMLA 109(3):432

Shin E H, Cummings E, Ford K 2018 A qualitative study of new graduates' readiness to use nursing informatics in acute care settings: clinical nurse educators' perspectives. Contemporary Nurse 54(1):64–76

Terry J, Davies A, Williams C et al 2019 Improving the digital literacy competence of nursing and midwifery students: a qualitative study of the experiences of NICE student champions. Nurse Education in Practice 34:192–198

Theobald K A, Tutticci N, Ramsbotham J et al 2021 Effectiveness of using simulation in the development of clinical reasoning in undergraduate nursing students: a systematic review. Nurse Education in Practice 57:103220

Toews A J, Martin D E, Chernomas W M 2021 Clinical debriefing: a concept analysis. Journal of Clinical Nursing 30(11–12):1491–1501

Vabo G, Slettebø Å, Fossum M 2022 Nursing students' professional identity development: an integrative review. Nordic Journal of Nursing Research 42(2):62–75

World Health Organization (WHO) 2020 Digital education for building health workforce capacity. WHO, Geneva. ISBN 978-92-4-000047-6

Yan Z, Carless D 2022 Self-assessment is about more than self: the enabling role of feedback literacy. Assessment & Evaluation in Higher Education 47(7):1116–1128

Yeager D S, Dweck C S 2020 What can be learned from growth mindset controversies? American Psychologist 75(9):1269

CHAPTER 21

RESEARCH IN NURSING

Thomas Buckley and Andrea P. Marshall

KEY WORDS
methodology
methods
paradigm
qualitative
quantitative
research

LEARNING OBJECTIVES
After reading this chapter, readers should be able to:
- understand evidence-based clinical practice and the role of research in informing clinical practice
- appreciate the range of approaches to research in nursing
- describe the basic research processes in nursing and start to critically review research.

INTRODUCTION

In this chapter the basic concepts of research in nursing are introduced and the important role of research in developing nursing knowledge is highlighted. How research can enhance health outcomes for individuals, their families and communities and develop the nursing profession is also discussed. While nurses might not always see a direct connection between research and their clinical work, the focus of this chapter will be how research can enrich nursing practice, policy, education and the workforce. The value-add of research to clinical practice and importance of clinical and academic partnerships in undertaking research will be emphasised. How nurses can engage in research as a distinct endeavour or one which is integrated with clinical practice and education is also discussed.

Research in nursing is not a new phenomenon. Florence Nightingale was an active researcher in the early nineteenth century. While perhaps best known for her work around sanitation, Nightingale was a passionate statistician, a pioneer of survey instruments and graphical data presentation for systematic data collection and using evidence to guide health and social policy (McDonald 2020). Nightingale identified key research issues, such as differential mortality between population sub-groups, the impact of care provided by trained and untrained nurses and childbirth mortality

(McEnroe 2020). Despite these early advances, nursing research did not progress substantially before the 1940s. Indeed, government support for nursing research in the US was not initiated until the 1950s (D'Antonio 1997) and it was not until 1963 that the first UK government-funded position for nursing research was established (Mulhall 1995). Finally, in 1972, the Briggs report recommended that UK nursing should develop an evidence base upon which to base clinical practice (Briggs 1972).

In Australia and New Zealand (Aotearoa), nursing was established as an academic discipline with a significant presence in universities in the 1980s (Bessant 1999). Prior to this, nurses were trained in an apprenticeship model within the hospital setting. Postgraduate education is common in Australia and often has a specialty-specific focus. Postgraduate research training is less common but increasing, although like other countries there is an increased need for doctoral-prepared nurses working in education, research and clinical practice (Dobrowolska 2021). Postdoctoral support and mentorship are also required as nurses transition from research training and into independent researcher roles.

Contemporary nursing has become accepted as a highly skilled profession in its own right. One of the key characteristics of a profession is that it has 'special knowledge and skills in a widely recognised body of learning derived from research, education and training at a high level' (Australian Council of Professions 2025). The importance of developing the nursing body of knowledge has been recognised by various professional organisations. The International Council of Nurses' Charter for Change highlights the need to recognise, value and promote nurses' skills, knowledge, attributes and expertise highlighting their varied roles as clinicians, scientists, researchers, educators and leaders (International Council of Nurses 2023). Nursing research is broad, incorporating research to optimise care delivery and promote quality health outcomes, as well as a range of issues affecting nurses and nursing and the general delivery of healthcare.

Within Australia and New Zealand (Aotearoa), the importance of research for all nurses is evidenced by the inclusion of relevant statements within the standards for practice for all nurses (New Zealand Nurses Organisation 2012, Nursing and Midwifery Board of Australia 2016). These standards define how nurses are expected to identify relevant research, apply evidence-based practice principles in clinical practice, evaluate the quality of evidence and support/contribute to nursing and health research.

What is research?

Research is a rigorous process of inquiry designed to answer questions about phenomena of concern within an academic discipline or profession. Research is the systematic collection of information which is planned and carefully organised to address a specific question (Tappen 2023). Developing and conducting an original study, where data is collected to answer a research question, is called 'primary research'. The collation and/or synthesis of existing research, such as occurs in literature, integrated or systematic reviews, is considered to be 'secondary research'.

Nurses are concerned with a range of important issues that can be the foci of research. Of prime importance is improving the quality of nursing practice, patient care and the health outcomes of individuals, families and communities. However, nurses are also concerned with a range of related issues such as establishing and evaluating best clinical practice, improving nurse education, monitoring and exploring nursing workforce issues, and understanding concepts around nursing education and management. Nursing research is necessarily diverse to address these various problems. So, while some studies are designed to directly inform clinical practice by describing a clinical activity, or comparing various ways of performing an intervention, other studies may shed light on individuals, family/community or nurses' experiences of phenomena that are poorly understood, such as a particular disease process, or specific concepts such as hope or suffering.

In the same way that nursing education and management are underpinned by adult learning principles, pedagogy and management theory, research too is underpinned by a series of principles and well-established but diverse traditions. In a chapter such as this, it is possible to present only a broad overview to familiarise the reader with the language of research and highlight its key underpinnings. Developing detailed knowledge and understanding of nursing research in general, or any one of the research traditions, methodologies and/or methods, will require further study and reading from a variety of sources as well as intellectual engagement with the materials.

Nurses' involvement in research

The degree of involvement a nurse has in conducting research will vary between individuals; however, all nurses will use research in their career. This is reflected in Glasziou's triangle (Stehlik et al 2020), which depicts the different levels of engagement in research to include users of research, participation in research and leaders of research (Fig. 21.1).

During their undergraduate preparation, nursing students will gain an awareness of the research literature and develop key skills in appreciation of the language of research and research critique. While some may perceive learning of clinical skills to be more valuable than research skills, positive views of clinical research are generally held by undergraduate nursing students who see the value of research to professional nursing practice (Ross & Burrell 2019). A grounding in understanding the language of research and critiquing research is vital to support the use of research in clinical practice. Using research is a powerful tool to ensure that our clinical practice, education, management and

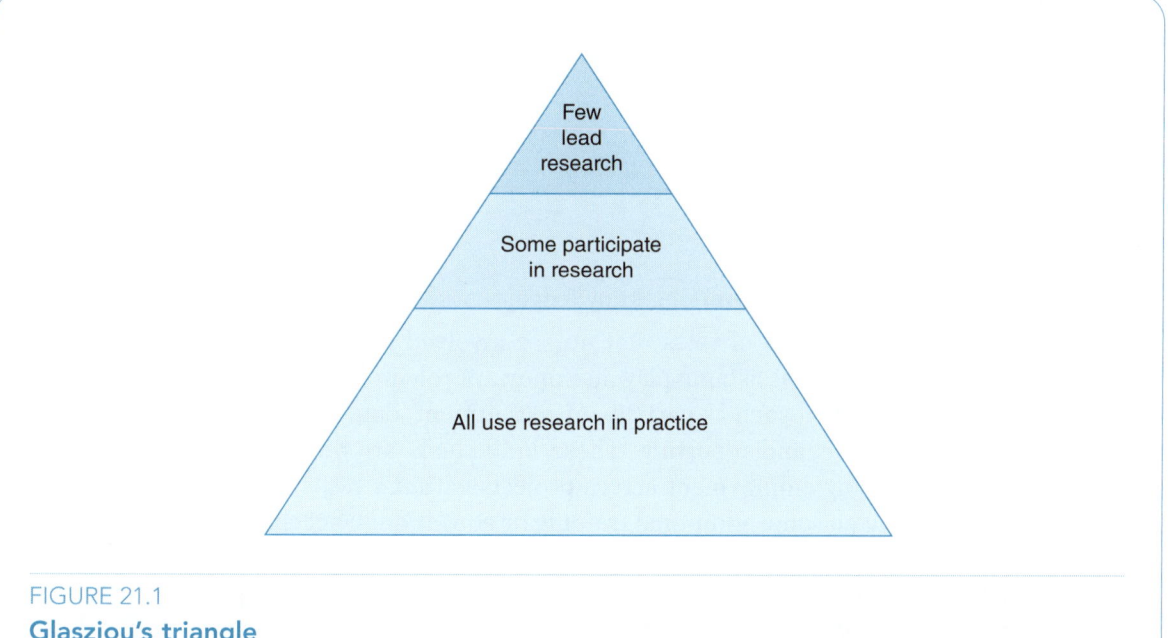

FIGURE 21.1
Glasziou's triangle

Source: Reproduced with permission from The Royal Australian College of General Practitioners from: Del Mar C. Publishing research in Australian Family Physician. Aust Fam Physician 2001;30:1094–95.

TABLE 21.1
Research terminology

TERM	DEFINITION
Paradigm	A way of viewing the world, an overarching framework of values, beliefs and assumptions
Methodology	The approach to the research process taken by the researcher (e.g. phenomenology, grounded theory, randomised controlled trial)
Design	The overall plan for collecting data within a specific study
Methods	The specific strategies used to collect data within a study (e.g. interviews, surveys, observation)

Source: Polit & Beck 2020

workforce activities are effective both in terms of being a responsible allocation of finite resources and optimising the health outcomes for individual patients, their families and communities. To ensure that nurses can appropriately critically appraise research it is vital that they have a good knowledge of research terminology (Table 21.1) and the research process as well as an understanding of research design considerations.

As a user of research, it is important to ensure that the research being used to inform clinical practice is based on the best available evidence.

Sometimes sufficient high-quality research is lacking to inform clinical decisions and original research might be needed. Nurses can and should take on active roles in conducting research. As a dynamic profession with our own body of knowledge, nurses need to take responsibility for designing and conducting high-quality research within our discipline. Such research is necessary to:

- test commonly held knowledge or assumptions
- increase understanding
- stimulate self-action/study
- develop best practice
- explain behaviours
- test predictions, and
- assist in the development of new nursing knowledge.

Generally, there are two kinds of roles that nurses involved in undertaking research perform. First, research nurses/research assistants play an important role in supporting the practical aspects of conducting a research study, such as participant recruitment, data collection, data entry, project administration, data analysis and reporting. These individuals are often employed for a specific project or may have ongoing employment across projects within a research centre or team. These nurses may have undertaken some additional training or education in specific aspects of data collection, project management or analysis techniques. Second, nurse researchers are leaders or members of the research team who are responsible for the conceptualisation, design and planning of the study, as well as managing the overall project, data analysis and dissemination of study findings. Nurse researchers are usually either undergoing or have completed a Bachelor of Nursing (Honours) course or a Higher Research Degree, such as a Master of Philosophy or Doctor of Philosophy, which has prepared them to undertake independent research.

In addition to being involved in conducting or leading nursing research, nurses with research skills have an important contribution to make to interdisciplinary or multidisciplinary research teams. Different disciplinary perspectives can help strengthen the research ensuring greater relevance and applicability. Nurses' clinical experience and expertise can also be used to guide the practicalities of conducting research in the clinical setting by identifying potential barriers that may be encountered.

> ### REFLECTION
> 1. Since the beginning of your university studies, what research papers have you accessed and read?
> 2. What, if any, nursing contribution was there to the conduct of the research reported in one of these papers?

Nursing research approaches

Research traditions can be investigated in relation to their philosophical underpinnings. In the course of your reading of research you will encounter a number of different paradigms. A research paradigm is an overarching framework that is based on values, beliefs and assumptions. This framework contains theory about the nature of reality and guidelines for the methods to be used in carrying out research within the paradigm (Corry et al 2019). In addition, the ideas within the paradigm have implications for the type of knowledge being sought in a study, the way in which the study will be carried out and the way in which outcomes from the work will be used. The nature of the specific research *problem* and scope of the research question determine the most appropriate research paradigm to use in the given situation.

Two major paradigms in nursing research are Positivism and Naturalism/Interpretivism (Kelly et al 2018). While a detailed discussion of the underpinnings of these paradigms is beyond the scope of this chapter, some of the key differences are summarised in Table 21.2. A third key paradigm is Pragmatism, which involves a combination of approaches to best design research that answers complex research questions. Pragmatism is designed to help address real-world problems and accommodates the use of multiple data sources and is a helpful approach when addressing complex social problems in healthcare (Allemang et al 2022).

QUANTITATIVE RESEARCH

Quantitative research includes studies that seek to objectively measure a concept or phenomenon of interest (e.g. blood pressure, pain level or quality-of-life score). The quantitative research paradigm is also called positivist, reductionist or empirical. It is referred to as reductionist as it reduces the concept under investigation to a numerical value. Quantitative research uses deductive reasoning, which means that the thinking leads from a known principle to an unknown, and is used to either test a particular research hypothesis or objectively describe a concept or occurrence.

Quantitative research encompasses a range of research designs and associated methods; the most common designs used in nursing research are outlined in Table 21.3. Selection of an appropriate design is undertaken based on the specific research question being posed.

TABLE 21.2
Differentiating paradigms

	POSITIVISTIC PARADIGM (QUANTITATIVE RESEARCH)	NATURALISTIC PARADIGM (QUALITATIVE RESEARCH)
Approach	• Reductionist	• Holistic
Focus	• Focus is specific	• Focus is broad and complex
Nature of data	• Objective	• Subjective
Reasoning	• Deductive reasoning	• Inductive reasoning
Emphasis	• Cause and effect	• Meaning, discovery
Purpose	• Tests theory	• Develops theory
Methodology	• Control	• Shared interpretation
Tools	• Instruments	• Communication, observation
Data type	• Numbers	• Words
Outcome	• Generalisability	• Uniqueness

TABLE 21.3
Common quantitative research designs

DESIGN	PURPOSE
Descriptive study	Examines characteristics of a single sample; clarifies concepts; generates questions about potential relationships between variables (e.g. case study, cross-sectional analysis)
Correlation study	Examines (describes, predicts or tests) relationships between two or more variables, but does not infer a cause-and-effect relationship
Quasi-experimental study	Tests a cause-and-effect relationship, but without either a control group or randomisation (e.g. case control, intervention only)
Experimental study (randomised controlled trial)	Tests a cause-and-effect relationship using randomisation of subjects to groups, manipulation of an intervention and a control group

QUALITATIVE RESEARCH

Qualitative research is a broad term encompassing a range of research drawn from subjective human experiences. These data are derived from either narrative, observational or non-numerical sources in naturalistic settings. Qualitative research often involves close, sustained contact between the researcher and participant(s) as data are commonly collected through the conduct of interviews (Doyle et al 2020). This approach uses inductive reasoning, whereby theory is developed out of the participants' experiences. The term 'qualitative research' spans a range of methodological approaches and research designs (Table 21.4). This field of research has its origins in the humanities disciplines, such as philosophy, anthropology, history and sociology (Renjith et al 2021). The qualitative researcher approaches research with a different set of values and beliefs from the quantitative researcher. In qualitative research, value is placed on individual subjectivity, multiple truths are accommodated

TABLE 21.4
Common qualitative designs

DESIGN	DEFINITION
Phenomenology	Exploration of the lived experience of the phenomenon of interest
Ethnography	Derived from anthropology, ethnography is a study of cultures and sub-cultures
Grounded theory	Develops theoretical explanations for an occurrence and generates hypotheses for future research
Case study	An in-depth examination of a 'case' or specific environment
Descriptive qualitative	Explores a phenomenon of interest from a distinctly human perspective
Participatory action research	Researchers work with participants in cycles of Planning, Acting, Observing and Reflecting to achieve change
Feminist research	Researcher attempts to see the world from the vantage point of specific groups of women to reduce their oppression

and individuals who participate in the study are regarded as active participants and partners in the research (Tomaszewski et al 2020).

Qualitative research can either be interpretative or critical. Interpretative methods are richly descriptive in nature (Renjith et al 2021). They seek to explain, describe, generate meaning and make sense of the phenomenon of interest. These methods allow exploration of a range of human experiences that are of interest to nursing from the perspective of individuals, their family and community and/or nurses themselves. Interpretative methodologies include phenomenology, grounded theory, ethnography, and descriptive qualitative research (Tomaszewski et al 2020).

In contrast, critical qualitative research involves researchers working collaboratively with participants to effect change in the status quo (Shaw et al 2022). It is the explicit intent of critical qualitative research for social or political change to occur as a result of the research. Critical methodologies include participatory action research and feminist research.

MIXED METHODS RESEARCH

Mixed methods research is most often associated with the pragmatic paradigm, whereby the choice of methods is made based on the most appropriate means to answer the specific research questions (Halcomb et al 2023). A mixed methods study combines both qualitative and quantitative methods of data collection in a single study. Such broad data collection provides multiple perspectives of the topic of interest, thus allowing a deeper exploration than would be revealed by either qualitative or quantitative methods alone (Dawadi et al 2021). Just because you could collect both qualitative and quantitative data within a single study does not mean that you should (Younas et al 2019). Mixed method designs have significant implications for resources required, project duration and skills needed and, therefore, should only be used when the deeper insight assists in answering the research question more adequately (Dawadi et al 2021).

Mixed methods research studies can broadly be categorised into either sequential or concurrent designs (Halcomb et al 2023) (Table 21.5). In sequential studies one method of data collection follows the other, with the second method usually either taking data from or building on the first method. Concurrent studies, on the other hand, collect qualitative and quantitative data

TABLE 21.5
Common mixed methods research designs

DESIGN	PURPOSE
Sequential explanatory	Quantitative data are collected first and then qualitative data are collected to explain the quantitative findings
Sequential exploratory	Quantitative data are collected to build on qualitative findings
Convergent parallel	Quantitative and qualitative data are collected concurrently to obtain different but complementary data to answer a single research question
Embedded or nested	Quantitative data collection within a qualitative study or qualitative data collection within a quantitative study. The embedded data set answers a complementary but discrete research question

Source: Halcomb & Hickman 2015

simultaneously. The choice of a sequential versus a concurrent design must consider both the purpose of the research and any time constraints on the project (Halcomb & Baille 2018).

THE RESEARCH PROCESS

Regardless of the paradigm, methodological approach or design, the research process generally follows a series of basic systematic steps (Box 21.1). Following the identification of a problem, the researcher will need to know what is already known about the problem (via a critical literature review) and identify what is not known (the research gap). Conducting a literature review involves the development and conduct of a robust search strategy and the appropriate critical synthesis of identified literature. Health librarians are well placed to assist in identifying appropriate search terms and suitable databases to be included in the search. In terms of the critical literature synthesis, various review methods have been described in the literature (Aveyard & Bradbury-Jones 2019, Cronin et al 2023, Garritty et al 2021, Peters et al 2021, Shaffril et al 2020, Stern et al 2021). A suitable review method should be selected based on the topic, resources and purpose of the review. An overview of the main literature review methods is summarised in Table 21.6.

BOX 21.1
Overview of the research process

1. Identify research problem
2. Review literature
3. Develop a research question
4. Design study proposal
5. Recruit participants
6. Collect data
7. Analyse data
8. Report and disseminate findings
9. Translate findings to practice

TABLE 21.6
Literature review methods

Critical review	Aims to demonstrate writer has extensively researched literature and critically evaluated its quality. Goes beyond mere description to include degree of analysis and conceptual innovation. Typically results in hypothesis or model
Literature review	Generic term: published materials that provide examination of recent or current literature. Can cover wide range of subjects at various levels of completeness and comprehensiveness. May include research findings
Mapping review/ systematic map	Map out and categorise existing literature from which to commission further reviews and/or primary research by identifying gaps in research literature
Meta-analysis	Technique that statistically combines the results of quantitative studies to provide a more precise effect of the results
Mixed studies review/ mixed methods review	Refers to any combination of methods where one significant component is a literature review (usually systematic). Within a review context it refers to a combination of review approaches, for example combining quantitative with qualitative research or outcome with process studies
Overview	Generic term: summary of the [medical] literature that attempts to survey the literature and describe its characteristics
Qualitative systematic review/qualitative evidence synthesis	Method for integrating or comparing the findings from qualitative studies. It looks for 'themes' or 'constructs' that lie in or across individual qualitative studies
Rapid review	Assessment of what is already known about a policy or practice issue, by using systematic review methods to search and critically appraise existing research
Scoping review	Preliminary assessment of potential size and scope of available research literature. Aims to identify nature and extent of research evidence (usually including ongoing research)
State-of-the-art review	Tends to address more current matters in contrast to other combined retrospective and current approaches. May offer new perspectives on issue or point out areas for further research
Systematic review	Seeks to systematically search for, appraise and synthesise research evidence, often adhering to guidelines on the conduct of a review
Systematic search and review	Combines strengths of critical review with a comprehensive search process. Typically addresses broad questions to produce 'best evidence synthesis'
Systematised review	Attempts to include elements of systematic review process while stopping short of systematic review. Typically conducted as postgraduate student assignment
Umbrella review	Specifically refers to review compiling evidence from multiple reviews into one accessible and usable document. Focuses on broad condition or problem for which there are competing interventions and highlights reviews that address these interventions and their results

Adapted from Grant M J, Booth A 2009 A typology of reviews: an analysis of 14 review types and associated methodologies. Health Information and Libraries Journal 26:91–108

Once the literature review is completed, the researcher will next formulate the research question that they will seek to answer through their study. The specific research question will determine which research design and method will most effectively answer that question. Once the project proposal has been developed and the study has received approval from an ethics committee (where human participants are involved), participants are recruited and data are collected. Data collection and analysis may occur concurrently or sequentially depending on the type of study. The specific analysis strategies will be determined by the kind of data collected. Once the data has been analysed, the researcher(s) need to communicate their findings. While this step in the research process often receives limited attention, dissemination of the findings is vital if others are to learn from the research. Findings should be made available to researchers, clinicians and end-users. This may require a range of dissemination strategies, including peer-reviewed papers, conference presentations, stakeholder meetings, policy briefs and dissemination through social media. Arguably, the most difficult step occurs last, which is for the results of the findings to be incorporated into usual care (translation). To truly achieve translation of findings into practice requires commitment from the researcher(s) and sustained engagement with stakeholders.

EVIDENCE-BASED PRACTICE

Evidence-based practice (EBP) has become a commonly used term in nursing and healthcare circles. The notion of EBP was first introduced into medicine by Archie Cochrane in the 1970s (Straus et al 2019). Since this time, it has been translated across the healthcare system.

In 1996, D.L. Sackett, a Canadian medical practitioner and founder of the department of clinical epidemiology at McMaster University in Ontario, proposed that EBP is the conscientious, explicit and judicious use of current best evidence in making decisions about the care of individual patients (Sackett et al 1996). Therefore, the practice of evidence-based medicine means integrating individual clinician expertise and the patient's unique values and circumstances with the best available evidence from systematic research (Straus et al 2019). Clearly, from this definition, EBP can only be achieved via the combination of the best available clinical evidence, individual clinician expertise to apply this evidence to the individual situation and preferences of the individual, family and/or community around resource allocation and care choices. An often stated major criticism of EBP is that it is a 'cookbook' practice that seeks to reduce clinicians to following guidelines to make decisions about service provision. However, this criticism often comes from those who forget to incorporate the clinician's clinical expertise and the patient's values and circumstances into the EBP equation. As a clinician, it is your clinical expertise that decides whether a particular piece of research evidence applies to the individual patient and if it does, how this evidence should be integrated into clinical decision making.

CRITICAL APPRAISAL

Determining best available evidence requires nurses to be able to critically evaluate research effectively. To assist in comparing various types of research evidence, the Australian National Health and Medical Research Council provides a hierarchy of evidence to guide decision making (Table 21.7). This hierarchy identifies that the evidence obtained from more rigorous research designs should be weighted more strongly than the evidence from less rigorous designs. However, critical appraisal of research needs to go beyond this and critically interrogate the conduct of the specific research project. Today there are many established tools to facilitate a structured critique of research. In particular, organisations such as the Joanna Briggs Institute (https://jbi.global/) and the Cochrane Collaboration (www.cochrane.org) provide clear guidance around specific strategies for critical appraisal. These organisations also provide training courses and online modules/resources to help develop critical appraisal skills. Regardless of which critical appraisal tool is used, good critique of research is a skill that requires knowledge of the research process and practice to develop and maintain.

TABLE 21.7
National Health and Medical Research Council (NHMRC) evidence hierarchy

LEVEL OF EVIDENCE	TYPE OF STUDY
I	A systematic review of level II studies
II	A randomised controlled trial
III-1	A pseudo-randomised controlled trial (i.e. alternate allocation or some other method)
III-2	A comparative study with concurrent controls: • non-randomised, experimental trial • cohort study • case-control study • interrupted time series with a control group
III-3	A comparative study without concurrent controls: • historical control study • two or more single arm study • interrupted time series without a parallel control group
IV	Case series with either post-test or pre-test/post-test outcomes Descriptive study

Source: NHMRC 2009 (CC BY 3.0 Australia)

THE 5 STEPS OF EVIDENCE-BASED PRACTICE (STRAUS ET AL 2019, NISHIKAWA-PACHER 2022)

1. **Ask the clinical question.** Step 1 is to formulate a clear, detailed and answerable question. Some clinical questions lead themselves to using the PICO method to help convert the need for information into an answerable question. PICO stands for patient/population, intervention, comparison and outcomes:
   P - Population or Patient/client group
   I - Intervention or Indicator (Intervention, prognostic factor or exposure)
   C - Comparator or Control (note: your clinical question may not always need a specific comparison)
   O - Outcome (What are you trying to accomplish, measure, improve, effect, achieve?)
2. **Acquire the evidence.** Search for the best possible evidence to answer the question from high-quality, peer-reviewed sources
3. **Appraise the evidence.** Critically appraise the evidence for validity, impact and applicability
4. **Apply the evidence.** Apply the evidence in combination with clinical experience and patient values and circumstances
5. **Assess the process.** Assess the effectiveness and efficiency of your process and find ways to improve for next time.

REFLECTION

Identify a clinical practice guideline relevant to your clinical practice or current studies. What features of this practice guideline help you to identify the evidence that informed the guideline?

WHERE DO WE FIND RESEARCH?

Research can be found in many places. High-quality research is largely published in academic peer-reviewed journals; however, the grey literature provides important research findings in the form of research reports, project and literature summaries and resources. The growth of social media and the internet has led to a concomitant growth in electronic dissemination of research findings (Roberts-Lewis et al 2023). Such strategies can now rapidly disseminate research to a large geographically dispersed audience. These various dissemination channels also have the advantage of using different levels of language and pitch that can increase the reach of the findings to the broad group of stakeholders, including lay people, policy makers and managers.

PEER-REVIEWED JOURNALS

Peer-reviewed journals are an important vehicle for the dissemination of research findings and discussion about research methodology and methods within the profession. The term 'peer-reviewed' means that each paper that is published has been subjected to a review process involving peer reviewers and editorial oversight to ensure the quality of the work. Peer reviewers are individuals with expertise, knowledge and skills in the topic area. Criteria that must be met before a paper is accepted for publication in a peer-reviewed journal vary; however, editors hold responsibility to ensure that a standard of excellence in regard to scientific merit, the literary standard of the paper and the relevance of the paper in terms of its potential to contribute to knowledge development is maintained. Although the reader can have a degree of confidence in the quality of the work published in the peer-reviewed literature, they should still critically appraise the research described in a peer-reviewed paper before applying findings into practice.

PREDATORY JOURNALS

In recent years there has been a growth in predatory journals, also called fraudulent, deceptive or pseudo-journals, in nursing and many other disciplines (Elmore & Weston 2020, Watson 2019). These journals make money by charging authors fees to publish their papers but do not use the same quality processes for evaluating research prior to publication or have robust production and curation practices commonly seen with legitimate journals. In the digital era where papers are often sourced online, these publications can appear deceptively similar to legitimate journals, particularly where journal names have very similar wording. However, care should be taken to avoid these sources as there is no peer-review process and papers are included regardless of their quality.

GREY LITERATURE

The term 'grey literature' refers to information produced outside of traditional publishing processes and can include reports, policy documents, newsletters, government reports, speeches, white papers etc. Grey literature is so named because of the uncertain quality of the information (Hoffecker 2020). These documents have not necessarily been reviewed for either accuracy or quality and, with the growth of the internet, can be widely disseminated with limited oversight of the standard or accuracy of the content. While high-quality grey literature can be found on the websites of reputable organisations (e.g. the Australian Institute of Health and Welfare, the Heart Foundation, Ministry of

Health NZ, Te Whatu Ora – Health New Zealand), the reader should always carefully critically analyse the document and its source before accepting the findings.

ONLINE PORTALS

Traditionally, research findings were only available in scientific journals and in presentations at scientific meetings, so they were largely unavailable to end-users including patients, researchers and clinicians from low-income countries who may not have access to traditional academic journals. Today, thanks to the growth of the internet, researchers are able to publish their findings to a much broader audience (Ross & Cross 2019). Platforms such as X (formerly Twitter), LinkedIn, and news websites like The Conversation are increasingly being recognised as important tools for communication and dissemination (Roberts-Lewis et al 2023). Like all other sources, information gathered from online portals should always be critically analysed before the information is accepted and used.

REFLECTION
What strategies can you use to assess the quality of peer-reviewed journals and grey literature?

CONCLUSION

An understanding of basic concepts and processes in research is central to professional nursing practice. Quality nursing care is based on applying the best available evidence, using professional clinical judgment and incorporating individual and community preferences. All nurses require research utilisation skills in order to make judgments about how relevant and applicable research findings are to practice. Nursing is a complex, practice-based discipline in which researchable questions will require answers to extend our knowledge base. For this reason, some nurses will move beyond using research to inform their work and become involved in the conduct and development of nursing and/or interdisciplinary research. This is an exciting career path that can open a range of opportunities.

An array of research paradigms, methodologies and methods are available to appropriately answer the range of questions facing the nursing profession. As the content of this chapter is introductory, you can expect to learn more about the various research traditions, paradigms, methodologies and methods during your undergraduate education. It is important that as nurses we take responsibility for ensuring that we are sufficiently skilled in research to enable us to meet regulatory requirements and optimise our contribution to the nursing profession and the individuals, families and communities who rely on our work.

Recommended readings

Gray J, Grove S 2020 Burns and Grove's the practice of nursing research, appraisal, synthesis, and generation of evidence. Elsevier, United States

Jackson D, Halcomb E, Walthall H 2023 Navigating the maze of research: enhancing nursing and midwifery practice, 6th edn. Elsevier Health Sciences, Sydney

Polit D F, Beck C T 2020 Nursing research: generating and assessing evidence for nursing practice, 11th edn. Lippincott Williams & Wilkins, Baltimore

References

Allemang B, Sitter K, Dimitropoulos G 2022 Pragmatism as a paradigm for patient-oriented research. Health Expectations 35(1):38–47

Australian Council of Professions 2025 What is a profession? Online. Available: https://professions.org.au/what-is-a-professional/ 23 January 2025

Aveyard H, Bradbury-Jones C 2019 An analysis of current practices in undertaking literature reviews in nursing: findings from a focused mapping review and synthesis. BMC Medical Research Methodology 19(1):105

Bessant B 1999 Milestones in Australian nursing. Collegian 6(4):i–iii

Briggs A 1972 Report of the committee on nursing. Cmnd 5115, HMSO, London

Corry M, Porter S, McKenna H 2019 The redundancy of positivism as a paradigm for nursing research. Nursing Philosophy 20(1):e12230

Cronin M A, George E 2020 The why and how of the integrative review. Organizational Research Methods 26(1):168–192

D'Antonio P 1997 Toward a history of research in nursing. Nursing Research 46(2):105–110

Del Mar C 2001 Publishing research in Australian Family Physician. Australian Family Physician 30:1094–95.

Dawadi S, Shrestha S, Giri RA 2021 Mixed-methods research: a discussion on its types, challenges and criticisms. Journal of Practical Studies in Education 2(2):25–36

Dobrowolska B, Bhrusciel P, Markiewicz R et al 2021 The role of doctoral-educated nurses in the clinical setting: findings from a scoping review. Journal of Clinical Nursing 30(19–20):2808–2821

Doyle L, McCabe C, Keogh B et al 2020 An overview of the qualitative descriptive design within nursing research. Journal of Research in Nursing 25(5):443–455

Elmore SA, Weston EH 2020 Predatory journals: what they are and how to avoid them. Toxicologic Pathology 48(4):607–610

Garritty C, Gartlehner G, Nussbaumer-Streit B et al 2021 Cochrane rapid reviews methods group offers evidence-informed guidance to conduct rapid reviews. Journal of Clinical Epidemiology 130:13–22

Halcomb E, Massey, D, Gunowa N O 2023 Mixed method research. In: Jackson D, Power T, Walthall H, et al (eds) Navigating the maze of research: enhancing nursing and midwifery practice, 6th edn. Elsevier Health Science, Sydney

Hoffecker L 2020 Grey literature searching for systematic reviews in the health sciences. The Serials Librarian 70(3-4):252–260

International Council of Nurses 2023 International Nurses Day 2023 Report: Our nurses. Our future. Online: Available: https://www.icn.ch/sites/default/files/2023-07/ICN_IND_2023_Report_EN.pdf 3 January 2023

Kelly M, Dowling M, Millar M 2018 The search for understanding: the role of paradigms. Nurse Researcher 25(4):9–13

McDonald L 2020 Florence Nightingale: the making of a hospital reformer. Health Environments Research and Design Journal 13(2):25–31

McEnroe N 2020 Celebrating Florence Nightingale's bicentenary. The Lancet 395(10235):1475–1478

Mulhall A 1995 Nursing research: what difference does it make? Journal of Advanced Nursing 21(3):576–583

National Health and Medical Research Council (NHMRC) 2009 NHMRC levels of evidence and grades for recommendations for developers of guidelines. Online. Available: https://www.mja.com.au/sites/default/files/NHMRC.levels.of.evidence.2008-09.pdf 21 December 2024

New Zealand Nurses Organisation 2012 Standards of professional nursing practice. New Zealand Nurses Organisation, Wellington. Online. Available: https://www.nzno.org.nz/Portals/0/publications/Standards%20-%20Standards%20of%20professional%20nursing%20practice,%20N2012.pdf

Nishikawa-Pacher A 2022 Research questions with PICO: a universal mnemonic. Publications 10(3):21

Nursing and Midwifery Board of Australia 2016 Registered Nurse Standards for Practice. Online. Available: https://www.nursingmidwiferyboard.gov.au/Codes-Guidelines-Statements/Professional-standards/registered-nurse-standards-for-practice.aspx January 2024

Peters M, Marnie C, Tricco A H 2021 Updated methodological guidance for the conduct of scoping reviews. JBI Evidence Implementation 19(1):3–10

Renjith V, Yesodharan R, Noronha J A et al 2021 Qualitative methods in health care research. International Journal of Preventative Health 12:20

Roberts-Lewis S F, Baxter H A, Mein G et al 2023 The use of social media for dissemination of research evidence to health and social care practitioners: protocol for a systematic review. JMIR Research Protocols 12:e45684

Ross J G, Burrell S A 2019 Nursing students' attitudes toward research: an integrative review. Nurse Education Today 82:79–87

Ross P, Cross R 2019 Rise of the e-Nurse: the power of social media in nursing. Contemporary Nurse 55(2–3):211–220

Sackett D L, Rosenberg W M C, Gray J A M et al 1996 Evidence based medicine: what it is and what it isn't. British Medical Journal 312(7023):71–72

Shaffril H A M, Samsuddin S F, Samah A A 2020 The ABC of systematic literature review: the basic methodological guidance for beginners. Quality & Quantity 55:1319–1346

Shaw J, Gagnon M, Carson A et al 2022 Advancing the impact of critical qualitative research on policy, practice and science. International Journal of Qualitative Methods 21 https://doi.org/10.1177/16094069221076929

Stehlik P, Noble C, Brandenburg C et al 2020 How do trainee doctors learn about research? Content analysis of Australian specialist colleges' intended research curricula. BMJ Open 10:e034962

Stern C, Lizarondo L, Carrier G et al 2021 Methodological guidance for the conduct of mixed methods systematic reviews. JBI Evidence Implementation 19(2):120–129

Straus S E, Glasziou P, Richardson W S, et al 2019 Evidence based medicine, how to practice and teach EBM, 5th edn. Elsevier, Edinburgh

Tappen R 2023 Advanced nursing research from theory to practice. Jones and Bartlett Learning, Burlington

Tomaszewski L E, Zarestky J, Gonzalez E 2020 Planning qualitative research: design and decision making for new researchers. International Journal of Qualitative Methods 19 https://doi.org/10.1177/1609406920967174

Watson R 2019 Predatory journals and the pollution of academic publishing. Journal of Nursing Management 27(2):223–224

Younas A, Pedersen M, Tayaben J L 2019 Review of mixed methods research in nursing: methodological issues and future directions. Nursing Research doi: 10.1097/NNR.0000000000000372

CHAPTER 22

BECOMING A NURSE LEADER

Patricia M. Davidson and Kelly Lewer

KEY WORDS

clinical leadership
clinical management
evidence-based practice
transformational leadership

LEARNING OBJECTIVES

After reading this chapter, readers should be able to:

- describe the social, economic and political trends influencing nursing practice globally
- identify the differences between the terms 'leadership' and 'management'
- recognise strategies for undergraduate nurses to develop to become nurse leaders
- appreciate the importance of evidence-based practice in facilitating optimal patient outcomes
- leverage your personal experiences to inform your leadership journey
- identify professional and organisational factors that facilitate effective leadership and strategic management.

INTRODUCTION

Leadership is an attribute that defines the capacity to motivate and inspire others (Anders et al 2021). Contemporary health systems are increasingly embedded in complex social, political and economic ecosystems. We live in a global environment, and this has implications not just for health but also for professional practice. The recent coronavirus (COVID-19) pandemic emphasised that we are highly interconnected across the planet and need to consider health in a global context. Evolving geopolitical conflicts and an escalating climate crisis increase the complexity of healthcare delivery and increase the importance of nursing leadership (Daly et al 2020).

Expert nursing practice extends beyond knowledge, skills and competencies to translation and implementation and also advocacy for human rights, diversity, equity and inclusion as well as care of our planet (Catton 2023). Nursing leadership is critical for implementing evidence-based practice, promoting patient outcomes and optimising the value of healthcare within ethical frameworks. Although individual countries have discrete issues, across the globe healthcare systems and nurses are facing similar challenges in delivering quality, high-value and accessible healthcare. Increasing geopolitical instability globally underscores the importance of considering healthcare within a social, political and economic context. The growing burden of chronic illness and ageing of the population increases the importance of coordinated care led by competent, credentialed and capable nurses practising to the full extent of their education and training. Importantly, promoting quality and excellence in nursing care and ensuring safe and effective work environments is important in providing high-quality patient care. Achieving these goals is very challenging in the context of a global nursing workforce shortage. The International Council of Nurses (ICN) projected in 2021 that over 13 million nurses worldwide are required to bridge the gap in the nursing shortage by 2030 (Adhikari & Smith 2023). We also need to increase diversity in our workforce and ensure that our profession reflects the cultural diversity and pluralism of contemporary society and the communities we serve (National Academies of Sciences, Engineering and Medicine et al 2021).

Deplorable health outcomes of Indigenous peoples emphasise the importance of recognising sovereignty and the adverse impact of colonisation on First Nations peoples. Consequently, there is a call for increasing the voices of Indigenous nurses (Geia et al 2020). This chapter will discuss the desirable attributes of nurse leaders in the workplace and the role of expert clinical practice in forging a professional identity. The chapter will also provide insights into the way expert practitioners, functioning as leaders in a range of practice settings, can face challenges and successfully implement strategies to improve patient care and advance nursing practice. We also emphasise the increasing need to engage meaningfully with communities to provide acceptable and efficacious interventions. The first section of the chapter sets the scene in describing contemporary trends influencing clinical practice, models of nursing care delivery and aspects of leadership in the clinical setting, and the latter part of the chapter focuses more specifically on becoming a nurse leader.

As you read this chapter, it is important as a nurse starting your professional journey that you consider the attributes that you will need to develop to become a leader. It is never too early to focus on developing your leadership style, evaluating others' leadership styles and preparing to transition from being a student to a registered nurse. You will soon learn that you will manage care and provide leadership for critical patient care issues quickly after becoming a registered nurse. Anticipating this transition is critically important.

Effective leaders cultivate a self-reflective appraisal of their strengths and weaknesses as part of a lifelong learning process. Your experiences, both personal and professional, will shape the nurse you will become. Nurse leaders also engage in activities to develop competencies and skills in their personal and professional life. Leadership is crucial at all levels of nursing practice—from novice to expert. Becoming a leader requires focused time to reflect on your performance and continue to learn and evolve. You will observe leadership styles that are positive and enabling as well as dominating and destructive. You will probably experience many leadership styles in your career. Learning to work with a range of leadership and managerial styles as well as clinical practice settings is an important part of your personal and professional development. Maintaining your personal equilibrium, engaging in self-care and seeking help when necessary are critical skills.

As you observe the behaviours of your peers, you can probably see the emergent characteristics of future nursing leaders; for example, how your colleagues deal with challenges in both the classroom and the clinical setting. Increasingly, we are aware that the level of nursing competence, staffing and communication as well as the quality of working environments influence patient outcomes (Ullman & Davidson 2021). Even in your early days of practice, you can shape the future of patient care and the nursing profession through engaging in critical discussion, student leadership, reflective practice and providing a voice for patients and their families. This will require focusing on both your personal and professional development as well as forging your nurse identity.

> ## REFLECTION
> 1. What do you consider are the attributes of an effective leader?
> 2. How do different leadership styles contribute to clinical effectiveness and improving patient outcomes?
> 3. What are the strategies needed to promote physical and emotional health of a leader?

Internationally, clinical, administrative and policy environments in healthcare generate challenges to both professionals and consumers. Increased demands for clinical services, rising healthcare costs and health workforce shortages are just some of the issues you will face as you begin your nursing career. In spite of these challenges, the healthcare setting has never been so welcoming for dynamic nurse leaders and managers. Data suggests that contemporary healthcare systems should shift from hierarchical leadership models to those that are more inclusive and interdisciplinary (O'Donovan et al 2021). Moreover, never have nurses been so well educated and prepared to lead clinical practice (Ullman & Davidson 2021).

Nurses make a unique contribution to patient care. Nurses need to be empowered to provide leadership and direction for models of care development and delivery in policy, practice and research. At many levels, you will see nurse leaders functioning in organisational, policy and nursing-specific leadership. The growth of nursing research and scholarship has demonstrated the unique and valuable contributions of nurses to health-related outcomes, particularly related to promoting continuity and coordination of care.

A number of strategic reports globally have emphasised key recommendations to promote the role of nurses and drive equity (Wakefield et al 2021). These can be summarised as:

- Nurses should practise to the full extent of their education and training.
- Nurses should achieve higher levels of education and training through an improved education system that promotes seamless academic progression.
- Nurses should be full partners with physicians and other healthcare professionals, in redesigning healthcare.
- Effective workforce planning and policy making require better data collection and information infrastructure.

- There should be close collaboration between the clinical and practice communities.
- Health equity should be an important focus of healthcare interventions.
- The self-care of nurses is critical in achieving a sustainable workforce.

The increasing recognition of advanced practice creates an exciting opportunity for nurses to work in an interdisciplinary context. These new opportunities create increased responsibility to work with evidence-based, ethical and collegial frameworks. Accountability, integrity, ethical and expert practice are core values of all professions. For nursing, this should be the essence of our work and manifest in our practice and interactions. For nurses to function effectively in dynamic clinical environments and exert influence to optimise patient care, there is a need to appreciate the multiple factors that impact nursing practice and healthcare delivery. These factors are as diverse as the nature of nursing practice. It is also important to consider that, regardless of the healthcare system in which you will work, healthcare delivery is provided in a political context that is strongly influenced by economic factors and prevailing cultural and social values.

Healthcare in context

Contemporary healthcare settings are often portrayed as systems in crisis as they battle increasing demands and diminishing resources. These issues are common in both high- as well as lower- and middle-income countries. Across the globe, an ageing population and the increasing burden of chronic conditions challenge healthcare delivery and professional practice. Currently, many healthcare systems are designed for acute procedural care where current epidemiological trends emphasise the importance of population and community-based care.

The worldwide nurse staffing shortage continues to attract government and public comment. Nurses, along with many other professional groups, are experiencing workforce shortages exacerbated by increasing demand and an ageing workforce. This emphasises the importance of coordinated human resources for health strategy and of considering nursing workforce issues within the context of global economies.

Increasing challenges facing healthcare are global and strongly mediated by factors such as epidemiological transitions, climate change, increased migration and geopolitical instability. Taking the time to consider these forces is critical in assessing current clinical situations and planning for your future and the nursing profession's future. Given the increasing globalisation of health and emphasis on internationalisation, there is an emphasis on global competencies for health professionals. Across the world, there is an increasing number of refugees, many of whom are forcibly displaced (Alharthi et al 2024). The World Bank predicts that nearly half of the world's poor will live in fragile and conflict-affected states by 2030. Often, nurses are working within refugee communities and encampments, and so nurses along with other health professionals are powerful advocates for health and human rights.

> ### REFLECTION
> What is the role of nursing leadership in upholding human rights such as the care of refugees and the care of children in detention camps?

As you begin your nursing journey and come to terms with the necessary skills and terminology, words such as 'leadership' and 'mentorship' can appear distant, remote and have limited relevance. However, it is important to consider that you and your colleagues are the nurse leaders of the future and have a personal and professional responsibility to develop the necessary skills and competencies. Leadership is rarely a historical accident; rather, it is associated with a set of knowledge, skills and attributes that are developed over time and enacted in particular situations (Wallace et al 2021). As you read this chapter and reflect on the exercises, consider the knowledge and skills that you will need to develop to prepare yourself for a leadership role.

The skill mix of nursing in the clinical setting is increasingly diversifying, particularly with growing numbers of enrolled nurses and technical and assistant roles. The registered nurse will increasingly take on a role of leadership and coordination. No matter how small or large your clinical team is, you will need to inspire, motivate and lead your team to achieve negotiated goals and deliver effective clinical care. Skills such as effective communication, reflection, listening and critical thinking are crucial in developing these roles. Take the time to develop these skills and to seek feedback from your peers.

STORY

Jackie's first clinical appointment was in the cardiothoracic intensive care surgical unit following a 12-month new graduate placement program. Following this program, Jackie was starting to feel confident in clinical skills and mastering time management. Starting in the intensive care unit propelled her back to the feelings of inadequacy and anxiety of her first few weeks of practice. These emotions were exacerbated by a particularly busy day in the unit and the patient she was assigned having a postoperative bleed following cardiac bypass surgery, requiring a return to the operating room. Unfortunately, this patient died on the operating table and Jackie had to deal with distraught family members and the devastation of the clinical team.

Going home after that shift Jackie felt awful, racking her brain trying to consider if she should have identified any clinical signs earlier, or if she could have done any more or anything better. She had a sleepless night and returned to work the next day with fear and trepidation. The second day was much less eventful, but she still felt scared. The pace and intensity of the work were daunting and getting used to the new equipment and staff was challenging.

On her shifts she avoided taking breaks, taking extra time to catch up on her work. At night she was not sleeping well. On day 5 of the week, when the supervisor asked her when she expected to discharge a patient from the intensive care unit (ICU), she burst into tears.

Reflective questions

Please consider both Jackie's situation and that of the ICU and nursing leadership.
1. How could Jackie have coped better with this difficult week?
2. What strategies could the unit have implemented to ensure a less stressful transition?
3. What is the role of the nurse leader in this setting?

> **REFLECTION**
> The story above is a complex scenario reflecting the reality of the clinical setting with many important messages, but four key points to make are:
> 1. All clinical units should have effective orientation programs and it is the role of clinical leaders to ensure their colleagues have access to adequate support
> 2. Debriefing after critical incidents is important for both continuous quality improvement as well as team cohesion
> 3. Clinical leaders (e.g. shift supervisors and nursing unit managers) should monitor new employees for their coping and adjustment
> 4. As a new staff member, Jackie should have spoken out earlier about her fears and anxieties. Seek mentors and role models early and be comfortable asking for help

Opportunities for clinical nursing leaders

A commitment to equity and access is driving healthcare reforms in many countries, such as Australia, New Zealand (Aotearoa), the US, the UK, Thailand and Malaysia. Nurses undertake a crucial role in these reforms, from the primary to tertiary care sectors. Technological innovation has improved clinical outcomes for many non-communicable diseases (NCDs) and, in particular, we are entering an era of multimorbidity requiring innovative models challenging traditional organ-specific models (Koirala et al 2023).

Within a climate of healthcare reform, nurses now also have increasing opportunities to influence healthcare policy and practice globally (Ferguson & Davidson 2023). Nurses are working in advanced practice roles such as nurse practitioners (NPs). NPs are trained to comprehensively assess the needs of patients, order and interpret diagnostic and laboratory tests, provide diagnoses as well as formulating and prescribing treatment plans. Significant barriers may exist in advancing nursing roles, such as opposition from powerful groups, including medical organisations (De Raeve et al 2023). However, these challenges are not insurmountable and stewardship by effective nurse leaders is necessary. Demonstrating outcomes that show the quality and safety of nursing care is critical in gaining acceptance and endorsement.

There are examples across a range of nursing practice areas where innovative models of care have improved patient outcomes by challenging traditional views and perspectives. For example, nurses involved in the management of chronic heart failure have demonstrated their ability to influence patient outcomes and policies through nurse-coordinated programs and advanced practice nursing roles (Sokos et al 2023). Recognising that the greatest power base for nurses exists within the practice domain is important. The demonstration of clinical excellence and innovation is an important factor in overcoming scepticism surrounding an innovative practice.

Clinical leadership in the practice setting is an important tool and strategies to achieve this are discussed below. A clinical leader is a nurse who demonstrates the ability to influence and direct clinical practice. This clinical leader also has an ability to forecast the direction of practice and healthcare delivery as well as the knowledge, skills and competencies to develop a strategy and the ability to execute it. The vision of clinical leaders is informed by expert knowledge, credible evidence and an analysis of the social, political and economic trends influencing healthcare as well as ethical principles.

> ### REFLECTION
> Consider the barriers and facilitators impacting on the implementation of the nurse practitioner role in your practice setting.

Policy frameworks for nursing practice

Directing change and asserting leadership in an organisational system requires an appreciation of barriers and facilitators to achieving desired outcomes. This observation is relevant at both a macro- and a micro-level of operation. Politics and organisational strategy can be just as intriguing and complex within a hospital ward or community health centre as at the bureaucratic or parliamentary levels. However, at all levels, it is important to be aware of social, political and economic factors that influence healthcare delivery. Politics in nursing is discussed in more detail in Chapter 10.

As outlined above, the working environment of nurses is influenced by the social, economic and political systems of the healthcare system. These factors influence practices and trends in healthcare delivery. In some instances, policy can be either a barrier to or a facilitator of clinical leadership. The emerging role of the NP in Australia, Thailand and New Zealand (Aotearoa) is an example where significant policy and legislative reform has created a context to promote advanced nursing practice in spite of opposition and scepticism from some medical professional groups.

Policy initiatives in the UK have seen the embedded nature of practice nurses working in general practice, whereas in Australia this is an emergent and evolving role (Halcomb 2020). Internationally, healthcare professionals strive to ensure the delivery of safe and effective evidence-based care. Frameworks to monitor the quality and safety of healthcare are important in monitoring the efficacy and effectiveness of nurse-led models of care.

Strategies for promoting the quality and safety of patient care are mechanisms through which healthcare organisations are held accountable for adhering to evidence-based practice standards, continuously improving the quality of their services and ensuring high standards of care (for more on safety and quality, see Chapter 8 of this text). As you engage in your clinical placements and nursing studies, consider the factors of nursing care which can shape the outcomes of patients. Measuring nurse-sensitive patient outcome indicators, which are nursing activities that influence patient outcomes, is of increasing importance (Steel, Seaton et al 2021).

> ### REFLECTION
> Identify a nurse-sensitive patient outcome indicator (e.g. falls prevalence) appropriate to monitor in your clinical setting.

Changing models of care delivery

A variety of care delivery models are used in healthcare—some relate to nursing only and are historic, while others are interdisciplinary and responsive to emerging practice trends. The changing healthcare environment—characterised by increasing short-stay surgery, decreasing lengths of stay and numbers of acute beds, combined with increasing patient acuity related to comorbidities—requires vastly different models of care delivery from even a decade ago. Novel models of care are commonly developed in response to actual or perceived deficits in existing care delivery.

A description of common nursing models is provided in Table 22.1. It is important to note that to date the majority of investigations of nursing care have been undertaken in the acute care setting. Patients are admitted to acute care hospitals primarily for collaborative or independent nursing care, as many medical diagnostic and therapeutic procedures can now be conducted in ambulatory care settings, except in critical or emergency circumstances. However, efficient and effective care also requires continuity of patient management beyond the traditional hospital admission period to encompass the entire episode of care, particularly for those with continuing chronic disease. So, as healthcare shifts to the community, these models will likely need to be adapted.

TABLE 22.1
Common care delivery models

CARE DELIVERY MODEL	CHARACTERISTICS
Functional nursing	Ward-based care with allocation of specific clinical tasks, such as medication administration, to nursing personnel
Team nursing	Ward-based care where a small team of nurses (perhaps with different educational preparation, skills and competencies) provides care to a designated number of patients
Patient allocation/total patient care	Ward-based care provided by a registered nurse (RN) on a shift-by-shift basis to a defined number of patients
Primary nursing	Ward-based care with an RN assigned to patients for their entire admission period. Within this model a plan of care is developed, implemented and evaluated by the 'primary' nurse, with 'associate' nurses continuing the plan in the absence of the 'primary' nurse
Care management/clinical pathways	Ward- or hospital-based multidisciplinary coordinated patient care for a specific case type (e.g. patients with total hip replacement). This model frequently incorporates a 'critical' or 'clinical path' tool to 'map' and document care, including the sequence and timing of interventions and variances from expected outcomes
Case management	Hospital, outreach and/or community-based multidisciplinary care that provides continuity of care for a specific case type of patients (e.g. patients with heart failure and chronic obstructive pulmonary disease) across the entire episode of care from hospital to community
Interprofessional practice	Models of care where two or more professional groups work synergistically and collaboratively to achieve shared goals to improve patient care
Telehealth	Telehealth is the application of digital information and communication technologies, such as computers and mobile devices, to provide healthcare

Source: Adapted from Davidson P M, Hickman L 2012 Managing client care. In: Crisp J, Taylor C (eds) Fundamentals of nursing, 4th edn. Elsevier, Sydney, p 129

Programs that promote nurse coordination of care are emerging across many conditions, including cancer, diabetes, heart disease, arthritis and chronic obstructive pulmonary disease. As you consider your options for nursing in the future, it is important to remember that most nursing care occurs in community and primary care settings. Many countries around the world are adopting primary healthcare approaches to decrease health disparities and the lack of dependence on the acute care setting.

Increasing adoption of technology will see nursing interventions delivered by telehealth and web-based media. This is likely to require the development of a suite of skills and resources to work in this setting effectively. Performing effective interventions over the phone or internet is likely to be of increased importance. This will also have implications for the regulation of professional practice and the monitoring of health outcomes (Al-Alawy & Moonesar 2023).

Leadership in action

An important attribute of a leader is to formulate an action plan and support their team in achieving negotiated goals. There is an increasing discourse and discussion of leadership within the nursing profession. The concepts that make nursing leadership unique are the requisites for evidence-based healthcare: responsibility for the care and safety of patients and the need for evaluation of clinical practice. Leadership has long been an important part of the function of any organisational structure. Leadership styles vary along a continuum from authoritative to participatory, although common characteristics for leaders include being a visionary and having a plan to take individuals and services into the future. Leadership is influenced by the values of individuals and organisations, as well as society. Values are a set of beliefs and concepts derived from knowledge, experience and aspiration.

Values can be: *personal*, such as the importance placed on honesty and integrity; *professional*, such as the emphasis placed on reflective practice, accountability and continuing professional development; and *organisational*, such as the emphasis placed on patient outcomes and adherence to policy. In order to function effectively and avoid role conflict, there needs to be a congruency between the values and beliefs of the individual and the organisation in which they work. A mismatch is often a recipe for discord, conflict and low work satisfaction.

As you choose your work setting, it is important that you take the time to understand the mission and values of the organisation and ensure that these are congruent with your own belief system. The confluence between personal, professional and organisational values and leadership styles can often determine not only successful leadership but also your 'fit' within an organisation. That is, how committed you are personally to the direction of the organisation and how happy you are within the organisation. The power of nursing to drive social change cannot be underestimated. The Social Change Model for leadership promotes equity, social justice, self-knowledge, service and collaboration in nursing students and is one model of increasing personal potential for leadership (Read et al 2016). From the origins of contemporary nursing in the work of Florence Nightingale, nurses have been advocates for improving access and quality of care. It is for this reason that nurses are consistently voted the most trusted professional group across the globe. In order to promote leadership, communication strategies are important. Emerging strategies, such as social media, increase the capacity of nurses to engage in advocacy and advancing patient care (Wright et al 2020).

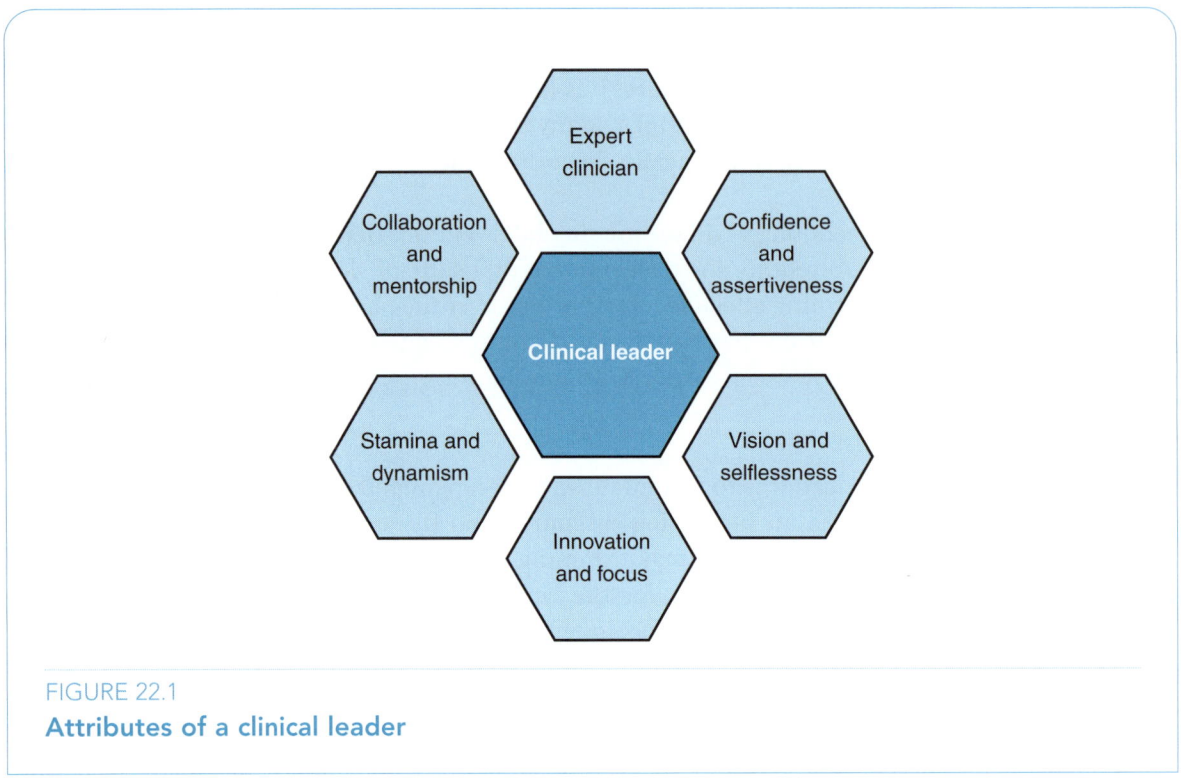

FIGURE 22.1
Attributes of a clinical leader

Figure 22.1 describes the desirable attributes of an effective clinical leader. This leadership is linked to the cultural values of the systems, resources and support available. A distinction of leadership characteristics is made between transactional, transformational, connective, renaissance and other leadership styles (Jackson & Hutchinson 2015). Transactional leadership focuses on transactions or exchanges between leaders and others, with self-interest the key motivator. In contrast, transformational leaders create a culture of leadership for all stakeholders, generating empowerment, open dialogue and inclusive decision making. An additional concept, 'breakthrough leadership', incorporates role modelling, clarification of own values and respect for others' views. Role modelling, mentoring and succession planning are vital aspects in preparing current and future nursing leaders. Jackson (2008) described servant leadership as an important trend where the servant-leader does not work in isolation, but rather actively searches for opportunities to build connections to promote creativity and thus enabling mutually beneficial relationships (Jackson 2008). Regardless of the leadership style, it needs to be a good fit with broader organisational contexts to promote quality and safety of patient care and the work satisfaction and retention of nurses in the workplace.

What makes a clinical leader?

In organisations such as hospitals and community health settings, there are different nursing leaders functioning at all levels. The individuals who readily come to mind are often those who are very visible in organisations, such as directors of nursing. However, it is important to differentiate

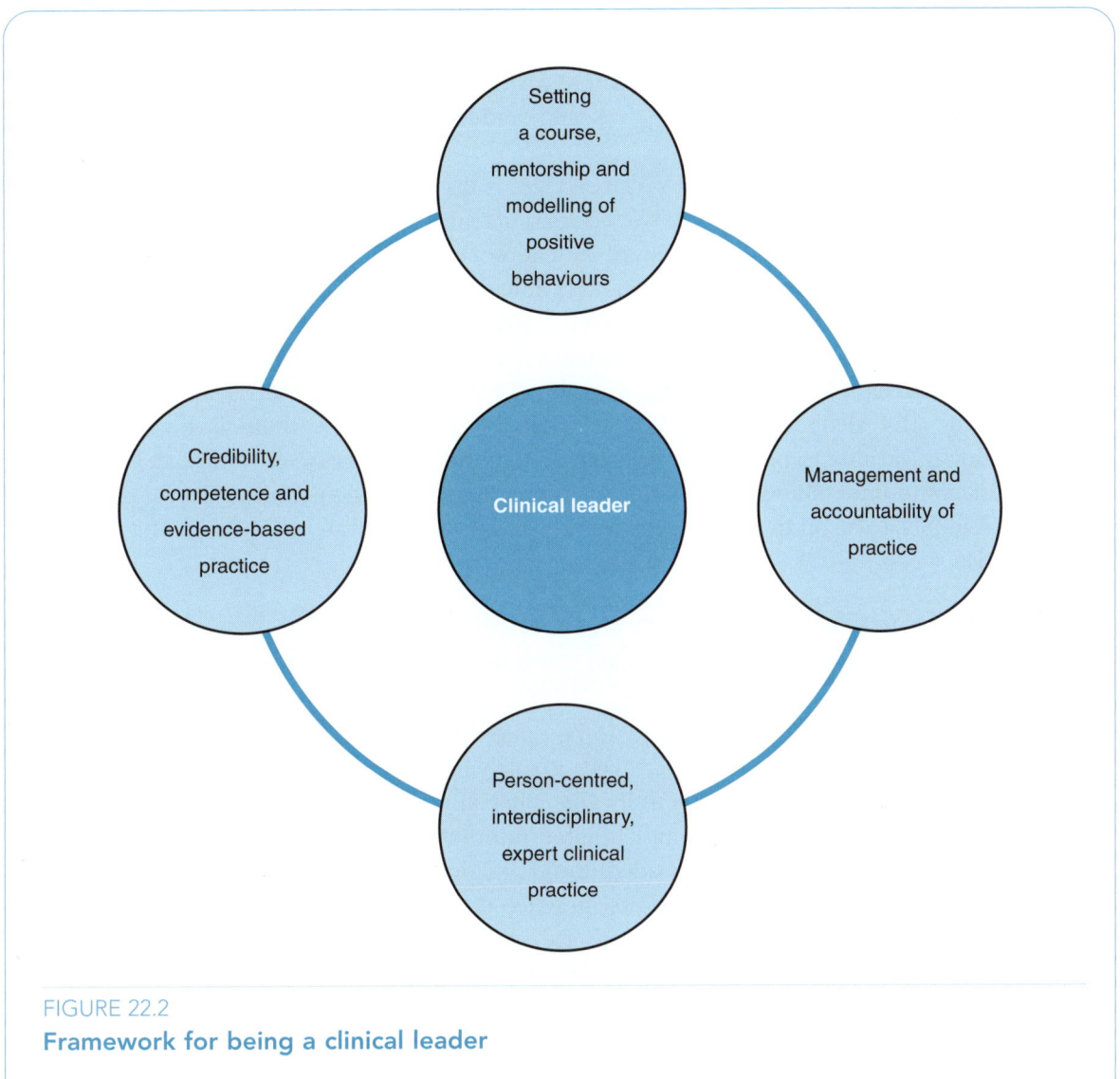

FIGURE 22.2
Framework for being a clinical leader

between management and leadership. Management refers to the planning and organisation of services. The term 'leadership' infers that an individual is visionary and pivotal in directing and shaping clinical practice. Implicit in functioning as a clinical leader in nursing is a significant mentoring role, as shown in Figure 22.2. It also means that the nurse leader lives and models their values.

These attributes show that the clinical leader is not only an expert clinician but applies a range of skills to address the needs of patients and colleagues. In discussing clinical leadership, it is important to challenge the assumption that the leader making the difference to care is at the hierarchical apex of the organisation. Clinical leaders are involved in providing and directing patient care and are experts in their field. Often a differentiating focus between vibrant research-inspired, evidence-based practice cultures and those based upon historical and hierarchical practice is the nursing leader (Cummings et al 2021). Organisations that foster nursing leadership by involving personnel in decision making and promoting nursing research and innovative practice frequently have better patient outcomes.

The intersection between health and social services is becoming more critical (Singh et al 2022). Nurses have demonstrated their ability to work as part of teams and be collaborative and participatory in their actions and decision making (for more on teamwork, see Chapter 12).

There are two critical factors in healthcare as clinicians face the complexities of current patient care: the need for clinical expertise and the need for these professionals to collaborate. Interdisciplinary healthcare teams with members from many disciplines increasingly work together to optimise patient care. Examples of these teams are found in trauma, neonatal retrieval, geriatric assessment and drug and alcohol areas of clinical practice. Increasingly, there is an emphasis on interprofessional learning to promote interprofessional practice (Aldriwesh et al 2022). Promoting nursing students to understand their own professional identity while gaining an understanding of other professionals' roles on the healthcare team is an important strategy for preparing for professional practice.

Promoting leadership in the practice setting

Given the challenges facing contemporary health systems, focusing on clinical leadership development strategies is of crucial importance. Empowering nurses to have control and influence over their practice is critical. This leadership role has to be undertaken within the complexity of healthcare systems. It is important that nurses undertake this role with credibility, competence and capability and interact with their colleagues respectfully and collegially.

A number of strategies have been implemented internationally to promote nursing leadership and in particular the links between the academic and practice settings. These include clinical professoriate positions, clinical development units, practice development strategies, clinical leadership programs and initiatives focusing on promoting evidence-based practice. The outcomes of these approaches are variable and commonly influenced more by local contextual and management factors than the overarching value of the approach. Regardless of the model undertaken, the following factors are critical: 1) increasing the voice of nurses at the decision-making table; 2) encouraging nurses' control over their practice; 3) promoting science and scholarship in nursing practice; 4) fostering an emphasis on patient outcomes and nurse-sensitive measures; 5) ensuring healthcare interventions are co-created with patients; and 6) working more effectively and efficiently in interprofessional practice environments.

An example of successful leadership models can be seen in the 'Magnet' programs, which have been widely implemented in the US and in several Australian sites and are currently being introduced in the UK. Magnet status is an award status administered by the American Nurses' Credentialing Center (ANCC), an affiliate of the American Nurses Association, to hospitals that satisfy a set of criteria designed to measure the strength and quality of their nursing. This ranges from a focus on specific nursing tasks to the quality of functional relationships within the organisation.

Many Magnet-accredited facilities have demonstrated optimal outcomes in respect of nurse-sensitive patient outcome indicators, such as pressure areas and falls. These programs have a

> **BOX 22.1**
> **An innovative nurse-led model of practice**
>
> Nurse-led care is delivered using a comprehensive approach to patient care using the best available evidence. Advanced practice nurses work in collaboration with physicians and offer a valuable contribution to the clinical care of acute and chronically ill patients. In the community there are many nurse-led models in chronic care, such as heart failure. There has also been an increase in the nursing role in procedural techniques, such as gastroscopy and vascular access devices. Often dedicated positions can lead to higher procedural volume and technical expertise. Nurse leaders in Australia have led the evidence base for nurse-led vascular access devices through technical competence, expertise and monitoring of patient outcomes, with Alexandrou and colleagues having led studies in vascular access insertion and management (Rickard et al 2021). This is an exciting approach to improving the quality and safety of patient care through nursing leadership and advanced practice.

strong influence across all levels of the organisation, from human resources to customer relations. Programs that employ such an approach are likely to have a greater chance of sustainable integration of strategies to promote clinical leadership. Strategies that foster clinical leaders within interdisciplinary care models espouse and profile the important role of nurses in improving health outcomes (Mezzina et al 2021).

As you move through practice areas during your clinical placements, observe and critically evaluate strategies that you consider enabling for clinical leaders. Strategies that support a culture of collaborative clinical decision making, as well as an emphasis on education and reflective practice, are just some examples. See Box 22.1 for an example of an innovative nurse-led model of practice.

PROFESSIONAL SOCIETIES AND ORGANISATIONS TO PROMOTE CLINICAL LEADERSHIP

Professional societies play an important role in terms of providing not only an environment of collegiality but also leadership, advocacy, mentorship and promotion of clinical excellence. These aims are achieved through the development of policy documents, publication of professional journals, conduct of scientific meetings and sponsorship of research and attendance at professional meetings. Some organisations serve the nursing profession broadly, focusing on an array of nursing issues, while others maintain a specialty focus. Examples of this in Australia are specialty groups such as the Australian College of Critical Care Nurses (ACCCN) and the Australasian Cardiovascular Nursing College (ACNC) and more generic organisations such as the Australian College of Nursing and, internationally, Sigma Nursing and the International Council of Nursing (ICN). Sigma Nursing is an international organisation promoting leadership globally through scholarship, knowledge and technology to improve the health of the world's people.

Increasingly, professional nursing organisations are playing a role in terms of social advocacy and also mentoring and supporting nursing colleagues in emerging economies. The importance of social determinants of health in moderating health outcomes underscores the importance of advocacy and

> **BOX 22.2**
> **Examples of professional nursing and midwifery organisations**
>
> - Australasian College of Cardiovascular Nurses: www.acnc.net.au
> - Australian College of Mental Health Nurses: http://www.acmhn.org/
> - Australian College of Critical Care Nurses: www.acccn.com.au
> - Australian College of Midwives: https://www.midwives.org.au/
> - Australian College of Nursing: www.acn.edu.au
> - Australian College of Nurse Practitioners: www.acnp.org.au
> - College of Nurses Aotearoa (NZ): http://www.nurse.org.nz/
> - International Council of Nursing: www.icn.ch/
> - Sigma: https://www.sigmanursing.org/

engagement (Gray et al 2023). What is increasingly apparent in a variety of settings is that a united voice can be a powerful force. For example, the ICN has taken strategic stances on issues such as ethical recruitment and women's health.

Take the time to view the information and resources on the professional nursing organisation's websites presented in Box 22.2. Many resources are available to support professional development, and opportunities for advocacy and influencing healthcare policy. These sites can also provide an opportunity to reach out to other nursing colleagues globally.

Leadership in evidence-based practice

The assessment of the cost-effectiveness and efficacy of nursing interventions and the relationship to patient outcomes is becoming increasingly important. Patient outcomes are largely dependent on implementing the best available evidence. As you study nursing, you will hear a lot of discussion about evidence-based practice. This term refers to the implementation of the best available evidence within the context of the patient's needs, knowledge and belief systems, and using the clinician's expertise (Sackett et al 1996). There is also an increasing emphasis on translational science to ensure that optimal models are translated into practice change (Chan et al 2023). Therefore, nurse leaders focus not only on assessing the needs of the patients and their families but also on measuring outcomes of nursing care.

Outcome evaluation continues to be an important way in which nurses demonstrate their influence, not only to others but also to each other. This underscores that to be an effective clinical leader, you need to reach beyond charismatic personal attributes to implement clinical evidence and evaluate the efficacy of nursing interventions. Clinical leaders know that strategies to support research and scholarship are important to develop the evidence base for advancing nursing practice.

> **REFLECTION**
> What is the role of evidence-based practice in influencing health outcomes?

SIGNIFICANCE OF EXPERT CLINICAL PRACTICE

Expert clinical practice remains the foundation of the nursing profession's standing in communities. Clinical practice, informed by nursing science, is what makes nursing exceptional and unique, and is the key to our autonomous, professional practice. This underscores the importance of emphasising expert nursing within models of professional practice, education and research. Nursing roles such as clinical nurse specialists, clinical nurse consultants and NPs are crucial in advocating for expert nursing care. Internationally and even nationally, the names for these roles may differ, but the fundamental attributes are similar.

Nurses who function as leaders in these roles carry not only the privilege but also the professional responsibility to direct healthcare practices to optimise the health of the populations they serve and also to foster the professional development of their colleagues. This is achieved through promoting evidence-based practice, nursing scholarship and developing and delivering care that is tailored to the needs of patients and their families.

Take the time to review the code of conduct of peak nursing organisations, such as the Australian Nursing and Midwifery Accreditation Council, the Nursing Council of New Zealand, the Thailand Nursing and Midwifery Council and the Philippine Board of Nursing. The recommendations of these peak bodies should provide the blueprint for your professional actions and professional practice.

Looking to the future

In this chapter, we have discussed the challenges, strategies and progress for clinical leadership. Contemporary health systems are facing considerable challenges because of the increasing burden of chronic conditions, population ageing and fiscal constraints. Yet never before has the importance of nursing care and the evidence to support nursing interventions been so strong. The COVID-19 pandemic has provided many exemplars.

It is an exciting time to embark on a nursing career and never before has leadership been so crucial. As you begin your nursing career, it is important to try to turn challenges into opportunities. You will be working in rapidly evolving settings, and the practice environments you enter in the next few years are likely to be radically different on the 10th anniversary of your graduation. Focusing on the needs of patients and their families is important in shaping care models for the future and also in setting your compass for the future.

The test remains to influence nursing practice through positive and enabling leadership strategies and to develop innovative approaches to dealing with challenges facing current clinical environments. In order to achieve this, a system of mentoring, career progression and succession planning in the clinical setting needs to be created and nurtured. Clinical and academic settings require a culture that develops innovation and fosters leadership potential.

CONCLUSION

At every level of an organisation, and regardless of whether nurses work in policy, practice, education or research settings, they have the potential to influence and direct patient care by exemplary leadership and evidence-based clinical practice. The potential for nurses to influence clinical outcomes is an empowering and motivating concept. As you embark upon your nursing career, seek enabling clinical environments and mentors who will guide you along your professional journey.

Taking the time to develop your interpersonal, communication and leadership skills will be critical for you having a productive and satisfying nursing career.

REFLECTIVE QUESTIONS

1. How can leadership in the clinical setting influence the quality and safety of patient care? Please identify both positive and negative leadership behaviours and styles and formulate a model for what you consider an effective leader to be
2. What are nurse-sensitive patient outcome indicators? Identify an indicator from one of your clinical practice settings and consider how nursing leadership can influence the capacity to achieve optimal outcomes
3. Identify a professional nursing organisation, and review their activities relating to leadership. Why are professional organisations important in formulating a professional identity and advocating for quality and safety in healthcare environments?
4. Can you identify some of your personal characteristics that will enable you to undertake a leadership position? How have your personal experiences influenced your leadership journey? Once you have identified these factors, what are some strategies for fostering your leadership from what you have read in this chapter?

Recommended readings

Sorensen C, Campbell H, Depoux A et al 2023 Core competencies to prepare health professionals to respond to the climate crisis. PLOS Climate 2(6):e0000230 https://doi.org/10.1371/journal.pclm.0000230

Meese K A, Colón-López A, Singh J A et al 2021 Healthcare is a team sport: stress, resilience, and correlates of well-being among health system employees in a crisis. Journal of Healthcare Management 66(4):304–22

Vogt K S, Simms-Ellis R, Grange A et al 2023 Critical care nursing workforce in crisis: a discussion paper examining contributing factors, the impact of the COVID-19 pandemic and potential solutions. Journal of Clinical Nursing 32(19–20):7125–34

References

Adhikari R, Smith P 2023 Global nursing workforce challenges: time for a paradigm shift. Nurse Education in Practice 69:103627

Al-Alawy K, Moonesar I A 2023 Perspective: telehealth–beyond legislation and regulation. SAGE Open Medicine 11: 20503121221143223

Aldriwesh M G, Alyousif S M, Alharbi N S 2022 Undergraduate-level teaching and learning approaches for interprofessional education in the health professions: a systematic review. BMC Medical Education 22:1–14

Alharthi A, Al-Rousan T, Commodore-Mensah Y 2024, World Refugee Day 2024: a call to action for nurses. The Journal of Advanced Nursing https://doi.org/10.1111/jan.16282

Anders R L, Jackson D, Davidson P M et al 2021 Nursing leadership for 21st century. Revista Latino-Americana de Enfermagem 29:e3472

Catton H 2023 Nursing our planet. International Nursing Review 70(1):7–9

Chan R J, Knowles R, Hunter S et al 2023 From evidence-based practice to knowledge translation: what is the difference? What are the roles of nurse leaders? Seminars in Oncology Nursing 39(1):151363

Cummings G G, Lee S, Tate K et al 2021 The essentials of nursing leadership: a systematic review of factors and educational interventions influencing nursing leadership. International Journal of Nursing Studies 115:103842

Daly J, Jackson D, Anders R et al 2020 Who speaks for nursing? COVID-19 highlighting gaps in leadership. Journal of Clinical Nursing 29(15-16):2751–2752

De Raeve P, Davidson P M, Bergs J et al 2023 Advanced practice nursing in Europe—results from a pan-European survey of 35 countries. Journal of Advanced Nursing 80(1):377–386

Ferguson C, Davidson P M 2023 Moving from rhetoric to real climate action making a difference for a sustainable planet. Heart Lung and Circulation 32(1):4–7

Geia L, Baird K, Bail K et al 2020 A unified call to action from Australian nursing and midwifery leaders ensuring that Black lives matter. Contemporary Nurse 56(4):297–308

Gray T F, Henderson M D, Barakat L P et al 2023 Advancing family science and health equity through the 2022–2026 National Institute of Nursing Research strategic plan. Nursing Outlook 71(5):102030

Halcomb E J 2020 General practice nursing. In: Wilson N J, Lewis P, Hunt L et al (eds) Nursing in Australia. Routledge, pp 254–260

Jackson D 2008 Servant leadership in nursing: a framework for developing sustainable research capacity in nursing. Collegian 15(1):27–33

Jackson D, Hutchinson M 2015 Leadership ethics and nursing work environments. In: Daly J, Speedy S, Jackson D (eds) Leadership and Nursing Contemporary Perspectives, Churchill Livingstone Elsevier, p 51

Koirala B, Badawi S, Frost S et al 2023 Study protocol for Care cOORDInatioN And sympTom managEment (COORDINATE) programme a feasibility study BMJ Open 13(12):e072846

Mezzina P, Agbozo D, Hileman P 2021 Leveraging Magnet® principles leadership during the COVID-19 pandemic. Nursing Management 52(12):22

National Academies of Sciences, Engineering and Medicine 2021 The future of nursing 2020–2030: charting a path to achieve health equity. Flaubert J L, Le Menestrel S, Williams D R et al (eds) The National Academies Press, Washington, DC doi:10.17226/25982

O'Donovan R, Rogers L, Khurshid Z et al 2021 A systematic review exploring the impact of focal leader behaviours on health care team performance. Journal of Nursing Management 29(6):1420–1443

Read C Y, Pino Betancourt D M, Morrison C 2016 Social change: a framework for inclusive leadership development in nursing education. Journal of Nursing Education 55(3):164–167

Rickard C M, Marsh N M, Larsen E N et al 2021 Effect of infusion set replacement intervals on catheter-related bloodstream infections (RSVP): a randomised controlled equivalence (central venous access device)–non-inferiority (peripheral arterial catheter) trial. The Lancet 397(10283):1447–1458

Sackett D L, Rosenberg W M, Gray J M et al 1996 Evidence based medicine what it is and what it isn't. British Medical Journal 312:71–72

Singh G K, Ivynian S E, Davidson P M et al 2022 Elements of integrated palliative care in chronic heart failure across the care continuum; a scoping review. Heart Lung and Circulation 31(1):32–41

Sokos G, Kido K, Panjrath G et al 2023 Multidisciplinary care in heart failure services. Journal of Cardiac Failure 29(6):943–958

Steel M, Seaton P, Christie D, Dallas J, Absalom I 2021 Nurse perspectives of nurse-sensitive indicators for positive patient outcomes. A Delphi study. Collegian 28(2):145–156

Ullman A J, Davidson P M 2021 Patient safety: the value of the nurse. The Lancet 397(10288):1861–1863

Wallace D M, Torres E M, Zaccaro S J 2021 Just what do we think we are doing? Learning outcomes of leader and leadership development. The Leadership Quarterly 32(5):101494

Wright R, Ferguson C, Bodrick M et al 2020 Social media and drug resistance in nursing training: using a Twitterchat to develop an international community of practice for antimicrobial resistance. Journal of Clinical Nursing 29(13–14):2723–2729

CHAPTER 23

NURSING AND THE ENVIRONMENT

Kim Usher and Naomi Tutticci

KEY WORDS

climate change
climate health
environment
first peoples
health
health industry
health services impacts
health systems
nursing
One Health
priority populations
the anthropocene

LEARNING OBJECTIVES

After reading this chapter, readers should be able to:

- understand the history of the environment in nursing
- understand the relevance of environmental health to nursing
- describe the role of nurses in promoting environmental health
- identify environmental hazard risks in the community
- identify how and why climate change is a public health emergency
- define the concept of 'One Health' and how this concept informs nursing care
- examine the relationship between climate change and human health
- reflect and critically think about how the health industry can mitigate its impact on the environment and human health.

INTRODUCTION

Nursing has long recognised the importance of the environment to human health. It is probable, however, that those early exponents of the importance of the environment to nursing and human health did not in their wildest dreams consider the impact that climate change would have on the environment. What we mean by the environment is the air we breathe, the water we drink, the food we eat, and the places where we live, work and play. Nurses recognise the connection between the environment and the health of individuals and communities. A health hazard caused by the environment is a substance or pathogen that can cause an adverse health event in individuals or communities. Environmental hazards include air contaminants, toxic waste, radiation, disease-causing microorganisms and plants, pesticides, heavy metals, chemicals in consumer products, and extreme temperatures and weather events. Nurses have long appreciated the importance of a healthy environment to the health of individuals, families and communities. All nurses will at some time in their career find themselves caring for someone affected by an environmental hazard or disaster. As the impacts of natural, man-made and infectious disease disasters increase globally, nurses have a frontline role in supporting individuals and communities (Usher et al 2023).

Nursing organisations have more recently delivered specific position statements on the role of nursing in addressing the impacts of human-caused climate change on the environment and human health. One such statement was delivered by the International Council of Nurses (2018), *Nurses, climate change and health*, which calls on nursing groups and nurses to raise awareness of the health implications of climate change, how it impacts on the environment and how these issues can be addressed. Nurses have also been actively engaged in collecting evidence to support the need for interventions to address climate change and improve the health of the environment. Nurses, as the largest sector of the health workforce, are seen to have an important role in advocating for changes that improve the health of the environment and help overcome some of the health issues related to climate change. For example, they play a key role in helping patients and families to not only reduce personal greenhouse gas emissions but also to influence the adoption of better lifestyles and strategies for climate efficiency in healthcare facilities as well as climate preparedness in the community (Sayre et al 2010). Nurses are also involved in the development of strategies to avoid the excessive use of travel for patients from rural and remote areas to attend specialist appointments through the increased use of virtual health technologies, such as telehealth, which have been used in different formats by nurses for some time (Rutledge & Gustin 2021). What is evident is that when disasters occur, it is nurses who are there in large numbers to help all who are in need. Nurse graduates must be well informed and prepared to manage environmental disasters that affect human health and to undertake strategies to reduce the impact of health service delivery on GHG emissions. Unfortunately, the current nursing education undergraduate curriculums fail to adequately prepare nurse graduates for these roles (Rutledge & Gustin 2021). This chapter will provide an overview of the issues of relevance to nursing and the environment. It is presented in four sections.

The history of environmental awareness in nursing

Nursing has always had an environmental focus. Florence Nightingale recognised the importance of the environment to human health in her text *Notes on Nursing* (1860), where she established environment theory. In that theory, Nightingale outlined 10 factors that influence health of which she believed nurses should remain aware. The theory included both indoor and outdoor pollutants such as light and noise, cleanliness, psychosocial support, food security and ventilation (Alliance of Nurses for Healthy Environments 2016). Nightingale was an avid researcher and gathered data that helped her demonstrate the importance of a clean environment during her work with soldiers in the Crimean War, where she established that soldiers were dying because of complications related to poor sanitary conditions rather than from the wounds they had acquired in battle. While environmental threats have remained since the time of Nightingale, and in many cases worsened, nurse scientists have continued Nightingale's work related to environmental threats to human health (McCauley & Hayes 2021). For example, nurse scientists have taken up the challenge to respond to environmental threats as they arise. Issues such as the impacts of smog on communities, the unregulated use of substances such as hydrochlorofluorocarbons (HCHCs) depleting the ozone layer, rivers and lakes impacted by sewerage, the impacts of wastewater and industrial runoff on soils and farms, worker vulnerability to coal, asbestos, dichlorodiphenyltrichloroethane (DDT) and other cancer-causing chemicals, fetal exposure to chemicals, asthma related to environmental hazards, lead poisoning, health issues for low-socioeconomic areas, and more, have all been targeted by nurse scientists (McCauley & Hayes 2021). More recently, as we experience the environmental threats related to climate change, nurse scientists are ramping up their research on issues of concern, including the impacts of disasters on mental and physical health (Fatema et al 2023), especially concerning those considered most vulnerable (Usher et al 2023), the need for nursing disaster competencies and preparedness (Chegini et al 2022), the impacts of bushfires and other environmental events on Indigenous peoples (Usher et al 2023, Upward et al 2021, 2023), heatwave impacts on emergency departments (Mayner et al 2010), earthquake impacts on the mental health of locals (Warsini et al 2014), anxiety related to environmental changes caused by climate change (Coffey et al 2021), the impact of COVID-19 on workers (Kabir et al 2020) and the impacts of hospital environments on patient outcomes (Jamshidi et al 2020).

Climate change is a public health emergency

In 2021, the World Health Organization (WHO) identified climate change as the '*single biggest threat facing humanity*' (WHO 2021). Anthropogenic, or human-caused, climate change is occurring due to harmful pollutants, overconsumption and other human actions that lead to the emission of millions of tonnes of greenhouse gases (GHGs) into the environment every day (IPCC 2023a). These gases cause heat to be trapped in the atmosphere and, as a result, the Earth's average temperature is increasing. The rising temperatures are causing global warming, which is causing significant changes, some of which put human health at risk. The GHGs that retain heat in the atmosphere include carbon dioxide, and the largest source of carbon dioxide pollution is the burning of fossil fuels including natural gas, gasoline, oil, propane, jet fuel and diesel. In addition, gases used in health services such as anaesthetic agents also contribute to this problem. Other causes of the climate crisis come from plastics, chemicals and deforestation. When people seek health services because of environmental-related illness, this contributes to more pollution of the environment and leads to an environment–health services cycle.

Public health initiatives act to prevent disease, prolong life, and promote health through the organised efforts of society (Winslow 1920). Fast forward 100 years from when Winslow's paper was written (1920) and these same public health goals are found in the Sustainable Development Goals (SDGs), but with a global focus on preventing, mitigating, adapting and promoting planetary health, alongside human health. Equity is central to public health, and the United Nations (UN) SDGs (WHO 2023b) can advocate for primary healthcare at a population level. Health equity is realised when everyone can attain their full potential for health and wellbeing (WHO 2023b). How is this relevant to climate change and emerging climate health-related emergencies? SDG #3 (Fig. 23.1) highlights the surge in global malaria cases. Malaria is a vector-borne disease (mosquito) that thrives in warmer, wetter climates. These changing climatic and ecological conditions optimise the range and behaviour of mosquitoes that carry malaria and other diseases. With the planet's temperature now 1.1°C warmer than in 1800, the threat of increased malaria transmission is already evident (Samarasekera 2023). Effective management of malaria is reliant on universal primary healthcare, which has at its core quality comprehensive care inclusive of promotion, prevention, treatment, rehabilitation and palliation, as close as possible to

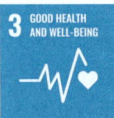
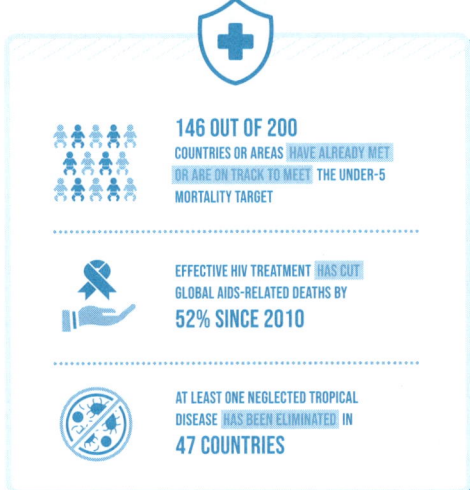
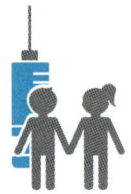
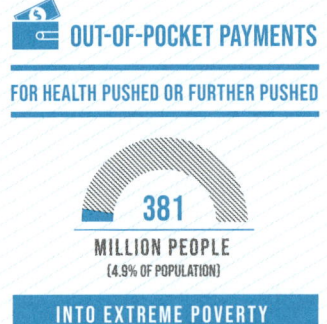
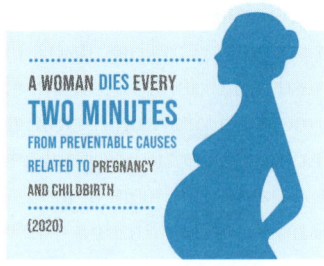

FIGURE 23.1

Sustainable Development Goal 3: Ensure healthy lives and promote wellbeing for all at all ages

Source: From Infographic: Good Health and Well-Being. https://www.un.org/sustainabledevelopment/health/. © 2023 United Nations. Reprinted with the permission of the United Nations.

people's everyday environment. Effective access to and delivery of primary healthcare is hampered when people are displaced due to climate-mediated emergencies, such as rising sea levels, flooding, fire and vector-borne diseases.

> REFLECTION
>
> Take a moment to view the UN's Sustainable Development Goals (SDG): https://sdgs.un.org/goals. Which SDGs do you think align with public health policy and practice? Why?

Public health emergencies are not limited to people becoming ill due to vector-borne diseases. The ripple effect is that illness can disrupt livelihood/earning capacity/food security, which can lead to large-scale population displacement. Human migration can lead to increases in malaria presentations within populations that have low immunity to malaria, or these same people relocating to a malaria-endemic area (Samarasekera 2023).

Climate change and extreme weather events

Climate change is worsening and is expected to significantly impact human health in the future (Centers for Disease Control and Prevention [CDC] 2024, IPCC 2023b, Lindsay et al 2023). Acute and chronic conditions are worsened by extreme heat, bushfires, bushfire smoke, flooding, extreme weather events, intense allergens and an increase in vector-borne diseases such as malaria and dengue fever (Butterfield et al 2021). Mental health is also at risk with vulnerable populations most affected (Usher et al 2023). Vulnerable groups include Indigenous people, poor and homeless people, older and younger groups, and other minority groups (Benevolenza & DeRigne 2019, Fatema et al 2021). As climate change accelerates there is an increase in the extremity and frequency of weather events, which has led to widespread adverse impacts and associated losses and damage to nature and people (high confidence). Vulnerable communities who have historically contributed the least to current climate change are disproportionately affected (high confidence; IPCC 2023b).

Why are humans and animals experiencing more frequent and extreme weather events, such as heatwaves, wildfires, floods, droughts, tropical storms and hurricanes? Science is attributing climate-related extremes to anthropogenic climate change (Clarke et al 2022, Ebi et al 2021). The rate and intensity of heat extremes are increasing with a downward trend in cold extremes, with formerly 'rare' heat events having significant societal consequences. The IPCC Report (2021) is certain that average and extreme heat is increasing on every continent, and this is due to human-induced climate change.

The cost associated with climate emergencies is increasing and has been doing so for several decades. Beyond the damage to infrastructure, extreme weather events and disasters negatively impact on individual health and wellbeing and cause catastrophic harm to communities and health systems (Ebi et al 2021).

CLIMATE CHANGE SCIENCE 101

To understand climate emergencies, we first need to recap Climate Change Science 101. You may be familiar with the greenhouse effect, caused by greenhouse gases (carbon dioxide, methane, nitrogen oxide) that trap the sun's radiation as they bounce off the planet's surface, causing the planet to heat.

As the volume of greenhouse gases increases, less radiation passes through the atmosphere, further enhancing the greenhouse effect. Visualise a glasshouse full of plants; the glass ceiling allows sunlight to pass through, for photosynthesis to occur. The sun's radiation warms both the plants and the air inside. The glass walls and ceiling trap the heat keeping the plants warm, even overnight (Fig. 23.2).

All systems seek a balanced state; for example, the human body works to maintain a state of homeostasis. The planet relies on plants and oceans to absorb carbon dioxide and produce oxygen. As the volume of greenhouse gases increases, plants cannot compensate for the increased carbon dioxide, and ocean waters become more acidic, harming marine ecosystems (Fig. 23.3).

Before the industrial revolution of the nineteenth century (Samarasekera 2023), countries were characterised by low carbon emissions, agrarian, artesian and craftsman-based economies. Mass production of high carbon emission products, which could be transported significant distances by carbon-based fuels, were not the mainstay of developed countries. Since the industrial revolution of the late 1800s, there has been a rapid increase in the use of fossil fuels, which correlates with the rapid rise in global temperatures (Masson-Delmotte et al 2021). The Earth is now 1.1°C hotter than it was in the late 1800s (IPCC 2022). As a result, post-industrial rates of extreme weather events in most land regions are observable as:

- intense and heavy precipitation globally
- more frequent and intense droughts in some regions
- desertification in some dryland areas and decreased precipitation
- increased and more intensive dust storms due to over-farming/deforestation in dryland areas (Ebi et al 2021).

Phasing out fossil fuels is now imperative, with countries shifting from a reliance on carbon-based energy sources to renewable energy (solar, wind, hydrogen). SDG#7 Ensuring Access to Affordable, Reliable, Sustainable, and Modern Energy for All (Fig. 23.4) highlights trends in energy

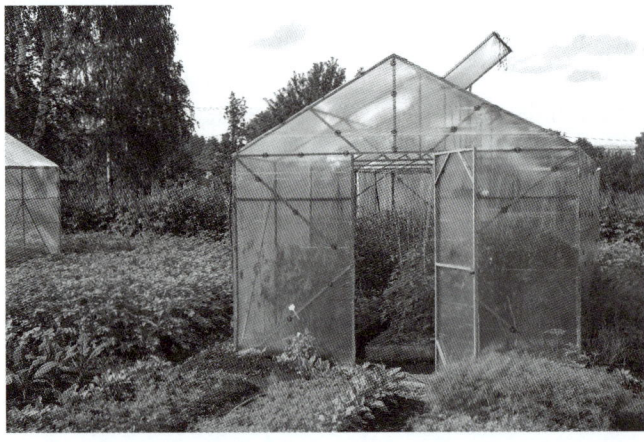

FIGURE 23.2
Glasshouse

Source: ANATOLii SAVITSKii at www.iStockphoto.com/.

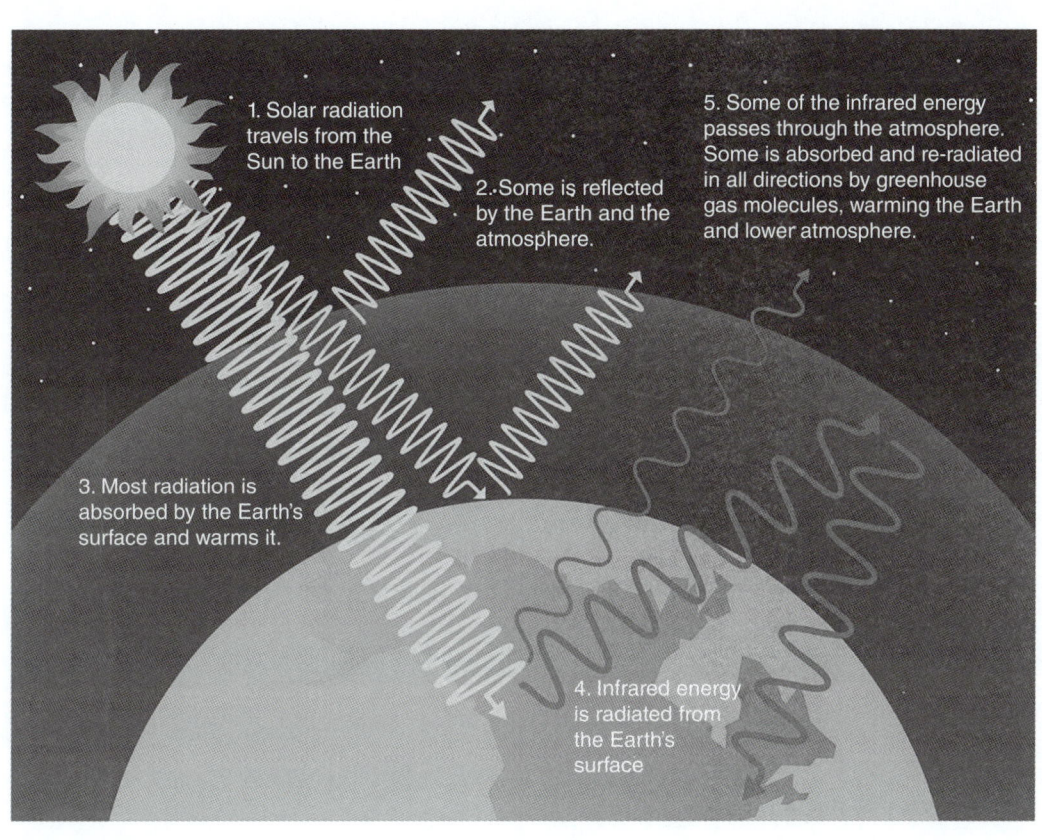

FIGURE 23.3
Greenhouse effect

Source: Adapted from the Environmental Protection Agency greenhouse effect. https://commons.wikimedia.org/wiki/File:Earth%27s_greenhouse_effect_(US_EPA,_2012).png#filehistory.

inefficiencies and the lagging use of renewable energy to power heating and transportation. A positive trend has been the uptick in modern renewables overall with an increase of 30% in electricity generated from renewables (UN n.d.).

Climate crisis

You possibly have grown up with the term climate change, which has overtaken global warming in the English language, yet the term 'climate crisis' is now being increasingly used. WHO (2023a) expanded on the term climate crisis to include a trifecta of pollution, climate change and biodiversity loss. This shift in language matches the trend in climate warming and our proximity as a planet to the 'tipping point' of 1.5°C (OECD 2022). This tipping point is a threshold, which if reached will lead to significant, rapid and often irreversible changes to climate and ecosystems. If the tipping point of 1.5°C above pre-industrial levels is crossed, the ability of the planet to stabilise the climate and maintain equilibrium will be severely compromised. Figure 23.5, produced by the Climate Council

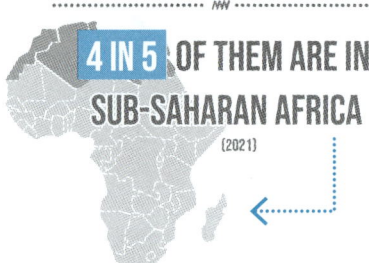

FIGURE 23.4
Sustainable Development Goal 7: Affordable and clean energy

Source: From The Sustainable Development Goals Report 2023: Special Edition. https://unstats.un.org/sdgs/report/2023/. © 2023 United Nations. Reprinted with the permission of the United Nations.

DIRECT IMPACTS	1.5°C	2°C	2°C IMPACTS
EXTREME HEAT Global population exposed to severe heat at least once every five years	14%	37%	**2.6X** WORSE
SEA-ICE-FREE ARCTIC Number of ice-free summers	AT LEAST 1 EVERY **100 YEARS**	AT LEAST 1 EVERY **10 YEARS**	**10X** WORSE
SEA LEVEL RISE Amount of sea level rise by 2100	**0.40** METERS	**0.46** METERS	**0.06m** MORE

SPECIES	1.5°C	2°C	2°C IMPACTS
SPECIES LOSS: VERTEBRATES Vertebrates that lose at least half of their range	4%	8%	**2X** WORSE
SPECIES LOSS: PLANTS Plants that lose at least half of their range	8%	16%	**2X** WORSE
SPECIES LOSS: INSECTS Insects that lose at least half of their range	6%	18%	**3X** WORSE

LAND	1.5°C	2°C	2°C IMPACTS
ECOSYSTEMS Amount of Earth's land area where ecosystems will shift to a new biome	7%	13%	**1.86X** WORSE
PERMAFROST Amount of Arctic permafrost that will thaw	**4.8** MILLION KM²	**6.6** MILLION KM²	**38%** WORSE
CROP YIELDS Reduction in maize harvests in tropics	3%	7%	**2.3X** WORSE

OCEANS	1.5°C	2°C	2°C IMPACTS
CORAL REEFS Further decline in coral reefs	70–90%	99%	UP TO **29%** WORSE
FISHERIES Decline in marine fisheries	**1.5** MILLION TONNES	**3** MILLION TONNES	**2X** WORSE

FIGURE 23.5
The difference in projected climate impacts between 1.5°C and 2°C of warming

Source: Climate Council (https://www.climatecouncil.org.au/resources/impacts-degrees-warming/)

(2023), graphically demonstrates the impact of a difference between 1.5°C and 2°C of warming on the Earth's ecosystems, species and humans. Mitigation will become increasingly difficult with the rise in global temperatures. Human societies will be overwhelmed if the Earth's systems can no longer compensate for rising temperatures.

The climate crisis is a health crisis

Extreme weather events contribute to health emergencies, overwhelming health systems, including the health professionals who are providing care. Today, the healthcare system is permanently in disaster response mode (Australian College of Nursing [ACN] 2023). Globally, human health is being directly impacted by this climate crisis, either directly or indirectly by climate-driven diseases, caused by extreme weather events, global climate change and seasonal abnormalities (Lindsay et al 2023). Sobering statistics from WHO (2023a) about the human and economic impact of this climate crisis is a call to action:

- Research findings report that 3.6 billion people already live in areas highly susceptible to climate change. Between 2030 and 2050, climate change is expected to cause approximately 250,000 additional deaths per year, from undernutrition, malaria, diarrhoea and heat stress alone
- The direct damage costs to health (excluding costs in health-determining sectors such as agriculture, water and sanitation) are estimated to be between US$2 billion and US$4 billion per year by 2030
- Areas with little health infrastructure—mostly in developing countries—will be the least able to cope without assistance to prepare and respond
- Despite a minimal contribution to global emissions, low-income countries and small island developing states (SIDS) suffer the harshest health impacts. In vulnerable areas, the death rate from extreme weather events in the last decade was 15 times higher than in less vulnerable ones.

Vulnerable populations are especially at risk for poorer health outcomes due to climate change attributed to weather extremes and diseases. Figure 23.6 lists factors that increase the likelihood of individuals and/or communities being affected by climate change. Do you notice how many of these vulnerability factors are the same as health determinants? Climate change is now considered a social determinant of health (Ragavan et al 2020). Children particularly are at risk now and into the near future of experiencing less than optimal health due to climate change. Reframing climate change as a social determinant of health could activate a large group holding differing ideologies to work collaboratively to improve healthcare access for children and their families (Ragavan et al 2020). Unfortunately, climate change is also undermining many of the social determinants of **good** health such as earning capacity, equality and access to healthcare and social support structures (WHO 2023a).

Climate resilience development is a necessary adaptation human individuals and communities need to embrace. This requires targeted action to address existing constraints such as poverty, inequity, injustice, economic and institutional barriers, trade-offs with SDG and 'greenwashing'.

Some examples of how climate change and health are interconnected and intersecting are the impact of wildfires and air pollution on human and planetary health (Fig. 23.7). As the climate warms, the frequency and intensity of wildfires increase, further contributing to air pollution and diversity loss, exacerbating respiratory diseases and deforestation. It is a no-win situation for both human and planetary health.

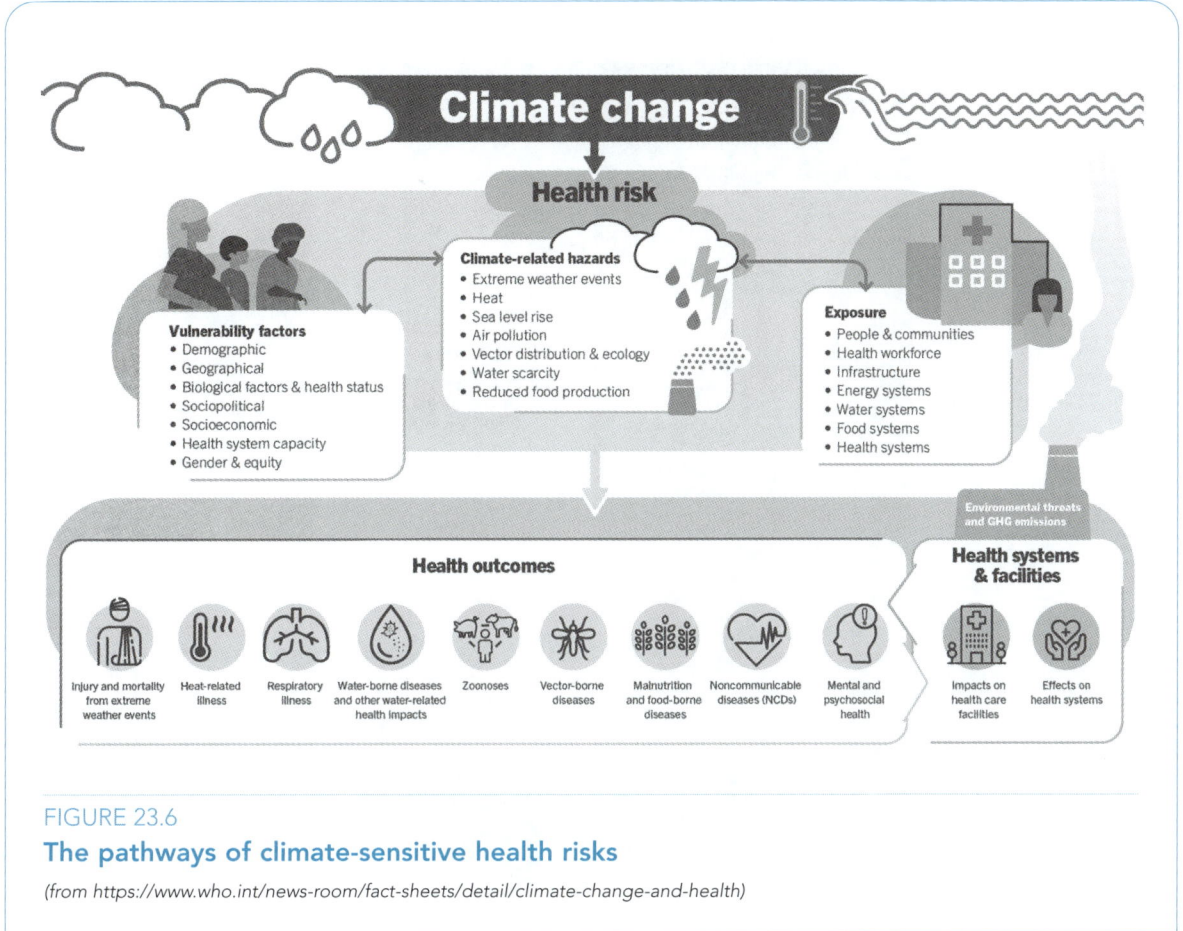

FIGURE 23.6
The pathways of climate-sensitive health risks
(from https://www.who.int/news-room/fact-sheets/detail/climate-change-and-health)

Climate change, the environment and health services

While we work hard to care for patients affected by environmental changes, we must realise that health services have their own environmental footprint that adds to environment-related threats to human health (Lenzen et al 2020). Health services are one of the largest contributors to GHG emissions and global warming (Vasilevski et al 2023); the footprint of health services varies between countries (Lenzen et al 2020). For example, patients use air and road travel to attend appointments, health workers use road and air travel to attend clinics, especially in remote locations, and health services use many disposable and other resources that add to GHG emissions. Tsagkaris et al (2020) outlined many important learnings from the COVID-19 pandemic; during the COVID-19 pandemic, GHG emissions reduced significantly due to reductions in travel, including travel to attend healthcare services. The COVID-19 pandemic provided evidence to support the need for virtual health technologies and showed how virtual healthcare technologies such as telemedicine offer a viable alternative to face-to-face health visits for many patients, thus reducing the need for travel. In addition, the use of digital devices such as wearable and implantable devices, remote imaging and mobile apps allows patients to be assessed and monitored at home (Rodriguez-Jiménez et al 2023). Healthcare services have a variety of

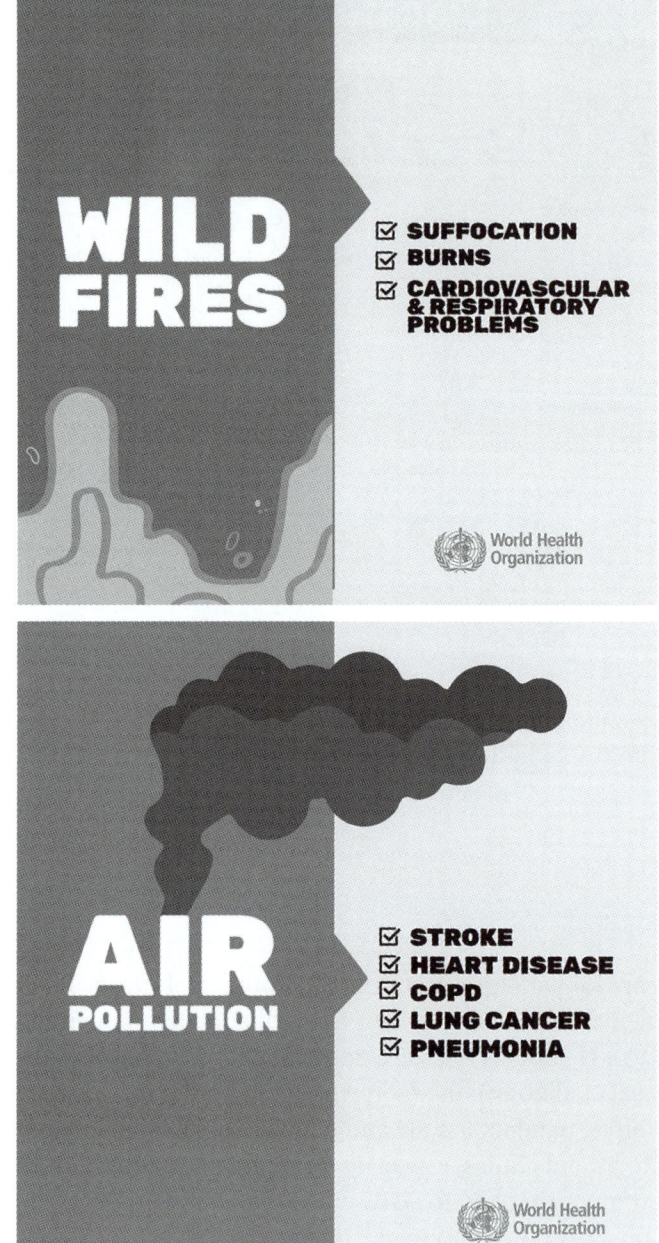

FIGURE 23.7
Wildfires and air pollution health impacts
Source: https://www.who.int/teams/environment-climate-change-and-health/climate-change-and-health/advocacy-partnerships/talks/cop27

practices that harm human health (Lenzen et al 2020). There is an urgent need to look for ways to address these practices and find less harmful ways of delivering healthcare in the future.

Nurses today have a unique opportunity to influence decisions that protect the environment. Unfortunately, many nurses lack awareness of knowledge about the effects of climate change on health and health services (Cook et al 2019) and lack the required knowledge and skills at graduation to effectively deliver virtual health services such as telehealth or digital assessment and monitoring techniques (Rutledge & Gustin 2021). This is an important concern that needs to be addressed urgently by those responsible for the education of nurses.

The following case study highlights the impact of climate change emergencies on health systems and how action now to better prepare nurses for these types of emergencies could improve health outcomes:

> In 2016, a high pollen count combined with an unusually severe thunderstorm cell contributed to a high level of respiratory distress in Victoria, Australia. This resulted in a 73% increase in demand for health services over six hours, with a 58% (9090 presentations) increase in emergency department presentations. This amounted to a 672%-increase in respiratory-related presentations. There was a fivefold increase in telehealth demand. A total of nine people died due to the climate event. Ambulance resources were stretched with resultant delays in dispatch and hospital wait times. The event was directly linked to poor awareness and planning for predictable climate events. Better planning could have anticipated and provided surge capacity.
>
> (ACN 2023)

As healthcare service environmental impacts vary between countries, the need for strategies to address these impacts must occur at a local level. We know that high-income countries' health services account for much higher environmental impacts than those of low-income countries. Hence, strategies to manage this issue must be at the country level (Lenzen et al 2020). In any situation, there is a need to reduce waste and reduce emissions. These goals must be at the forefront of all health service delivery professionals in the future.

THE EMOTIONAL IMPACTS OF CLIMATE CHANGE AND HOW WE RESPOND AS HEALTH PROFESSIONALS

With the future of our planet looking grim, hope is precarious and despair is prevalent (Frumkin 2022). Media is regularly reporting on climate emergencies, the delayed response by humanity to the climate crisis and on the toll on human life and infrastructure. This constant message of distress and despair can reduce individual and community resilience (Frumkin 2022). Concerns about climate change usually bring thoughts of environmental impact and physical health concerns, but climate change also affects people's mental health (Usher et al 2019). Climate change has led to concerns about the future of the planet for many people. Anxiety related to climate change has been reported and many terms have been used to describe it, including eco-anxiety, eco-grief, eco-angst and others (Coffee et al 2021). Climate change-induced weather events and natural disasters cause issues including sleep disorders, stress, anxiety, depression, and the development of posttraumatic stress disorder and suicidal ideation (Warsini et al 2014).

Anecdotal evidence suggests that climate anxiety can result in people wanting to avoid media about climate change and the consequent risk to human health. Pessimistic attitudes, particularly held by young people, about climate change, do not help in mitigating climate change (Ratinen 2021). The mental toll of environmental change is emotional distress (Duggan et al 2021). As nurses, we are frequently exposed to individuals in our care who are emotionally distressed while needing to manage our own mental and physical wellbeing. This balancing act can be challenging when we are feeling anxious about the climate, and our sense of hope can be eroded.

Burnout in nursing is a well-documented experience, recently compounded by the global pandemic of COVID-19 and the intense pressures this global pandemic placed on nurses to provide care, often at the expense of their own health and safety (Galanis et al 2021). Nurses have been adjusting to competing pressures to provide care in increasingly challenging circumstances; we are seeing a similar tipping point with health professionals and their capacity to increasingly accommodate physical and mental stressors, while functioning and 'being present' in frontline duties of care. The risk of adding climate crisis and the emotional distress and grief of climate-related emergencies to this workload is that thresholds for stress become lower. The nursing workforce may not be able to continue to mobilise when climate-related emergencies result in increased hospital admissions, whether due to traumatic injury or diseases acquired via polluted water sources, reduced air quality, heat stress or vector-borne.

Hope is important when all seems lost or unattainable, such as our current and projected climate state. For nurses, we need to develop a 'high-hope' state of thinking, to moderate some of the effects of negative climate messaging. With many real and potential barriers to mitigating climate change and adapting to changing environmental conditions, nurses can adopt a high-hope state of practice and outlook by developing plausible routes to implausible problems (Snyder 2002). For our health and wellbeing, constructive hope should not be overlooked; in fact, hope may be an underrated health asset (Frumkin 2022). Hope can be defined as 'the perceived capability to derive pathways to desired goals and motivate oneself via agency thinking to use those pathways' (Snyder 2002); simply put, self-belief combined with clear goals can determine outcomes. Let us look at an example that contrasts hope with hopelessness in the context of healthcare supply chains and nurses' potential to influence the current high-emission supply chains of consumables for our health systems. Briefly, supply chains are the pathway a product follows from development or manufacture to consumption and then disposal. It is a multilayered and multifactorial process of acquiring, using and eliminating consumables for high-quality healthcare. In 2014–2015 the carbon footprint attributed to healthcare was 7% of Australia's total emissions, with hospitals and pharmaceuticals the major contributors (Malik et al 2018). How can nurses be actively hopeful that they can influence the purchase, consumption and disposal of products (upstream and downstream of the supply chain) made using carbon-based fuels, and their disposal by burning or landfill?

> ### REFLECTION
> A high-hope state for the climate could be challenging to sustain in the workplace. How can you individually or within a team establish and maintain a positive, goal-focused approach to climate adaptation and mitigation?

One Health

A One Health approach to health recognises the link between human health, animal health and the environment. It is a somewhat emerging yet critical approach to managing health inequity and novel diseases. The wide and rapid spread of the COVID-19 pandemic recently revealed longstanding health inequalities related to the lack of health resources for some people in society, meaning people from low-income areas/regions/countries are less likely to be able to access affordable health services when required. One Health is premised on the understanding of the link between human and animal health and their interdependence. As many infectious diseases are shared with animals, and most emerging diseases are linked to wildlife, One Health focuses on the human–animal health connection. The focus of One Health is infectious diseases, including zoonotic diseases (those that pass between animals and people); however, other conditions, such as chronic disease, mental health, injury, occupational health and non-communicable diseases, can also benefit from a One Health approach (Riley et al 2023). A 'One Health' approach has recently been defined as:

> an integrated, unifying approach that aims to sustainably balance and optimize the health of people, animals, and ecosystems. It recognizes the health of humans, domestic and wild animals, plants, and the wider environment (including ecosystems) are closely linked and interdependent.
>
> (One Health High-Level Expert Panel [OHHLEP] et al 2022:2)

The 'One Health' approach claims that not only is the health of the environment and land and the health of humans and animals intrinsically interconnected, but also suggests that working on one of these elements has the potential to improve the other when the interconnectedness is acknowledged (Skinner 2022). The responsibility for the future of human health is not only the remit of health professionals; rather, the future health of people and the planet requires a transdisciplinary and multisectoral collaboration to confront threats to ecosystems and health (OHHLEP et al 2022). Until recently, the One Health approach predominantly focused on understanding and preventing the transmission of diseases between animals and humans within the environment (Skinner 2022). However, the recent global priority of implementing One Health action plans specifies the first action focus as 'enhancing One Health capacities to strengthen health systems' (World Health Organization [WHO] 2022:21). While this action area prompts systemic thinking about health service delivery with consideration of the environment and animals, the dominant application remains in the intersection of veterinary and medical sciences. This initiative is a global strategy that highlights the need for an initiative with the ability to recognise the need for a holistic and transdisciplinary approach that includes multidisciplinary professionals when dealing with the health of humans, animals and ecosystems (Destoumieux-Garzón et al 2018).

Nursing's role in environmental health

Our climate and our environment are changing. The impacts of climate change threaten the existence of human health and the environment (Butterfield et al 2021). Nurses have an important role to play in responding to the distress related to climate change and an important advocacy role in raising public awareness of climate change mitigation strategies (such as clean energy, water resilience and reducing health service GHGs; Usher et al 2019). Nursing is the largest group in the healthcare workforce and thus best placed to advocate for sustainable healthcare (Nicholas & Breakey 2017). Collectively, nurses can educate consumers and buyers on the bulk purchasing of low-emission products, provide evidence to support the use of lower-emission products as substitutes and act as role models for the environmentally responsible use of plastic products. Nurses are also obligated to ensure health is delivered in a clean and environmentally safe way. For this to occur, pre-registration nurses must be aware of climate change and its impacts on the environment. They must also realise the links between humans, animals and the environment. As we discussed earlier, this is not the case at present (Rutledge & Gustin 2021). Those responsible for the education of pre-registration nurses must ensure this content is adequately covered in all registered nurse education programs and that nurses not only understand the issues but can initiate change (Butterfield et al 2021). Nurses are also close to the people most vulnerable to climate change-related environmental impacts. Nurse staffing numbers have been associated with reduced mortality from climate-related diseases such as malaria, dengue fever and schistosomiasis (Butterfield et al 2021). Nurses will be increasingly called on to respond to the needs of vulnerable groups and to attend to the increasing needs of all communities (Usher et al 2023).

CONCLUSION

This chapter outlines the importance of recognising the role of environmental health in human health. Nurses must understand the connection between the environment and human health as well as their role in implementing strategies that help reduce GHGs and health service waste as one way to reduce the impact of health service provision on the environment. Nurses must also be well educated about the effect of climate change on the environment and able to initiate change when needed. These issues must be covered in all pre-registration nursing curricula. It is also essential for educators to develop innovative approaches to health education to help reduce the need for travel.

Recommended readings

Climate Action Nurses https://www.climateactionnurses.org/resources
Australian Nursing and Midwifery Federation, Climate change https://www.anmf.org.au/professional/professional-issues/climate-change
Alliance of Nurses for Healthy Environment, Climate change and health https://envirn.org/climate-change/

References

Alliance of Nurses for Healthy Environments (ANHE) 2016 Environmental health in nursing. Leffers J, Smith C, Huffling K et al (eds) ANHE, Mount Rainer, MD
Australian College of Nursing (ACN) 2023 The nursing response to the climate emergency. White Paper. ACN, Canberra
Benevolenza M A, DeRigne L 2019 The impact of climate change and natural disasters on vulnerable populations: a systematic review of literature. Journal of Human Behavior in the Social Environment 29(2):266–281 https://doi.org/10.1080/10911359.2018.1527739
Butterfield P, Leffers J, Vásquez M D 2021 Nursing's pivotal role in global climate action. BMJ 373:n1049 doi:10.1136/bmj.n1049
Centers for Disease Control and Prevention 2024 Effects of climate change on health. Online. Available: https://www.cdc.gov/climate-health/php/effects/index.html 15 January 2024
Chegini Z, Arab-Zozani M, Kakemam E et al 2022 Disaster preparedness and core competencies among emergency nurses: a cross-sectional study. Nursing Open. Online. Available: https://doi.org/10.1002/nop2.1172
Clarke B, Otto F, Stuart-Smith R et al 2022 Extreme weather impacts of climate change: an attribution perspective. Environmental Research: Climate 1(1) https://doi.org/10.1088/2752-5295/ac6e7d
Climate Council 2023 Impacts at 1.5 and 2 degrees of warming. The Climate Council. Online. Available: https://www.climatecouncil.org.au/resources/impacts-degrees-warming/

Coffey Y, Bhullar N, Durkin J et al 2021 Understanding eco-anxiety: a systematic scoping review of current literature and identified knowledge gaps. The Journal of Climate Change and Health 3:1000047 https://doi.org/10.1016/j.joclim.2021.100047

Cook C, Demorest S L, Schenk E 2019 Nurses and climate action: opportunities to lead national efforts. American Journal of Nursing 119(4):54–60

Destoumieux-Garzón D, Mavingui P, Boetsch G et al 2018 The One Health concept: 10 years old and a long road ahead. Frontiers in Veterinary Science 5:14 https://doi.org/10.3389/fvets.2018.00014

Duggan J, Haddaway N R, Badullovich N 2021 Climate emotions: it is ok to feel the way you do. The Lancet Planetary Health 5(12):855 https://doi.org/10.1016/S2542-5196(21)00318-1

Ebi K L, Vanos J, Baldwin J W et al 2021 Extreme weather and climate change: population health and health system implications. Annual Review of Public Health 42:293–315 https://doi.org/10.1146/annurev-publhealth-012420-105026

Fatema R, Rice K, Rock A et al 2023 Physical and mental health status of women in disaster-affected areas in Bangladesh. Natural Hazards 117:2715–2733 https://doi.org/10.1007/s11069-023-05964-5

Fatema S R, East L, Islam S et al 2021 Health impact and risk factors affecting south and southeast Asian women following natural disasters: a systematic review. International Journal of Environmental Research and Public Health 18(21):11068 https://doi.org/10.3390/ijerph182111068

Frumkin H 2022 Hope, health, and the climate crisis. The Journal of Climate Change and Health 5:100115

Galanis P, Vraka I, Fragkou D et al 2021 Nurses' burnout and associated risk factors during the COVID-19 pandemic: a systematic review and meta-analysis. Journal of Advanced Nursing 77(8):3286–3302

Intergovernmental Panel on Climate Change (IPCC) 2023a Summary for Policymakers. In: Climate Change 2023: Synthesis Report. Contribution of Working Groups I, II, and III to the Sixth Assessment Report of the Intergovernmental Panel on Climate Change [Core Writing Team, Lee H, Romero J (eds)]. IPCC, Geneva, pp 35–115 doi: 10.59327/IPCC/AR6-978929169164

Intergovernmental Panel on Climate Change (IPCC) 2023b Headline Statements. In: Climate Change 2023: Synthesis Report. A Report of the Intergovernmental Panel on Climate Change. Contribution of Working Groups I, II, and III to the Sixth Assessment Report of the Intergovernmental Panel on Climate Change [Core Writing Team, Lee H, Romero J (eds)]. IPCC, Geneva doi: 10.59327/IPCC/AR6-978929169164

International Council of Nurses 2018 Enfermeras, cambio climático y salud [Nurses, climate change and health.] Consejo Internacional de Enfermeras (pp 1–7) Online. Available: https://www.icn.ch/sites/default/files/2023-04/PS_E_Nurses_climate%20change_health_0.pdf

IPCC 2022 Climate change 2022: impacts, adaptation, and vulnerability. Contribution of Working Group II to the Sixth Assessment Report of the Intergovernmental Panel on Climate Change [Pörtner H-O, Roberts D C, Tignor M, et al (eds)]. Cambridge University Press. Cambridge University Press, Cambridge, UK and New York, NY, USA, 3056 pp doi:HYPERLINK https://dx.doi.org/10.1017/9781009325844"10.1017/9781009325844.

Jamshidi S, Parker J S, Hashemi S 2020 The effects of environmental factors on the patient outcomes in hospital environments: a review of the literature. Frontiers of Architectural Research 9:249–263

Kabir H, Maple M, Usher K 2020 The impact of COVID-19 on Bangladeshi readymade garment (RMG) workers. Journal of Public Health 43(1):47–52 https://doi.org/10.1093/pubmed/fdaa126

Lenzen M, Malik A, Li M et al 2020 The environmental footprint of health care: a global assessment. The Lancet Planetary Health 4(7):e271–e279

Lindsay S, Hsu S, Ragunathan S et al 2023 The impact of climate change related extreme weather events on people with pre-existing disabilities and chronic conditions: a scoping review. Disability and Rehabilitation 45(25):4338–4358

Mayner L, Arbon P, Usher K 2010 Emergency Department patient presentations during the 2009 heatwaves in Adelaide. Collegian: Journal of the Royal College of Nursing Australia 17(4):175–182

McCauley L, Hayes R 2021 From Florence to fossil fuels: nursing has always been about environmental health. Nursing Outlook 69(5):720–731

Mettenleiter T C, Markotter W, Charron D F et al 2023 The One Health High-Level Expert Panel (OHHLEP). One Health Outlook 5: 18 https://doi.org/10.1186/s42522-023-00085-2

Nicholas P, Breakey S 2017 Climate change, climate justice and environmental health: implications for the nursing profession. Journal of Nursing Scholarship 49(6):606–616 https:// doi.org/10.1111/jnu.12326

Nightingale F 1969 Notes on nursing. Dover Books on Biology. Dover Publications, New York, NY

OECD 2022 Climate tipping points: insights for effective policy action. OECD Publishing, Paris. Online. Available: https://doi.org/10.1787/abc5a69e-en

Ragavan M I, Marcil L E, Garg A 2020 Climate change as a social determinant of health. Pediatrics 145(5):e20193169

Ratinen I 2021 Students' knowledge of climate change, mitigation and adaptation in the context of constructive hope. Education Sciences 11(3):103

Riley T, Cumming B, Thandrayen J et al 2023 One Health and Australian Aboriginal and Torres Strait Islander Communities: a One Health pilot study. International Journal of Environmental Research and Public Health 20914:6416 https://doi.org/10.3390/ijerph20146416

Rodriguez-Jiménez L, Romero-Martin M, Spruell T et al 2023 The carbon footprint of healthcare settings: a systematic review. Journal of Advanced Nursing 79(8):2830–2844 https://doi.org/10.1111/jan.15671

Rutledge C M, Gustin T 2021 Preparing nurses for roles in telehealth: now is the time. Online Journal of Issues in Nursing 26(1) doi: 0.3912/OJIN.Vol26No01Man03

Samarasekera U 2023 Climate change and malaria: predictions becoming reality. Lancet 402(10399):361–362 https://doi.org/10.1016/S0140-6736(23)01569-6

Sayre L, Rhazi N, Carpenter H et al 2010 Climate change and human health: the role of nurses in confronting the issue. Nurse Administration Quarterly 34:334–342

Skinner T 2022 One health the future of rural health? Australian Journal of Rural Health 30:304–305 https://doi.org/10.1111/ajr.12893

Snyder C R 2002 Hope theory: rainbows in the mind. Psychological Inquiry 13:249–275

Tsagkaris C, Moysidis D V, Papazoglou A S, et al 2021 Detection of SARS-CoV-2 in wastewater raises public awareness of the effects of climate change on human health: the experience from Thessaloniki, Greece. The Journal of Climate Change and Health 2:100018

United Nations (UN) n.d. Ensure access to affordable, reliable, sustainable, and modern energy for all. Online. Available: https://sdgs.un.org/goals/goal7#targets_and_indicators

Upward K, Maple M, Saunders V et al 2021 Editorial: Mental health, climate change, and bushfires: what's colonization got to do with it? International Journal of Mental Health Nursing 30:1473–1475 https://doi-org.ezproxy.une.edu.au/10.1111/inm.12927

Upward K L, Usher K, Saunders V 2023 The impact of climate change on country and community and the role of mental health professionals working with Aboriginal communities in recovery and promoting resilience. International Journal of Mental Health Nursing 32(6):1484–1495 https://doi.org/10.1111/inm.13184

Usher K, Durkin J, Bhullar N 2019 Eco-anxiety: how thinking about climate change-related environmental decline is affecting our mental health. International Journal of Mental Health Nursing 28(6):1233–1234 https://doi.org/10.1111/inm.12673

Usher K, Rice K, Fatema S R et al 2023 Nurses on the frontline of health care in the escalating context of climate change: climate-related extreme weather events, injustice, mental health and eco-anxiety. Journal of Advanced Nursing https://doi.org/10.1111/jan.15838

Vasilevski V, Huynh J, Whitehead A et al 2023 The Green Maternity project: a midwife-led initiative to promote correct waste segregation on an Australian postnatal ward. Journal of Advanced Nursing 00:1–12 https://doi.org/10.1111/jan.15789

Warsini S, Buettner P, Mills J et al 2014 The psychosocial impact of the environmental damage caused by the Mt Merapi eruption on survivors in Indonesia. EcoHealth 11:491–501

Winslow C E A 1920 The untilled fields of public health. Science 51:23

World Health Organization (WHO) 2021 Climate change and health. WHO. Online. Available: https://www.who.int/news-room/fact-sheets/detail/climate-change-and-health 19 April 2023

World Health Organization (WHO) 2022 Mental health and COVID-19: early evidence of the pandemic's impact. Scientific brief. WHO. Online. Available: https://iris.who.int/bitstream/handle/10665/352189/WHO-2019-nCoV-Sci-Brief-Mental-health-2022.1-eng.pdf

World Health Organization (WHO) 2023a Climate change fact sheet. WHO. Online. Available: https://www.who.int/news-room/fact-sheets/detail/climate-change-and-health

World Health Organization (WHO) 2023b Primary health care fact sheet. WHO. Online. Available: https://www.who.int/news-room/fact-sheets/detail/primary-health-care

CHAPTER 24

GLOBAL HEALTH AND NURSING

Michele Rumsey

KEY WORDS

Chief Nursing and Midwifery Officer
climate impacts
data revolution
education
globalisation
governance
human resources for health
nurse migration
people-centred care
regulation
sustainable development goals
universal health coverage

LEARNING OBJECTIVES

After reading this chapter, readers should be able to:

▸ understand the context in which global and regional policies and strategies influence health system planning and leadership

▸ understand the role of major United Nations agencies in influencing global health priorities and planning

▸ discuss the governance role of the Chief Nursing Officer or Chief Nursing and Midwifery Officer

▸ explain the importance of global, regional and national human resources for health (HRH) inter-sectoral plans to achieve universal health coverage (UHC)

▸ explain the role that regulation, education, strategic partners (including associations) and governance play in shaping health workforce policy.

INTRODUCTION

This chapter describes the impact of global and regional policies on everyday nursing and healthcare outcomes. The ability of governments to improve outcomes for their citizens depends critically on their healthcare workforce. This chapter investigates approaches to building an effective international nursing workforce, discussing how nursing leaders can influence high-level decisions. It also explores the importance of effective continuing education and good governance, and the role major international agencies such as the World Health

Organization (WHO) play. This discussion highlights the importance of maintaining accurate, up-to-date data on the capacity and skill-mix of the nursing and midwifery workforce. This chapter draws on international experience, especially from Pacific Island nations, near neighbours of Australia and New Zealand (Aotearoa), to illustrate the relationship between nursing and global health.

Context

Global population health is affected by major social, political, economic and environmental trends; up-to-date relevant data are therefore necessary to plan effectively for future health needs. Globalisation, urbanisation and the influence of Western lifestyles on lower- and middle-income countries (LMIC) have brought previously unaffordable goods to new markets, contributing to dietary change, more sedentary lifestyles and increasing consumption of tobacco and alcohol (Casari et al 2022, Chen et al 2021). Together with increased life expectancy and population ageing, this has led to a shift in disease patterns. Incidences of chronic, non-communicable diseases (NCD), such as cancer and diabetes, have escalated with 41 million people dying each year, equivalent to 74% of all deaths globally; these deaths disproportionately impact LMIC where 31.4 million deaths occur each year (WHO 2023a). Changes in policy can, however, positively impact health outcomes. China, for example, witnessed an increase in NCD from the 1980s, attributed to rapid economic growth, increased life expectancy and lifestyle changes (Zhou et al 2024). China responded with major health reforms, including a universal health insurance scheme in 2009. Despite insufficient progress in NCD management and control, this has led to greater healthcare service coverage, substantially reducing inequality (Li et al 2023).

In addition to NCDs, infectious diseases remain a substantial challenge, especially in LMIC, as does the impact of climate change (see Chapter 23), unequal access to healthcare, antimicrobial resistance and public health emergencies. The migration of nurses and midwives further exacerbates global inequalities in health. Fuelled by huge international demand, healthcare professionals often leave their communities to pursue opportunities abroad, leaving source countries underserviced. This contributes to the dearth of skilled practitioners in LMIC where they are needed most (Buchan & Catton 2020, UNFPA et al 2021, WHO 2020b).

Nurses and midwives, so often on the frontlines of community engagement and healthcare responses, are key to providing people-centred care (Leyns et al 2023). The inability of many LMICs to achieve the previous health-related Millennium Development Goals (MDGs)—reducing child mortality, improving maternal health and eradicating malaria and HIV—can be directly linked to insufficient or under-skilled health workers (WHO 2021a). The nursing and midwifery professions therefore require leaders who can advocate for patients' needs and influence health policies, processes and health professional education. This influence can and should extend beyond national borders to international policy making through the World Health Assembly (WHA). This was seen in practice in May 2021, with the Global Strategic Directions for Nursing and Midwifery (SDNM) 2021–2025 initiative (WHO 2021a). The SDNM focuses on education, jobs, leadership and service delivery. Each strategic direction is underpinned by prioritised policy actions designed to achieve improved health outcomes.

COVID-19 emphasised the importance of nurses, who were central to the international response to the virus, but at a profound cost to the profession. Particularly early in the pandemic, limited availability of personal protective equipment meant many frontline workers became ill or died

(Buchan & Catton 2020). The pre-pandemic shortage of nurses has been exacerbated not only by continuing sickness and death, but from increasing nurse burnout and work-related stress (Buchan et al 2023). Data limitations mean the impact of nurse migration on human resources for health is unclear. Workforce attrition in LMIC may be intensifying as retirement, or moving overseas to better pay, career opportunities and working conditions become increasingly attractive (Buchan & Catton 2020).

The pandemic reinforced the global need to 'protect and invest in all occupations engaged in a preparedness and response capacity, in public health functions, and in the delivery of essential health services' (WHO 2021a:2). It takes an integrated approach, addressing governance, regulation, education and strategic partnerships to develop and sustain a strong, flexible and motivated health workforce (Rumsey et al 2022b, WHO 2020b, 2020c). Effective leadership and strategic planning are only possible once these areas are integrated within a health system (Rumsey et al 2022b).

Developing global health strategies and policies

The WHO is the Geneva-based United Nations (UN) agency that oversees global health agendas. It has 194 member states located across six regions: Africa, the Americas, Europe, South-East Asia, Western Pacific (including Australia and New Zealand [Aotearoa]) and Eastern Mediterranean. The WHA is the WHO's decision-making body with delegates from all WHO member states, as well as health professionals, non-government organisations (NGOs) and other UN agencies who gather annually to discuss responses to emerging global health agendas. Resolutions cover many areas including epidemics, pandemics, emergency disasters, chronic and acute medical issues, health workforce, universal health coverage (UHC) and WHO finances (WHO 2024a).

The Regional Health Innovation Strategy for the Western Pacific (WHO 2024d) outlines mechanisms to achieve its priorities based on five main principles (Fig. 24.1) that support equitable healthcare and enhance the health workforce. These are:

- Mission-oriented: recognising the problem, setting a direction and goals to achieve
- Collective intelligence: bringing together partners and stakeholders for collaboration in the mission
- Learning: from health innovation
- Evidence-based: assessing the impact of change, optimising resources, basing decisions on data
- Common good: prioritising equitable access to benefits.

To date, medical practitioners have dominated the representation of health professionals both within the ranks of WHO and at WHA debates (WHO 2024b). To meet the principles of collective intelligence and common good, the viewpoints of other stakeholder groups, including nurses and midwives, must not be ignored. In 2017, the WHO finally reappointed a Chief Nurse to provide leadership to nurses and midwives worldwide. Nursing and midwifery services are estimated to comprise over 59% of all healthcare services (WHO 2020b), including 69% in Western Pacific and 74% in Pacific regions (WHO 2020b). Nurses and midwives require high-level leadership and advocacy to engage in health policymaking and planning both in their own countries and internationally (Rumsey et al 2022a, 2022b).

In 2020, the International Council of Nurses (ICN) found that just 50% of countries had a Chief Nursing Officer. Of these, only half had authority to advise or influence at a strategic level

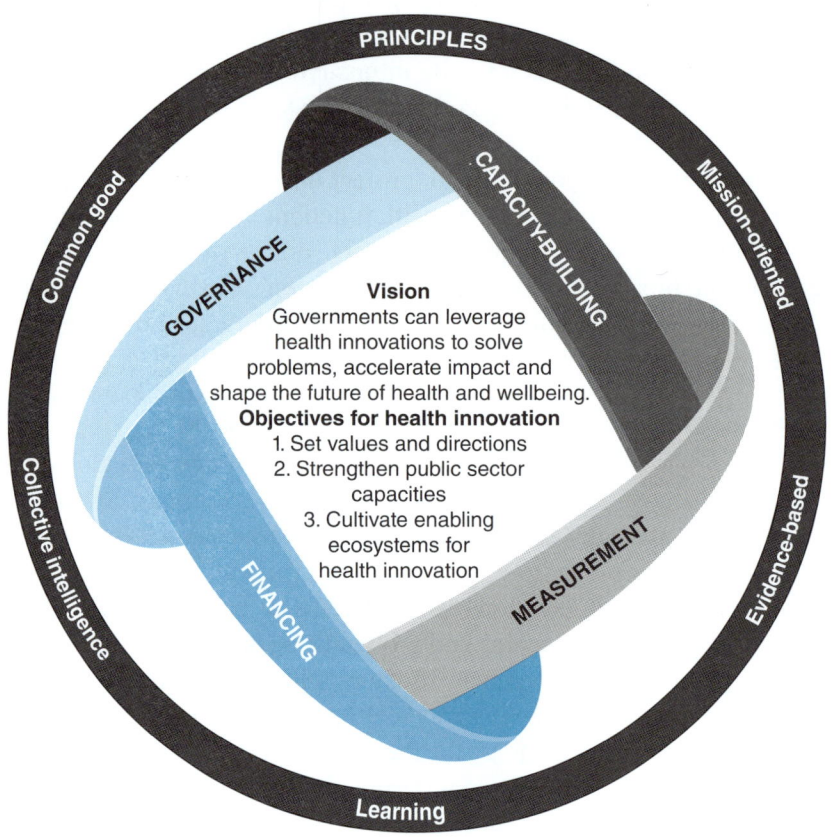

FIGURE 24.1
Action Framework – From WHAT and WHY to HOW: Health Innovation in PHC

Source: WHO 2024d:14

(ICN 2020). Similarly, there are limited leadership opportunities for midwives with access to their national health ministry (UNFPA et al 2021). Appointing a Chief Nursing Officer (CNO) or a Chief Nursing and Midwifery Officer (CNMO) with the authority to influence planning and developing and implementing health policies and systems are therefore critical for governments to ensure their own nursing and midwifery workforce is represented at the highest level both nationally and globally (WHO 2021). Nationally supported programs to develop nursing leadership, research or policy literacy skills are limited (Rumsey et al 2022a, WHO 2020a, 2021a).

> ## REFLECTION
> What unique insights do nurses and midwives bring to setting healthcare policy? Why is this important? How would their perspectives differ from other health professionals?

The Global Strategic Directions for Nursing and Midwifery

The Global Strategic Directions for Nursing and Midwifery (SDNM) 2021–2025 (WHO 2021a) set out strategic directions and policy priorities that will allow midwives and nurses to optimally contribute to achieving UHC and other health goals. The SDNM comprises four policy focus areas: education; jobs; leadership; and service delivery. Each policy priority is expressed through a human resource for health (HRH) lens designed to support the strategic direction (Fig. 24.2). The primary enactors of the SDNM will be health workforce planners and policymakers, although others will also deliver SDNM, including educational institutions, employers, professional associations, development partners, international organisations and civil society.

The SDNM and associated policy priorities seek to address the forces that drive nurse and midwife shortages and surpluses, geographical imbalances and suboptimal contributions by nurses and midwives in service delivery settings. They are supported by internationally agreed action plans on health resources that outline a progressive pathway to optimise and strengthen the global health workforce that all countries can follow to accelerate their progress towards UHC, emergency preparedness and response, and the Sustainable Development Goals (SDGs) (United Nations [UN] 2019). The action plan promotes using data to inform planning and investment decisions; engaging stakeholders; promoting equity; aligning investment and action with population needs and health systems; and empowering national governance and leadership.

THE NEED FOR DATA IN POLICY AND PLANNING

Effective planning and policy need to be underpinned by up-to-date and relevant data to provide evidence for global strategies, goals and policy priorities to meet UHC and achieve the SDGs. It is imperative to monitor critical indicators such as changing patterns of disease and population health needs related to shifts in lifestyle, climate change and poverty levels, and data on international migration and urbanisation of the health workforce especially in low-income countries or geographically isolated areas. HRH planning requires solid, accurate data on where health workers are, where they are most needed and where they are moving to and from; this allows hospitals, rural services

EDUCATION →

Strategic direction: Midwife and nurse graduates match or surpass health system demand and have the requisite knowledge, competencies and attitudes to meet national health priorities.

Policy priority: Align the levels of nursing and midwifery education with optimised roles within the health and academic systems.

Policy priority: Optimise the domestic production of midwives and nurses to meet or surpass health system demand.

Policy priority: Design education programs to be competency-based, apply effective learning design, meet quality standards, and align with population health needs.

Policy priority: Ensure that faculty are properly trained in the best pedagogical methods and technologies, with demonstrated clinical expertise in content areas.

JOBS →

Strategic direction: Increase the availability of health workers by sustainably creating nursing and midwifery jobs, effectively recruiting and retaining midwives and nurses, and ethically managing international mobility and migration.

Policy priority: Conduct nursing and midwifery workforces planning and forecasting through a health labour market lens.

Policy priority: Ensure adequate demand (jobs) with respect to health service delivery for primary healthcare and other population health priorities.

Policy priority: Reinforce implementation of the WHO Global Code of Practice on the International Recruitment of Health Personnel.

Policy priority: Attract, recruit and retain midwives and nurses where they are most needed.

LEADERSHIP →

Strategic direction: Increase the proportion and authority of midwives and nurses in senior health and academic positions and continually develop the next generation of nursing and midwifery leaders.

Policy priority: Establish and strengthen senior leadership positions for nursing and midwifery workforce governance and management and input into health policy.

Policy priority: Invest in leadership skills development for midwives and nurses.

SERVICE DELIVERY →

Strategic direction: Midwives and nurses work to the full extent of their education and training in safe and supportive service delivery environments.

Policy priority: Review and strengthen professional regulatory systems and support capacity building of regulators, where needed.

Policy priority: Adapt workplaces to enable midwives and nurses to maximally contribute to service delivery in interdisciplinary healthcare teams.

FIGURE 24.2
Summary of WHO strategic directions for nursing and midwifery, and policy priorities
Source: WHO 2021a

and clinics as well as health and education ministries to pre-empt staffing requirements. Knowing where the gaps and weaknesses are helps determine when and where to direct extra resources (Buchan et al 2023, WHO 2022).

In addition to monitoring baseline data to set targets, it is important to measure progress against these targets as action is taken. Measuring progress against, for example, the SDGs and SDNM is a huge challenge, but innovations in technology and approaches over the past decade have improved data collection and interpretation (UN 2023, WHO 2024c). While the WHO reports on the State of the World's Nursing (SOWN; WHO 2022b) and State of the World's Midwifery (SOWMy; WHO et al 2021b) provide extensive and valuable data, they were published during the COVID-19 pandemic. The data therefore do not reflect the pandemic's impact on global health needs and the health workforce, highlighting the need for continual data collection and analysis to promote responsive health policy and planning.

> ### REFLECTION
> As a student nurse, what data collections have you contributed to? How do you think these data might be used? What do you think are the challenges for collecting accurate data in low- and middle-income countries?

Global and regional priorities in health

THE HEALTH WORKFORCE

The WHO recommends that 4.5 doctors, nurses and midwives per 1000 people are necessary to meet population needs by 2030 (WHO 2022). Even pre-pandemic, many countries remained way below this WHO target, with a huge differential between countries. Figure 24.3 clearly shows, for example, Australia and New Zealand (Aotearoa) have over 10 times the proportion of health workers of Papua New Guinea (WHO 2020b). Further disparities remain between rural, remote, sub-national and hard-to-reach areas compared with capital cities and urban centres (UN 2023).

Almost 90% of the identified global shortage of 5.9 million nurses occurred in LMICs (WHO 2020b) with similar unequal distribution and shortages in midwifery (WHO et al 2021b). Many high-income countries are not only struggling to provide care for their ageing population but much of their health workforce is also ageing, especially nurses and midwives (Buchan et al 2023, WHO 2020b, UNFPA et al 2021). Worldwide, one in six (17%) nurses are aged 55 years or over and expected to retire within the next 10 years (WHO 2020b); a further 4.7 million nurses would be required simply to replace them. Addressing these HRH issues will require governments to implement globally endorsed strategies, to seek self-sufficiency in the supply of their health workforce and to invest in nursing jobs, education, leadership and service delivery (Catton & Iro 2021).

ETHICAL MIGRATION AND RECRUITMENT

A major contributing factor to the inequitable distribution of health workers is the so-called 'brain drain' where talented and skilled personnel leave their own countries or communities to pursue opportunities elsewhere, aiming to improve living standards or for professional development. The escalating health worker shortage in some middle- to high-income nations, arising from workforce

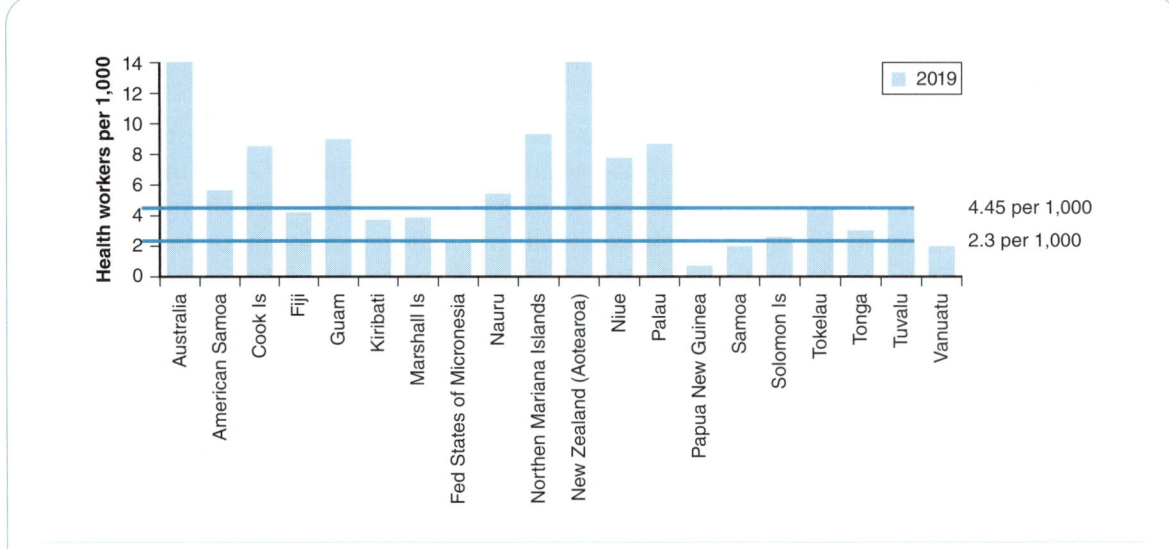

FIGURE 24.3
Pacific professional health workforce density

Source: Modified from Haakenstad A, Irvine CMS, Knight M, et al 2022. Measuring the availability of human resources for health and its relationship to universal health coverage for 204 countries and territories from 1990 to 2019: a systematic analysis for the Global Burden of Disease Study 2019, The Lancet 399, 2129-2154.

ageing, is increasingly being met by recruiting foreign health workers, often from LMICs. This can leave already vulnerable health systems in poorer countries even more depleted, particularly in times of medical emergency, undermining efforts to develop health systems. Accordingly, the WHA adopted the Global Code of Practice on the International Recruitment of Health Personnel (McQuide et al 2023, WHO 2023b), outlining ethical principles and practices for international recruitment, through discouraging active recruitment of health personnel from countries facing critical workforce shortages. Some argue for greater action to stem the flow of nurses from low-resource to high-resource countries, including calls for an international treaty enforcing legislation (Karan et al 2023, South Pacific Chief Nursing Midwifery Officers Alliance [SPCNMOA] 2021); others note that an individual's right to move between countries should be pre-eminent.

Managing international migration requires a considered, collective response from both 'source' and 'destination' countries and effective data on migratory flows. Data on trends and gaps can help countries develop considered measures to pre-empt damage to their health system through loss of health professionals (Buchan & Catton 2020). In 2019, only 40% of all countries signed up to the WHO Code had introduced or were developing national laws and policies consistent with the WHO Health Worker Migration Code (WHO 2023b).

During the COVID-19 pandemic, many countries turned to international recruitment to rapidly increase their health workforce capacity, simplifying inward migration and accepting foreign qualifications to facilitate international mobility. Increased international migration of nurses has continued apace, impacting progress to UHC and access to basic healthcare in many source countries. Fiji, for example, lost one-third of its nursing workforce to migration in a single year, 2022–23

(WHO 2023b). In a sample of 48 destination countries, approximately 12% of the foreign-trained nurses originated from countries on the WHO health workforce support and safeguards list; that is, countries whose limited health workforce made them unlikely to achieve the UN SDG target for UHC by 2030 (WHO 2023b).

Potential policies to promote ethical migration include high-income countries developing a more sustainable workforce; improved data on health workforce migration to monitor movement and identify unethical recruitment; clear delineation of fair recruitment and employment practices; bilateral agreements to ensure benefits to source countries; and stronger collaboration with the private sector (Stokes & Iskander 2021).

> ### REFLECTION
> Have you considered working overseas once you are qualified as a registered nurse or midwife? Reflect on some of the challenges related to this that you foresee.
> During your clinical placement experience, have you worked with health professionals from other countries? If so, what do you think are some of the challenges they faced when adapting to working in a different country?

Health policy at a country and regional level

So how do global development and health agendas and strategies filter down to regions and individual governments? And how do regions and individual countries promote their own health priorities to decision makers when global health agendas are being set?

The six WHO regional offices work semi-autonomously from headquarters in Geneva with their own budgets, and liaise and coordinate with local health ministers, NGOs and other partners to advocate for public health issues relevant to their region. The Western Pacific Regional Office works in 37 countries from China to New Zealand (Aotearoa) with a population of 1.9 billion people. It has headquarters in the Philippines and another 15 country offices (WHO 2024b). Australia and New Zealand (Aotearoa) sit within the South Pacific sub-region, based in Suva, Fiji, that coordinates forums such as the biennial Pacific Health Ministers Forum. This Forum debates the relevance of global policies to the region and allocates development funds to country and regional, bilateral or multilateral priority work (WHO 2024b); it also determines which local issues to highlight at the WHA (WHO 2024e).

How nursing leaders influence global health planning

Given the fundamental role nurses and midwives play in delivering people-centred health services, it is important their voices are heard in forums discussing global and regional health priorities. Governments can assist this by appointing a CNO or CNMO. To date, all South Pacific countries have a Chief Nursing and/or Midwifery Officer position, except Papua New Guinea (PNG). Of 37 countries in the Western Pacific region, 27 have a CNMO (Rumsey et al 2022a, 2022b, UNFPA et al 2021, WHO 2020b), and some (Korea, the Philippines, PNG, China and Mongolia) are working towards one.

A recent review of WHO documents highlighted common issues faced by the global nursing and midwifery community: management and leadership, service delivery, jobs, education and research. The most pressing issue was the nursing workforce—not only limited numbers but also the need for

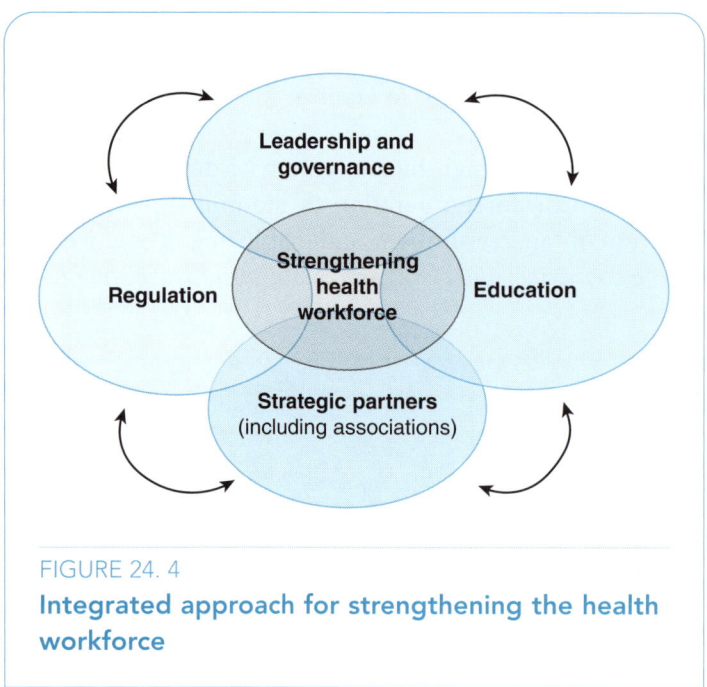

FIGURE 24. 4

Integrated approach for strengthening the health workforce

better planning. The review concluded that nursing leadership is critical to facilitate and improve nurse performance, which is essential for quality care and patient safety; nursing leaders need to 'think globally', sharing their expertise to stimulate mutual learning (Rumsey et al 2022a, WHO 2021a). The WHO Collaborating Centre for Nursing and Midwifery at the University of Technology, Sydney (WHO CC UTS) has adapted a model identifying four interdependent elements essential for leaders to effectively build collaborative health workforce policy: 1) leadership and governance; 2) regulation; 3) education; and 4) strategic partnerships (including associations) (Fig. 24.4).

LEADERSHIP AND GOVERNANCE

Strengthening the global nursing and midwifery workforce requires strong governance and leadership. Sound governance, policy and management are important to sustain the professional health workforce, ensure patient safety and continuous quality improvement, to maintain continuing professional development (CPD) and to deal with emergency situations. CPD and effective leadership programs for nurses and midwives are crucial to managing services and developing evidence-based programs (Roberts 2017, SPCNMOA 2021, WHO 2021a).

Nationally, nursing workforce governance is generally the responsibility of a country's health ministry. However, other departments also have a major stake in the governance of an effective health workforce (e.g. education authorities oversee nursing education standards and accreditation; immigration ministries monitor international recruitment and out-migration). The CNO or CNMO (Box 24.1) can articulate the concerns of the population from the nurses and midwives to policymakers and present policy decisions back to the workforce. They require negotiating and presentation skills and effective networks with their health ministry, national nursing associations, regulatory bodies and education institutes. The CNMO should have a direct line to their country's Minister for Health and/or the Health Secretary (who is not always a health practitioner). The nursing community should support the CNMO by ensuring they have accurate data about their national health workforce and population health issues. The CNMO also advises the government on strategic health policy, standards for primary care and midwifery, as well as promoting nursing and midwifery as careers of choice (White 2010, WHO 2015). Having a CNMO correlated significantly with a strong regulatory environment (WHO 2020b). Internationally, the CNMO attends specific CNMO meetings at the WHA. The WHO has had two Chief Nurses since 2017, providing a focus for many initiatives such as the State of the World's Nursing (SOWN) Report (WHO 2020b), increasing access to Basic

> **BOX 24.1**
> **Role of the Chief Nursing and Midwifery Officer**
>
> - Advise on nursing and midwifery's contribution to meeting population health goals and development of national health plans
> - Provide timely and accurate data-informed advice in relation to nursing and midwifery workforce, workforce capacity and skill-mix (including the maintenance of a minimum data set which is internationally comparable)
> - Oversee crisis response and emergency preparedness, planning and implementation
> - Professional regulation and policy in relation to nursing and midwifery and their interprofessional intersections
> - Service/care delivery quality, standards and patient safety
> - Inter-sectoral liaison, collaboration and networking
> - Educational program standards, accreditation and funding
>
> *Source: White 2010*

Emergency Care training for nurses and midwives from 25 countries by the end of 2025 (WHO 2024f), and the first global partners meeting to be held in Geneva in 2024.

The South Pacific Chief Nursing Midwifery Officers Alliance (SPCNMOA) links CNMOs in 22 Pacific Island nations, including New Zealand (Aotearoa) and Australia. New Zealand (Aotearoa) was the first nation to have a CNO, Elizabeth Grace Neil, who was instrumental in drafting her country's (and the world's) first Nurses Registration Act of 1901. In contrast, Australia finally appointed a CNMO in 2008 after many years of lobbying.

Research (Rumsey et al 2021, 2022b, 2022c) has concluded that contextualising leadership programs to country and health practitioner needs can result in positive career development changes. This was the case for 85% of 120 participants of the Pacific Leadership Program run at WHO CC UTS (Rumsey et al 2022b, WHO 2020a), with nine later appointed as CNMOs and two participants becoming Minister for Health in their respective countries (Rumsey et al 2022b, WHO 2020a).

> **REFLECTION**
>
> If you had the opportunity of a 30-minute meeting with your country's Chief Nursing and Midwifery Officer, what issues would you ask them to raise with your country's Health Minister or at the WHA?

Strategic partners

Strong relationships, common goals and partnership working between healthcare organisations can expedite effective changes to regulation, the development of agreed standards, service provision, decent work and improved education to ensure healthcare needs are met. Barriers between institutions or governments, conversely, will hinder change (Rumsey et al 2022a).

Partnerships can occur at multiple levels, from local through to international partnerships (Rumsey et al 2022c, SPCNMOA 2021, SPCNMOA et al 2020). Ensuring sustainable and scalable change is challenging, especially in countries with multiple dispersed organisations and limited resources and staff under pressure. Even in well-resourced environments, there is convincing evidence that many change initiatives fail, with an estimated failure rate of 60–70% consistently reported in the literature (Errida & Lotfi 2021, Jones-Schenk 2019).

A 'grounds-up' partnership methodology (Rumsey et al 2022c) describes the key principles of partnership working as: safety; respect; collaboration; beneficence and reciprocity; justice; and relationship-based. Using these as a basis ensures methods are collaborative, built on trust, commensurate with the local context and are sustainable, ethical and appropriate.

In addition to healthcare providers, strategic partners include civil society, non-governmental organisations, educational establishments, ministries and faith-based organisations. Partners should particularly consider how to involve the public and community in change. Other important partners are the professional associations, alliances, societies and unions that support the nursing and midwifery workforce; these play an important role in influencing CNMOs, Health Ministers and other power brokers in the health sector. Countries without strong nursing/midwifery associations lack a platform for relevant issues to be identified and considered at higher levels. Access to nursing industry information ensures Health Ministers involved in WHA decision making have a broad perspective on health workforce issues, not limited to medical practitioners' perspectives. International nursing and midwifery professional associations include the ICN and the International Confederation for Midwives (ICM), which provide regular forums for nursing and midwifery leaders to connect and engage with policy makers, advocacy for the professions and CPD opportunities for members. Not all countries have strong professional associations, minimising education opportunities and nursing and midwifery involvement in health policy making. Conversely, many nurses and midwives do not recognise the value of being involved in a professional association and the value it can add to their career development.

> ### REFLECTION
> Have you considered joining a professional nursing or midwifery association? What benefits might this bring? Do they offer student membership?

REGULATION

A modernised regulatory system is critical to strengthening the nursing and midwifery workforce. Health professional regulation creates a framework for safe and effective clinical practice; effective relationships between patients and health professionals; and patient confidence. Globalisation and increased migration of nurses and midwives call for internationally compatible standards of regulation. Yet, national regulation and accreditation of nursing and midwifery vary widely, with little international or even regional consensus (UNFPA et al 2021, WHO 2020b). There are four recognised elements of regulation: 1) registration; 2) standard setting; 3) accreditation and management of conduct; and 4) performance and fit-for-practice matters (Mahat et al 2023).

Nurses and midwives should be educated to a certain standard and the quality of their work maintained throughout their career through further qualifications and CPD. Standards in clinical practice can be maintained by Codes of Ethics and Conduct (ICN 2021).

The Global Strategy on Human Resources for Health: Workforce 2030 states that countries should have regulation and accreditation mechanisms for health workforce education by 2030 (WHO 2016). Most countries report having standards for nursing education, accreditation mechanisms for education institutions and a master list of accredited education institutions and 77% of countries report having standards for faculty qualifications (WHO 2020b). However, the existence of these regulatory processes or systems does not guarantee their quality or adequate function.

Regulation has been an ICN priority for many years. The ICN and WHO have published joint guidelines on regulation and resources (Mahat et al 2023). The ICM released Global Standards for Midwifery Regulation and developed a Midwifery Education Accreditation Programme and Global Standards for Midwifery Education (ICM 2011, 2024) in response to requests to improve quality from midwives, midwifery associations, governments, UN agencies and other stakeholders.

Given the huge diversity in population health needs and legislative processes the ICN favours a 'principle-based' approach to the development of international nursing regulatory guidelines.

> The role of health practitioner regulation in ensuring patient safety is well recognized. Less recognized is the role of regulation in addressing broader health system priorities. These goals include managing the costs, capacities and distribution of health professional education institutions; ensuring the competence and equitable distribution of health workers; informing workforce planning and mobilization; enabling the use of digital technologies; and addressing challenges related to the international mobility of health workers.
>
> (Mahat et al 2023:595)

Equally varied is the actual contribution of health practitioner regulation to UHC and health security (Mahat et al 2023). A review of regulation in the Western Pacific region found significant variation between countries in the systems and approaches used, the maturity of regulatory systems, regulation leadership (government or professional) and involvement of the wider community (SPCNMOA 2021). The review clearly articulates that weak regulation can negatively affect access to health services and healthcare efficiency, safety and quality. Ensuring equitable access to appropriately trained and skilled clinicians is therefore a priority in the Western Pacific.

The Australian Health Practitioner Regulation Agency (Aphra) is the national regulatory body for all health professionals. It was created in 2010 to streamline a system with over 90 authorities in health regulation in Australia. Ahpra works with national professional boards representing different groups of health practitioners (including the Nursing and Midwifery Board of Australia) to administer registration standards (Australian Health Practitioner Regulation Agency [Ahpra] 2024) and address the many multidisciplinary regulatory issues in Australia and internationally. New Zealand (Aotearoa) has a national regulatory body for nurses through the Nursing Council of New Zealand and is one of the few countries with a separate council for midwives—the New Zealand Midwifery Council.

> **REFLECTION**
>
> What are the benefits of international regulation and accreditation, if nurses and midwives are to be able to move smoothly between different countries?
> What are the practical difficulties in achieving international regulation for health professionals?

EDUCATION

The global drive for UHC demands a reliable, flexible, resilient and motivated workforce (WHO 2021a). Countries need well-trained nurses and midwives with flexibility to meet their communities' specific needs on a daily basis, and readiness to provide care in emergencies such as pandemics and increasing numbers of climate-related natural disasters (Pacific Islands Forum Secretariat 2022). Improving the performance of the health workforce is a vital component of HRH management (WHO 2020c), decision making and policy development, and will contribute to delivery of UHC.

Preparing nurses and midwives to practise in international settings poses a huge challenge as education standards vary greatly between countries (WHO 2020b). In some countries, nurses need only to complete high school to Grade/Year 12 to apply for a diploma, while in others, a university education is mandatory (SPCNMOA 2021, SPCNMOA & Rumsey 2020). The WHO strategic direction for education sets several priorities, including designing 'education programmes to be competency-based, apply effective learning design, meet quality standards, and align with population health needs' (WHO 2021a). WHO Education Standards (2009) also stipulate that nursing education should take place in an institution of higher learning such as a university. Although these global standards are over 15 years old, many educational institutes still fall short. Most countries set a minimum duration of 3 years for pre-practice nurse education (WHO 2020b). Variation in the curriculum can be compounded by faculty shortages, poorly trained educators, infrastructure shortages and restricted access to clinical training. This highlights the value of definitions, standards and accreditation to inform quality education, policy and practice.

More needs to be done to ensure an educational pipeline to create new graduates, then to support them plan a professional career (SPCNMOA 2021). Managers and leaders need to ensure opportunities for leadership and CPD so that health workers can continue to expand their skill set, post-registration (Buchan et al 2023, Rumsey et al 2022b, SPCNMOA 2021, SPCNMOA et al 2020). Research in the Western Pacific region (excluding Australia and New Zealand [Aotearoa]) found that many nurses report extremely limited CPD opportunities, with many never having received any professional development since registration (Rumsey et al 2021).

The SDNM calls for new approaches in health professionals' education and a move away from the traditional focus on tertiary care hospitals, to initiatives fostering community engagement. The strategy also requests:

> that faculty are properly trained in the best education methods and technologies, with demonstrated expertise in content areas.

(WHO 2021a:10)

The strategy promotes using accreditation findings, investments in information technology, incentives for high-performing faculties, and bridging programs to increase the number of expert clinicians eligible for graduate schemes (WHO 2021).

Educating nurses and midwives to a high level of professionalism with opportunities for research, management and leadership is important for population health outcomes, but also for improving career pathways, professional status and advancement. More highly educated nurses are needed to become educators, to oversee curriculum development, to advance practice, to conduct research and, ultimately, to become leaders in and advocates for the profession (WHO 2021a).

> ### REFLECTION
> How might the tertiary education you receive as a student nurse or midwife differ from a student in a Pacific Island country? How will these differences affect patient care in different countries?

CONCLUSION

The contribution of nurses and midwives has never been more crucial (WHO 2020b, 2021b, Catton & Iro 2021, UN 2023). Populations continue to grow and age. Patterns of disease fluctuate with multiple factors, including changes related to climate emergencies and economic and technological expansion. The COVID-19 pandemic clearly demonstrated the need to invest in nursing for global health and economic security with the quality of healthcare closely linked to the state of the nursing profession. Moreover, investment in nurses and midwives has a wider impact than simply improving health outcomes, with broader social benefits such as promoting inclusive and equitable growth, and positive macroeconomic impacts.

Health workforce shortages affect every corner of the globe. Urbanisation draws services and providers into cities, leaving those on the margins or in remote and isolated settings ever more vulnerable. International migration can aggravate this trend, restricting vulnerable communities' access to quality healthcare. Global shortages identified in SOWN and SOWMy (UNFPA et al 2021, WHO 2020b) have been exacerbated by the pandemic, leading to a health workforce crisis which is disproportionately impacting lower-income countries with already susceptible health systems.

As we know, nurses and midwives represent approximately 59% of the global workforce and 69% in the Western Pacific region (WHO 2020), yet leadership and career opportunities are still limited (Rumsey et al 2022a, 2022b, 2022c, UNFPA et al 2021, WHO 2020b). To benefit their patients and their professional status, nurses and nursing leaders must engage in health policy planning locally, nationally and globally. Nursing and midwifery leaders need to 'think globally and act locally'. Improved data literacy, analysis and management can strengthen health system performance, quality and sustainability by informing practice, management and policy decision making. Up-to-date data on health workforce flows is particularly vital.

Intersecting global pressures, including war, the COVID-19 pandemic and climate change, have stalled progress on many SDG indicators, including progress towards UHC. A renewed focus on

UHC and the SDGs demands a flexible and resilient, highly educated and motivated workforce. The SDNM provide a pathway to achieving such a workforce, but this will require significant investment. Achieving UHC will only be possible if the full potential of nurses and midwives is recognised, their full scope is utilised and measures are taken to ensure appropriate levels of recruitment and retention to address the global workforce shortages.

Dominating the frontline of health service delivery, nurses and midwives have a social responsibility. They need opportunities to report their experiences and articulate their requirements to policy makers, all the way up to the WHA. Appropriate channels of communication and empowered leaders are therefore required. National governments must instate a CNO or CNMO to ensure that the workforce experience and needs are appropriately considered in health policy deliberations. Well-briefed and informed ministers will enable senior health leaders to voice concerns and empower CNMOs to communicate with international policy makers. Leadership programs that are contextualised to country and regional needs and provide opportunities for succession planning, data literacy and policy development with a primary healthcare approach are urgently required (Rumsey et al 2022a, 2022b, WHO 2020b, 2021b).

Leadership and governance, regulation, strategic partnerships and education are the cornerstones of any health system (Fig. 24.4). To align the status of health professions with civil society's changing needs and to ensure best practice, the global nursing and midwifery community must shape itself around these key areas:

- Good **governance** ensures that health issues affecting populations are considered by ministerial policy makers. Equally, it ensures policies are relevant, communicated to and owned by the nursing and midwifery workforce. Empowered leaders such as CNOs and CNMOs are essential to promote policy dialogue across all health sectors to ensure sound governance.
- **Strategic partnerships** encourage stakeholder involvement, involve community and civil society, promote collaboration and ownership, and lead to sustainable change. Professional associations stimulate learning and offer information and advice to all health stakeholders. Associations also advocate for and support nursing and midwifery members with advice and CPD opportunities. Nurses and midwives should access and support these networks by joining associations/societies, seeking out CPD opportunities, contributing to debates and social media about regulatory and legislative issues, and supporting their leaders with information and advice.
- **Regulation** protects the public by developing, monitoring and maintaining standards to uphold health professional practice quality; it requires up-to-date legislation, reliable registration processes (including data), competencies and codes. It also supports equitable distribution of health workers and informs workforce planning and mobilisation. Accreditation of educational institutes and management of professional conduct are cornerstones of a well-regulated workforce.
- Quality **education** requires highly qualified educators, opportunities for CPD, research, regular institutional accreditation, and access to quality curriculums and resources. A sustainable source of well-trained nurses is critical to meet global demand. High-income countries should be self-sufficient in generating nurse graduates instead of relying on international migration.

Policy initiatives to strengthen the health workforce or contribute to the SDNM or WHO programs should integrate these four stand-alone yet interdependent areas.

Policy debates on health matters at country, regional and global levels must be informed by high-quality, accurate, timely and internationally comparable health data. The nursing and midwifery professions need a new wave of 'data literate' clinicians and leaders, trained in cutting-edge monitoring and evaluation methods. This will allow for better policy decisions promoting people-centred care with a primary healthcare focus, in partnership with civil society, nurses, midwives and other health professionals.

REFLECTIVE QUESTIONS

1. Why is it important that nurses/midwives and nursing/midwifery groups get involved in the development of global, regional and national policy?
2. How have WHO strategies for nursing and midwifery evolved post 2020?
3. Why is data collection so important to planning for human resources for health?
4. How do international policy decisions have an impact at our local clinical or practice level?
5. Why is a Chief Nursing and Midwifery Officer important in healthcare governance?
6. Why is nursing regulation important?

Recommended readings

Rumsey M, Iro E, Brown D et al 2022 Development practices in senior nursing and midwifery leadership: pathways to improvement in South Pacific health policy. Policy, Politics & Nursing Practice 23(3):195–206

Rumsey M, Leong M, Brown D et al 2022 Achieving universal health care in the Pacific: the need for nursing and midwifery leadership. The Lancet Regional Health – Western Pacific 19:1–10

Rumsey M, Stowers P, Sam H et al 2022 Development of PARcific approach: participatory action research methodology for collectivist health research. Qualitative Health Research 32(8-9):1297–1314

World Health Organization 2021 Global Strategic Directions for Nursing and Midwifery (SDNM) 2021–2025. World Health Organization, Geneva. Online. Available: https://www.who.int/publications/i/item/9789240033863

World Health Organization 2024 Regional health innovation strategy for the Western Pacific. WHO Regional Office for the Western Pacific, Manila. Online. Available: https://www.who.int/publications/i/item/9789290620341

World Health Organization 2023 WHO health workforce support and safeguards list 2023. World Health Organization, Geneva. Online. Available: https://www.who.int/publications/i/item/9789240069787

References

Australian Health Practitioner Regulation Agency (Ahpra) 2024 Information for international practitioners. Ahpra and the National Boards, Canberra

Buchan J, Catton H 2020 COVID-19 and the international supply of nurses. International Council of Nurses, Geneva

Buchan J, Catton H, Shaffer F A 2023 Sustain and retain in 2022 and beyond: the global nursing workforce and the COVID-19 pandemic. International Centre on Nurse Migration, Philadelphia

Casari S, Di Paola M, Banci E et al 2022 Changing dietary habits: the impact of urbanization and rising socio-economic status in families from Burkina Faso in sub-Saharan Africa. Nutrients 14(9):1782

Catton H, Iro E 2021 How to reposition the nursing profession for a post-covid age. BMJ 373

Chen L, Li J, Xia T et al 2021 Changes of exercise, screen time, fast food consumption, alcohol, and cigarette smoking during the COVID-19 pandemic among adults in the United States. Nutrients 13(10):3359

Errida A, Lotfi B 2021 The determinants of organizational change management success: literature review and case study. International Journal of Engineering Business Management 13 https://doi.org/10.1177/18479790211016273

Haakenstad A, Irvine CMS, Knight M et al 2022 Measuring the availability of human resources for health and its relationship to universal health coverage for 204 countries and territories from 1990 to 2019: a systematic analysis for the Global Burden of Disease Study 2019. The Lancet 399: 2129–2154

ICM 2011 Global Standards for Midwifery Regulation. International Confederation of Midwives, The Hague, The Netherlands

ICM 2024 Global Standards for Midwifery Education. International Confederation of Midwives, The Hague, The Netherlands

ICN 2020 ICN snapshot survey. International Council of Nurses, Geneva

ICN 2021 The ICN Code of Conduct for Nurses. International Council of Nurses, Geneva

Jones-Schenk J 2019 70% failure rate: an imperative for better change management. Journal of Continuing Education in Nursing 50(4):148–149

Karan A, Negandhi H, Kabeer M et al 2023 Achieving universal health coverage and sustainable development goals by 2030: investment estimates to increase production of health professionals in India. Human Resources for Health 21(1):1–14

Leyns C C, Stilma Memelink D, Bullinga L et al 2023 Integrated person- and people-centred primary care for diabetes in low- and middle-income countries: the nurses' perspective on patient needs. Journal of Advanced Nursing 79(10):4044–4057

Li Y, Zhang C, Zhan P et al 2023 Trends and projections of universal health coverage indicators in China, 1993-2030: an analysis of data from four nationwide household surveys. The Lancet Regional Health – Western Pacific 31:100646

Mahat A, Dhillon I S, Benton D C et al 2023 Health practitioner regulation and national health goals. Bulletin of the World Health Organization 101(9):595–604

McQuide P A, Brown A N, Diallo K et al 2023 The transition of human resources for health information systems from the MDGs into the SDGs and the post-pandemic era: reviewing the evidence from 2000 to 2022. Human Resources for Health 21:93

Pacific Islands Forum Secretariat 2022 The 2050 Strategy for the Blue Pacific Continent. Pacific Islands Forum Secretariat (PIFS), Suva

Roberts G 2017 Health Professions Education in the Pacific Region: standardisation and inclusion in the Regional Framework for Action. A discussion paper for the Heads of Health in the Pacific Region. Commissioned by WHO, not published

Rumsey M, Brown D, SPCNMOA 2021 Scoping study: improving the quality of nursing and midwifery education and regulation in Pacific Islands Countries and areas. WHO CC UTS, Sydney

Rumsey M, Iro E, Brown D et al 2022a Development practices in senior nursing and midwifery leadership: pathways to improvement in South Pacific health policy. Policy, Politics & Nursing Practice 23(3):195–206

Rumsey M, Leong M, Brown D et al 2022b Achieving universal health care in the Pacific: the need for nursing and midwifery leadership. The Lancet Regional Health – Western Pacific 19:100340

Rumsey M, Stowers P, Sam H et al 2022c Development of PARcific approach: participatory action research methodology for collectivist health research. Qualitative Health Research 32:1297–1314

South Pacific Chief Nursing and Midwifery Officers Alliance (SPCNMOA) 2021 Scoping roadmap: improving the quality of nursing and midwifery in education and regulation in Pacific Island countries. In: Pacific Heads of Nursing and Midwifery meeting, 25 November 2021. The Pacific Community (SPC), Suva

SPCNMOA, Rumsey M 2020 'Nursing leadership influencing global and regional policy: South Pacific Chief Nursing and Midwifery Officers Alliance (SPCNMOA) 2008-2018' Inaugural Pacific Heads of Nursing Meeting (PHoN), Nadi, Fiji 2020. WHO CC UTS, Sydney

SPCNMOA, Rumsey M, Brown D 2020 Accreditation and regulation standards and frameworks across the region. Online. Available: https://www.uts.edu.au/research/who-collaborating-centre/news/spcnmoa-meeting-november-2020

Stokes F, Iskander R 2021 Human rights and bioethical considerations of global nurse migration. Journal of Bioethical Inquiry 18(3):429–439

UNFPA, ICM, WHO 2021 State of the World's Midwifery Report – SOWMy. United Nations Population Fund, New York

United Nations (UN) 2019 Global indicator framework for the Sustainable Development Goals and targets of the 2030 Agenda for Sustainable Development. UN, New York

United Nations (UN) 2023 The Sustainable Development Goals Report 2023. Special edition. UN, New York

White J 2010 GCNMO consensus statement. Roles and responsibilities of the government chief nursing and midwifery officer (GCNMO). WHO CC UTS, Sydney

World Health Organization (WHO) 2009 Nursing and Midwifery Human Resources for Health: global standards for the initial education of professional nurses and midwives. WHO, Geneva

World Health Organization (WHO) 2015 Roles and responsibilities of chief nursing and midwifery officers: a capacity building manual. WHO, Geneva

WHO 2016 Global Strategy on Human Resources for Health: Workforce 2030. WHO, Geneva

WHO 2020a State of the World's Nursing Report – SOWN. Box 6.9. WHO, Geneva

WHO 2020b State of the World's Nursing Report – SOWN. WHO, Geneva

WHO 2020c Vital roles of nurses and midwives in the Western Pacific Region. WHO Regional Office for the Western Pacific, Manila

WHO 2021 Global Strategic Directions for Nursing and Midwifery (SDNM) 2021–2025. WHO, Geneva. Online. Available: https://www.who.int/publications/i/item/9789240033863

WHO 2022 Working for Health 2022–2030. Action Plan: education and employment. WHO, Geneva

WHO 2023a WHO fact sheet – Noncommunicable diseases. Online. Available: https://www.who.int/news-room/fact-sheets/detail/noncommunicable-diseases

WHO 2023b WHO health workforce support and safeguards list 2023. WHO, Geneva

WHO 2024a Fourteenth General Programme of Work, 2025-2028. WHO, Geneva

WHO 2024b Governance. Online. Available: https://apps.who.int/gb/gov/

WHO 2024c National Health Workforce Accounts (NHWA) Data Portal. WHO, Geneva

WHO 2024d Regional Health Innovation Strategy for the Western Pacific. Manila, WHO Regional Office for the Western Pacific. Online. Available: https://www.who.int/publications/i/item/9789290620341

WHO 2024e Dr Saia Ma'u Piukala, Regional Director for the Western Pacific, Opening Remarks at the Regional Nursing and Midwifery Forum in the Western Pacific. WHO Regional Office for the Western Pacific, Manila

WHO 2024f Initiative aiming to provide access to Basic Emergency Care training for nurses and midwives from 25 countries by the end of 2025. WHO Office of Chief Nurse, Geneva

Zhou Y, Wu Q, Li C et al 2024 Inequalities in non-communicable disease management in China and progress toward universal health coverage: an analysis of nationwide household survey data from 2004 to 2018. The Lancet Regional Health – Western Pacific Dec 26:44:100989

GLOSSARY

Aboriginal and Torres Strait Islander Health Services; Aboriginal Medical Services: Services that may be established and governed (controlled) by Aboriginal and Torres Strait Islander peoples in their communities or in partnership with Aboriginal and Torres Strait Islander peoples specifically to improve access to health services for Aboriginal and Torres Strait Islander peoples.

abuse of older people (AOP): *See* elder abuse.

artificial intelligence: The capability of machines or software to perform tasks that typically require human intelligence, such as learning from experience, recognising patterns, understanding language and making decisions.

acceptability: The test applied to a premise or reason. In order to have a sound argument, a premise must be acceptable to the person evaluating the argument.

accountability: Responsibility for one's own actions; this is a principle of professional practice that is obligatory for healthcare providers.

action: Anything done or performed; the process of doing something.

advocacy: Acting on behalf of, or in partnership with, a person and their family to ensure access to resources.

aesthetic: An abstract notion used in discussing the artistic aspect of nursing (and its creative expression). In this context, it relates broadly to theoretical and practical aspects of nursing art.

affective: Pertains to moods, feelings and attitudes.

agency: The ability of a person or community to act to exert or influence power.

altruism: Regard for others as a principle for action; unselfishness.

argument: A conclusion that is supported by a set of reasons intended to provide grounds for the acceptability of the conclusion.

art of nursing: Actions develop to create unique and deeply meaningful engagement with others that touch the commonality of the human experience.

autonomy: Personal or political independence, self-determination, self-sufficiency.

binary: Composed of two parts. *See also* dichotomy.

bioethics: An interdisciplinary field of inquiry characterised by a systematic and critical examination of the moral dimensions of healthcare and other associated fields (e.g. the life sciences) from the standpoint of various ethical perspectives.

biologism: A particular form of essentialism (see below) in which women's (or men's) essence is defined in terms of their biological capacities.

caring: Compassionate or showing concern for others. Can refer to behaviour used by those who belong to a profession such as nursing that involves looking after people's physical, medical and general welfare.

child abuse and neglect: Child abuse and neglect, also called child maltreatment, includes physical and emotional maltreatment, sexual abuse, neglect and negligent treatment and exploitation that harms or potentially harms a child's health, development and dignity. It also includes children's exposure to intimate partner violence (IPV).

clinical decision making: When making decisions, nurses draw from many sources, including their formal nursing education and/or from their experience gained over time in practice.

clinical decision support systems (CDSS): These systems use technology to assist healthcare providers in making clinical decisions. CDSS provides evidence-based recommendations, alerts and reminders to guide clinicians in diagnosing, treating and managing patient care. These tools help improve clinical outcomes by ensuring that decisions are based on the latest research and best practices.

clinical leadership: Leadership and management skills that nurses need to succeed in today's changing healthcare environment. A clinical nursing leader is one who is involved in direct patient care and who continuously improves the care that is afforded to such persons by influencing the treatment provision delivered by others.

clinical learning: Refers to the learning by which students have the opportunity to develop a wide range of skills through experience with patients and their problems. Its strengths are that it is highly relevant to future professional practice, integrates students into healthcare teams and provides role modelling by clinical teachers.

clinical management: Clinical management is the core of health services delivery—following best practice to deliver care and treatment to patients. As healthcare grows in complexity, as we move to models of care that are shared between clinicians, the challenges around access to information, decision processes and communication increase.

'close the gap': A campaign to reduce the gap in life expectancy, employment and educational opportunities between Aboriginal and Torres Strait Islander peoples and other Australians.

collaborative care: An environment where a range of healthcare professionals communicate and collaborate effectively with each other to improve health outcomes for patients; it can be multidisciplinary, interdisciplinary or transdisciplinary.

community assessment: A structured study of a specified community or targeted area that uses objective data to assess the current conditions and identify areas of strength and weakness.

community health: A major field of study within the nursing, medical and clinical sciences, which focuses on the maintenance, protection and improvement of the health status of population groups and communities as opposed to the health of individual patients.

community mental health: Community mental health is a decentralised pattern of mental health, mental healthcare, or other services for people with mental illnesses. Community-based care is designed to supplement and decrease the need for more costly inpatient mental healthcare delivered in hospitals.

community nursing: A field of nursing that is a blend of primary healthcare and nursing practice with public health nursing. The community health nurse conducts a continuing and comprehensive practice that is preventive, curative and rehabilitative. The philosophy of care is based on the belief that care directed to the individual, the family and the group contributes to the healthcare of the population as a whole.

compassion: A core professional value of caring is compassion and an ability to respond with humanity and kindness to others' pain, distress, anxiety or needs. It is also the possession of knowledge of assessed needs to identify ways in which to develop empathy, to give comfort and relieve suffering.

congruency: Agreement or consistency in two or more views or positions. For example, in examining two or more theoretical views, one may find that there are areas of agreement across the same ground; hence, there is evidence of congruency.

construct: 'A type of highly abstract and complex concept whose reality base can only be inferred. Constructs are formed from multiple less abstract or more empirical concepts' (Chinn & Jacobs 1983:200).

critical friend: A trusted colleague who provides feedback on your work.

critical incident analysis: The use of clinical or personal incidents as a reflective tool.

critical thinking: To stop and reflect on the reasons for doing things the way they are done or for experiencing things the way they are by focusing on what is frequently taken for granted and evaluating the values, beliefs and assumptions that are held, and asking whether what is done and thought is justifiable or not.

cultural competence: 'A set of behaviours, attitudes and policies that come together in a system, agency or among professionals to enable that system, agency or group of professionals to work effectively in cross cultural situations' (National Health and Medical Research Council 2005).

cultural safety: A philosophy of healthcare specific to working in a cross-cultural situation with Indigenous peoples. It is achieved by personal reflection and understanding of your own culture before you can meaningfully interact with Indigenous people (Ramsden 2002).

curriculum: A set of courses constituting an area of study or specialisation.

decision making: The process of making a choice between a number of options and committing to a future course of action.

deductive reasoning: The process of inferring particulars from general laws or principles.

dialectic: Defined in the Australian Concise Oxford Dictionary (1987) as the 'art of investigating the truth of opinions, testing of truth by discussion [or] logical disputation or criticism dealing with metaphysical contradictions and their solutions; existence or action of opposing forces'.

dialectical: A process or perspective involving a dialectic. For example, in theory development using a dialectical approach to generation of knowledge, the process could involve debate with presentation of an argument (thesis), which is considered critically and challenged by a counterargument (antithesis), which is considered critically in relation to the thesis and other knowledge, possibly leading to new areas of agreement and understanding (synthesis).

dichotomy: The term can be used to indicate a divide between two theoretical positions, which are polarised or incompatible.

digital health interventions: These are technology-based solutions designed to improve health outcomes. Examples include mobile health apps that track fitness or chronic conditions, wearable devices that monitor vital signs, and telehealth platforms that allow remote consultations with healthcare providers.

digital literacy: Ability to use digital technology to find, evaluate, apply and generate information.

discourse: An abstract notion used to label a collection of ideas or theoretical perspectives within an academic discipline. This may be composed of theses or arguments representing knowledge in the discipline, including areas of agreement and disagreement, fundamental assumptions, values and beliefs, expressed in disciplinary language and symbols. The notion reflects the idea of a conversation using language within these boundaries.

dissemination: The act of distributing or spreading something, especially information, for it to become widespread.

diversity: A variety of something, such as opinion, colour or style; can refer to ethnic variety, as well as socioeconomic and gender variety, in a group, society or organisation.

early intervention: The initiation of supportive therapeutic strategies as soon as a problem or challenge is identified. It is often associated with disability and involves longer-term engagement.

e-health: e-health is a broader term referring to the use of digital technology to access, store and exchange health-related information. This includes electronic health records (EHRs), online health portals and telemedicine. e-health systems allow for more efficient and accurate management of patient data, improving communication between patients and healthcare providers.

elder abuse: Abuse of older people involves a single or repeated act or an absence of care by a person(s) where a relationship of trust results in harm or distress to an older person (also known as Abuse of Older People [AOP]).

emotional competence: Emotional competence in nursing is to become self-aware, develop regard for yourself and work on ways to manage your emotional reactions. This includes moving beyond your own needs and working with another person's issues or needs, including recognising and managing conflict.

empathy: The ability to connect with the life of another person and to accurately perceive their current feelings and their meaning. Empathy begins with putting your own concerns and needs aside and being open to the other person's perspective and experience.

empiricist/logical positivist model: An approach grounded in the belief that the world can be viewed as a machine and that the task of science is to discover the laws by which the machine operates; emphasis on predictability, measurement and the quantification of observable data.

engagement: The ability of nurses to connect with patients as unique people. The process of engagement is built over time and includes recognising people as social beings with a need to connect and share experiences with others in order to give meaning to their situation and create a working partnership.

entrapment: Entrapment occurs at partner, social and systemic levels. It severely restricts a victim survivor's capacity to resist a partner's violence or to escape the situation, making it difficult to leave or keep themselves and their children safe.

epistemology: The theory of knowledge; the origins, nature, methods and limits of human knowledge.

essentialism: The attribution of a fixed essence to women; that there are given, universal characteristics of women, including biological, psychological and social characteristics, which are not readily amenable to change.

ethical principlism: The view that moral decisions are best guided by appealing to sound universal moral principles, such as the principles of autonomy, beneficence, non-maleficence and justice; ethical principlism is one of the most popular approaches used to examine ethical issues in healthcare.

ethical professional conduct: 'Conduct that accords with and upholds the accepted ethical principles and standards of a given profession and which is thereby deemed to be "right" and "correct"' (Johnstone 2016:4).

ethical universalism: The view that there exists one set of universal values/standards that is applicable to all people throughout space and time, regardless of their histories and/or cultural backgrounds (contexts).

ethics: A branch of philosophic inquiry concerned with understanding and examining the moral life. It seeks rational clarification and justification of basic assumptions and beliefs that people hold about what constitutes right or wrong/good or bad conduct. Can also be defined as a system of action guiding rules and principles that function by specifying that certain types of conduct are required, prohibited or permitted. The term 'ethics/ethical' may be used interchangeably with the term 'morality/moral'.

etiquette: A set of behavioural action guides concerned with the maintenance of style and decorum in social settings; often, although mistakenly, confused with ethics/morality.

evaluation: A critical appraisal or assessment; a judgment of the value, worth, character or effectiveness of something; measurement of progress. The purpose of the evaluation is to determine whether outcome criteria have been met and how care for the patient might be improved.

evidence: Something that gives a sign or proof of the existence or truth of something, or that helps us to come to a particular conclusion.

evidence-based practice: The conscientious, explicit and judicious use of current best evidence in making decisions about the care of the individual patient; integrating individual clinical expertise with the best available external clinical evidence. EBP is the integration of clinical expertise, patient values and the best research evidence into the decision-making process for patient care.

family violence: The physical, sexual, psychological and/or financial abuse or violence inflicted by one person against another person who is a family member. It is a cumulative pattern of harm over time that includes coercive control (such as manipulation, isolation, threats, imposing restrictions, surveillance and coercion), restricting a person's autonomy, agency and freedom.

feminisms: This term captures the variety of theoretical approaches to the support of equal rights for women, in all spheres of life, along with a commitment to improve the position of women in society; includes liberal feminism, socialist feminism, radical feminism, postmodern feminism and so on.

gender: A social construction that expresses the many areas of social life, as distinguished from biological sex; the socially learned behaviours and expectations that are associated with the two sexes.

generic: A characteristic that is 'general, not specific or special' (Australian Concise Oxford Dictionary 1987).

grounded theory: A research process designed to lead to generation of theory through study of a particular human situation or context.

grounds: The degree to which a set of reasons supports a conclusion.

habits of mind: The dispositions or inclinations of a thinker that influence the way in which a person uses or applies the cognitive skills of critical thinking.

health insecurity: The opposite of health security; the awareness of being (in)secure that health is good and if not there are ways to obtain care to return to good health. Whereas health security aims to guarantee a minimum protection from diseases and unhealthy lifestyles, there are no such guarantees in the case of health insecurity.

health literacy: The capacity to obtain, process and understand health information and services. A certain minimal health literacy capability is necessary to make appropriate health decisions and to take action on those decisions.

health policies: 'The strategies and courses of action adopted as being advantageous and expedient to provide within the resources available from a health system that at least maintains, and preferably improves, health' (Hennessy & Spurgeon 2000:6).

health promotion: 'Health promotion is a broad field of activity ranging from actions that are essentially medically focused and individual (such as individual risk-factor assessment and counselling) to actions aimed at helping people to change their behaviour, and further along to actions that seek to create supportive environments and settings that address a broad range of social and environmental determinants of health' (Marshall 2004:185).

hermeneutics: A process of interpretive analysis, which is concerned with uncovering meaning and a technique for interrogating text. Van Manen states that 'hermeneutics is the theory and practice of interpretation. The word derives from the Greek god Hermes whose task it was to communicate messages from Zeus and other gods to the ordinary mortals' (van Manen 1990:179). Hermeneutics was originally a technique used to interpret religious texts, which has made a transition into research activity in the social sciences and humanities. Hermeneutical refers to a process or perspective involving hermeneutics.

historical trauma: A collective trauma associated with a significant historical event(s), such as colonisation, that impacts individuals, groups and communities. It can result in lifetime trauma, chronic stress, physiological and epigenetic changes, and is associated with family violence and racism.

holism: A perspective in which people are seen as made up of biological, psychological, social and spiritual components, which are indivisible.

humanism: Suggested in nursing as a perspective on life that is centred on concern for human interests, meanings or values and safeguarding the person's dignity. Humanistic nursing is an experience lived between human beings, so nurses need to move beyond the technical *doing* of nursing, to become able to experience the feeling and *being* of nursing.

humanitarian concerns: Concerned with or seeking to promote human welfare; denoting an event or situation that causes or involves widespread human suffering, especially one which requires the large-scale provision of aid (English Oxford Living Dictionaries 2017).

hypotheses: Tentative statements of relationships between two or more variables, which have little empirical support. The repeated confirmation of hypotheses changes their status to empirical generalisations (statements with moderate empirical support) and thence to law (statements with overwhelming empirical support).

iconography: 'Illustration of subject by drawings or figures; book whose essence is pictures; treatise on pictures or statuary; study of portraits especially of an individual' (Australian Concise Oxford Dictionary 1987).

induction: The process of discovering a general principle from a set of facts.

inductive reasoning: The process of inference of a general law or principle from the observation of particular occurrences.

influence: The practice of expressing ideas and gaining support for those ideas and subsequent actions.

interprofessional education (IPE): The World Health Organization (WHO) defines interprofessional education as 'occasions when two or more professions learn with, from, and about each other to improve collaboration and the quality of care'. It emphasises the importance of collaboration, teamwork and effective communication among different health and social care professionals to improve outcomes.

intimate partner violence (IPV): Predominantly a gendered form of violence against women, sometimes referred to as domestic violence or partner violence.

journalling: The technique of recording thoughts and feelings after reflecting on an event.

magnet hospitals: Hospitals that have particular quantifiable features, each of which is based on recognition of the contribution of nurses to patient care and the overall environment. These features include: 'effective and supportive leadership; nursing staff decision making; commitment to professional clinical nurse qualities; participatory management; autonomy and accountability, and a supportive environment' (Buchan 1999).

managed care: A health management system that controls the resources and delivery of services to people who are enrolled in a specific type of healthcare plan.

masculinist: Pertaining to the masculine; the male gender characteristics derived from social construction and expectation.

megatrends: Literally a major or 'big' (mega) trend or movement that has a lasting impact on society, cultures and people's lives; may also be defined as 'an important shift in the progress of a society or of any other particular field or activity; any major movement' (English Oxford Living Dictionaries 2017).

mental healthcare: State and territory governments fund and deliver public sector mental health services that provide specialist care for people with severe mental illness. These include specialised mental healthcare delivered in public acute and psychiatric hospital settings, state and territory specialised community mental healthcare services, and state and territory specialised residential mental healthcare services. In addition, states and territories provide other mental health-specific services in community settings such as supported accommodation and social housing programs.

mental illness: Refers to a wide range of mental health conditions/disorders that affect mood, thinking and behaviour. Examples of mental illness include depression, anxiety disorders, schizophrenia, eating disorders and addictive behaviours.

meta: A prefix commonly encountered in theoretical literature. In this context it means 'beyond or higher order' (Australian Concise Oxford Dictionary 1987). A meta-paradigm of any discipline is a statement or group of statements identifying the relevant phenomena to the discipline (Fawcett 1984).

mHealth (mobile health): mHealth is a subset of e-health that specifically refers to health-related services and information provided through mobile devices, such as smartphones, tablets and wearable devices. Examples include apps that monitor chronic conditions (e.g. diabetes), fitness trackers and medication reminders.

model: A schematic representation of some aspect of reality, which may be empirical or theoretical. Empirical models are replicas of observed realities (e.g. a plastic model of the ear). Theoretical models represent the world in language or mathematical symbols (e.g. nursing's 'grand theories').

moral/morality: *See also* ethics.

moral duty: An act that a person is bound to carry out for moral reasons.

moral obligation: As above, an act that a person is obligated to perform for moral reasons; is generally regarded as being weaker than a moral duty and may be overridden by stronger moral duties.

moral principles: General standards of conduct that make up an ethical system of action guides and which carry particular imperatives (e.g. 'Do no harm').

moral right: A special interest that a person has and which ought to be protected for moral reasons (e.g. the right to life) (contrast with legal right, e.g. a special interest that a person has and which ought to be protected for legal reasons); moral rights generally entail correlative rights.

moral rules: Derived from principles and prescribed particular standards of conduct (e.g. 'Always tell the truth'). Rules have less scope than principles; they also do not have the same force and can be overridden by principles.

naturalism: A form of essentialism in which a fixed nature is assumed for women, not readily amenable to change.

nurse practitioner: A registered nurse who through advanced training is qualified to assume some of the duties and responsibilities formerly assumed only by a physician—abbreviation NP; also called a nurse clinician.

nursing ethics: The consideration of various ethical and bioethical issues from the standpoint of nursing theory and practice.

nursing roles: The role of the nurse refers to the main role (i.e. the core nursing role with the greatest number of hours) in the nurse's main job. Core nursing roles are divided into two main groups, clinical and non-clinical, with several categories in each group, such as registered or enrolled nurse, supervision and management. The non-clinical role may include education, research or industrial relations.

Occam's razor: The principle that the simplest explanation is most likely to be the right one.

organisational culture: The values and behaviours that contribute to the unique social and psychological environment of an organisation. Organisational culture includes an organisation's expectations, experiences, philosophy and values that hold it together, and is expressed in its self-image, inner workings, interactions with the outside world and future expectations. It is based on shared attitudes, beliefs, customs and written and unwritten rules that have been developed over time and are considered valid.

paradigm: A paradigm is a term used to describe accepted practices and techniques through which a discipline accumulates and refines its knowledge base.

patriarchy: The social system in which the masculine dominates, oppresses and exploits the feminine, within the spheres of reproduction, sexuality, work, culture and the state.

person-centred: A person-centred approach involves focusing on the elements of care, support and treatment that matter most to the patient, their family and carers. The priority is to identify what is most important to the person, without making assumptions. Person-centred nursing values the emotional and spiritual wellbeing of the person and reflects a person's values, relationships and need for self-expression. It is different to patient-centred care.

personal stress: The feeling of being overwhelmed or anxious when life's challenges start to feel like too much to handle. It can come from things like relationships, personal responsibilities or just the pressure of daily life.

phenomenology: A philosophy and descriptive research method designed to uncover the essence and meaning of lived experiences—for example, suffering or grieving (Parse 2001). In a phenomenological research study, the focus is on the meaning of the phenomenon under investigation for the research participants who participate in the study.

philanthropic: 'Loving one's fellow men, benevolent, humane' (Australian Concise Oxford Dictionary 1987).

philosophy (alternative view): 'A way of reflecting not so much on what is true and false but on our relationship to the truth' (Foucault, cited in Lotringer 1989).

philosophy/philosophic inquiry (conventional view): An argumentative intellectual discipline concerned with the discovery of 'truth' and meaning. Unlike science, which seeks answers to questions that can only be answered by empirical evidence, philosophy seeks answers to questions that cannot be answered by empirical evidence.

politics: The exercise and influence of power at both the micro and macro level.

population health: Population health has been defined as the health outcomes of a group of individuals, including the distribution of such outcomes within the group. It is an approach to health that aims to improve the health of an entire human population.

postmodernism: Relates to the critique of modern, capitalist, industrialised society; new political and social strategies, which embrace pluralism and diversity of cultures and values.

poststructuralism: Refers to a range of theoretical positions in which the mode of knowledge production uses particular theories of language, subjectivity, social processes and institutions to understand existing power relations and to identify areas and strategies for change.

power: The capability and expertise to perform a task in an appropriate way. Professional power comes from the law, regulation, professional code of conduct, common practice and consent.

praxis: Praxis can be seen as the link between reflection and action. Friere (1972) defines praxis as 'reflection and action upon the world in order to transform it' (Cox et al 1991:385).

premise: A reason offered in support of a conclusion.

pre-reflection: Preparatory reflection that occurs before the experience.

preventive ethics: The study and practice of ethics (including ethics education) aimed at preventing (as opposed to remedying) moral problems.

primary healthcare: Primary healthcare encompasses a large range of providers and services across the public, private and non-government sectors. At a clinical level, it usually involves the first (primary) layer of services encountered in healthcare and requires teams of health professionals working together to provide comprehensive, continuous and person-centred care. Primary healthcare providers include general practitioners, nurses, allied health professionals, midwives, pharmacists, dentists and Aboriginal health workers. Primary healthcare is the frontline of Australia's healthcare system. It can be provided in the home or in community-based settings (Australian Government Department of Health 2013).

professional development: Refers to skills and knowledge attained for both personal development and career advancement.

public health: 'The science and art of promoting health, preventing disease, and prolonging life through the organised efforts of society' (WHO 1998:3).

qualitative research: Research that focuses on human experiences, including accounts of subjective realities, and conducted in naturalistic settings, involving close, often sustained contact between the researcher and research participants (Denzin & Lincoln 2005, Sarantakos 2005).

quantitative research: Refers to research that seeks to measure some concept or phenomenon of interest (e.g. blood pressure, pain or student attitudes to learning about research). It is also called positivist, reductionist or empirical. Quantitative research is termed deductive, which means the thinking leads from a known principle to an unknown, and is used to test a particular research hypothesis.

racism: A 'form of oppression/privilege which exists in a dialectical relationship with antiracism ... societal system in which people are divided into races with power unevenly distributed, or produced based on their racial classification' (Paradies 2006:68).

rationalism: A philosophical position that argues that the only way to truth is through the deliberations of the rational human mind.

realism: An applied appreciation and acceptance of the authentic nature of the world, rather than an idealised view of it.

reflection (also reflection-on-action): Reflection that occurs after the experience.

reflective practice: The incorporation of reflection into practice.

regulatory authorities: Body responsible for regulating and maintaining the register of nurses.

relevance: A test applied to a premise or reason. If a premise or reason is relevant, it helps to support the conclusion of the argument.

science of nursing: Associated with technical capability and is underpinned by theories, concepts, models and frameworks. Scientific aspects of nursing help explain how to go about nursing relationships, the importance of the human health experience and contribute to nursing inquiry and evidence-based care.

self-awareness: Involves deliberately considering one's own values, beliefs and identity. This includes the ability to consider the values and beliefs of others.

shared governance: A concept based on the principles of partnership, equity, accountability and ownership (Porter-O'Grady 1991). It requires health professionals to be self-directive, effective decision makers, strongly involved in the activities of the organisation at every level of participation, and providing clinical leadership (Porter-O'Grady 1991).

social capital: 'Social capital represents the degree of social cohesion which exists in communities. It refers to the processes between people which establish networks, norms, and social trust, and facilitate co-ordination and co-operation for mutual benefit' (WHO 1998:19).

social class: A broad concept encapsulating objective material, position and subjective understandings, and incorporating differing access to power (Walter & Saggers 2007:88).

social determinants of health: The conditions in which people are born, grow, work, live and age, and the wider set of forces and systems shaping the conditions of daily life. These forces and systems include economic policies and systems, development agendas, social norms, social policies and political systems.

social justice: 'Justice in terms of the distribution of wealth, opportunities, and privileges within a society' (English Oxford Living Dictionaries 2017).

social support: 'That assistance available to individuals and groups from within communities which can provide a buffer against adverse life events and living conditions, and can provide a positive resource for enhancing the quality of life' (WHO 1998:20).

sound: An argument is sound when the premises are acceptable and provide adequate grounds for accepting the conclusion.

stereotype: A predetermined idea that ascribes particular characteristics to all members of a social group.

telehealth: Telehealth involves the use of telecommunications technology to provide remote clinical services. Through video consultations, remote monitoring and online diagnosis, telehealth enables patients to receive care without needing to visit a healthcare facility physically. This can be particularly useful for individuals in rural or underserved areas.

theory: A logically consistent set of propositions, which presents a systematic view of some aspect of reality.

theory–practice gap: Refers to the presence of lack in integration of theory into clinical practice which affects the patient care and satisfaction.

transformational leadership: A charismatic, motivating way of leading other individuals that generally comprises heightening followers' drive, satisfaction and confidence, bringing them together in the pursuit of mutual, challenging objectives, and altering their morals, beliefs and needs.

transition: A change from one form or type to another, or the process by which this happens.

unethical professional conduct: 'An umbrella term that incorporates the following three related although distinct notions: unethical conduct, moral incompetence and moral impairment' (Johnstone 2016:5).

universalism: Refers to the attributions of functions, social categories and activities to which women of all cultures are assigned; asserts what is shared in common by all women.

validity: An argument is valid when the premises that are offered provide adequate grounds for acceptance of the conclusion.

whistleblowing: Disclosure of information and/or actions that are unethical or illegal, by an employee.

whole-of-world scenarios: Situations or a sequence of events that have or stand to have a global impact; that is, have an impact on the whole world, not merely local communities (e.g. climate change).

workplace culture: This refers to the shared values, beliefs, behaviours and practices that define how employees engage with each other and across the organisation. It describes the 'personality' of a company and how it impacts employee experience.

References

Australian Concise Oxford Dictionary of Current English 1987 Oxford University Press, Melbourne
Australian Institute of Health and Welfare 2025 Primary health care. Online. Available: https://www.aihw.gov.au/reports-data/health-welfare-services/primary-health-care/overview
Buchan J 1999 Still attractive after all these years? Magnet hospitals in a changing health care environment. Journal of Advanced Nursing 30(1):100–108
Chinn P, Jacobs M K 1983 Theory and nursing: a systematic approach. Mosby, St Louis
Cox H, Hickson P, Taylor B 1991 Exploring reflection: knowing and constructing practice. In: Gray G, Pratt R (eds) Towards a discipline of nursing. Churchill Livingstone, Melbourne, pp 373–389
Denzin N K, Lincoln Y S 2005 (eds) Handbook of qualitative research, 3rd edn. Sage, Thousand Oaks
English Oxford Living Dictionaries 2017 Online. Available: https://en.oxforddictionaries.com/definition/ 07 March 2017
Fawcett J 1984 The meta-paradigm of nursing: present status and future refinements. Image: Journal of Nursing Scholarship 16(3):84–86

Friere P 1972 The pedagogy of oppression. Penguin, Harmondsworth
Hennessy D, Spurgeon P 2000 Health policy and nursing. Macmillan Press, London
Johnstone M 2016 Bioethics: a nursing perspective, 6th edn. Elsevier, Sydney
Lotringer S 1989 Foucault live (interviews, 1966–84). Semiotext(e), New York
Marshall B 2004 Health promotion in action: case studies from Australia. In: Keleher H, Murphy B (eds) Understanding health: a determinants approach. Oxford University Press, Melbourne
National Health and Medical Research Council (NHMRC) 2005 Cultural competency in health: a guide for policy, partnership and participation. NHMRC, Canberra
Paradies Y 2006 A systematic review of empirical research on self reported racism. International Journal of Epidemiology 35(4):888–901
Parse R R 2001 Qualitative inquiry: the path of sciencing. Jones and Bartlett, Boston
Porter-O'Grady T 1991 Shared governance for nursing. Association of Operating Room Nurses Journal 53(3): 691–703
Ramsden I 2002 Cultural safety and nursing education in Aotearoa and Te Waipounamu. Thesis, Victoria University, Wellington
Sarantakos S 2005 Social research, 3rd edn. Palgrave Macmillan, London
van Manen M 1990 Researching lived experience. State University of New York Press, New York
Walter M, Saggers S 2007 Poverty and social class. In: Carson B, Dunbar T, Chenhall R, Baillie R (eds) Social determinants of Indigenous health. Allen & Unwin, Sydney
World Health Organization (WHO) 1998. Online. Available: https://www.who.int/publications/i/item/WHO-HPR-HEP-98.1

INDEX

A

Aboriginal nurses, 26–27
Aboriginal people, in Australia, 62–63
abuse of older people (AOP), 231t
acceptable, sound argument and, 122
access, to healthcare, 326
accountability, for self-assessment, 295–296
accreditation standards, 92
action, 131
   developing influence through, 142t
   reflection and, 157, 158
active listening, 95
activity trackers, 205t
adaptability, in simulation, 275
adequate infrastructure, lack of, 206
adverse events, reporting of, 112
advice, negligent, 46
advocacy, 93t, 144–147, 147b
ageing, in rural and remote communities, 247
agency, 92, 143
AHPRA. *see* Australian Health Practitioner Regulation Agency
AIM. *see* Australian Inland Mission
air pollution, health impacts of, 350f
allocation, patient, 328t
American Nurses' Credentialing Center (ANCC), 332
ANCC. *see* American Nurses' Credentialing Center
Anglo-Boer War, second, 19–20
anthropocene, climate change and, 341
antimicrobial resistance, ethics in nursing, 39
AOP. *see* abuse of older people
application, in ethical thinking, 129
appraisal, 292
apprenticeship, 22
argument
   in clinical practice, 125f
   components of, 122f
   criteria of, 122
   critical thinking and, 121–124
   definition of, 121
   ethical, 129, 130f
   phases of clinical reasoning as, 126–127
   research as, 128f
   sound, 122–124, 124b
   structure of, 126f, 127f, 128f
   unsound, 124

artificial intelligence (AI)
   ethics in nursing, 39
   nursing and, 199
asceticism, 2
assault, 48
assessment, 143–144
assimilation, in Australian immigration policy development, 67t
associations, global health and, 368b
Asthma app, 205t
AsthmaCare, 205t
ASTHMAXcel, 205t
asylum seekers, 68
ATNA. *see* Australasian Trained Nurses' Association
augmented reality (AR), 270, 270f
Australasian Trained Nurses' Association (ATNA), 18
Australia
   correctional nurses in, 263
   cultural diversity in, 67t
   first people in, 64
   healthcare in early, 12–13
   immigration policy development of, 67t
   multicultural, 65–68
   nursing, milestones in, 19–23
Australian Commission on Safety and Quality in Health Care (ACSQHC), 89
Australian Government's Humanitarian Program, 68
Australian Health Practitioner Regulation Agency (AHPRA), 36, 54, 180, 369
Australian Inland Mission (AIM), 26
Australian National Disability Advocacy Program, 145
Australia's colonial administrations, 12
automated dispensing cabinets (ADCs), 202t
autonomy, 92
   in digital health, 207–208
availability, in simulation, 275
awareness, cultural, 69

B

'back-blocks' nursing, 21
Bangka Island massacre, 20
barcode medication administration (BCMA), 202t
beneficence, 130
   in digital health, 208
   ethical principles of, 190–191
Beyond Blue, 205t

biases, 91
biological hazards, occupational health nurses and, 262
biomedical model, 88
biopsychosocial model, 90
blood glucose level (BGL), remote monitoring of, 205t
Blue Knot Foundation, 205t
boundaries, setting, 82
brain drain, 363–364
Breath app, 205t
Bridging theory, 268–269
British Empire, 12
burnout, in nursing, 352
'but for' test, 47

C

CAN. *see* child abuse and neglect
care, 75–76
    challenges and impact on patient, 80–81, 81b
    in community, 13–14
    cultivating a culture of, 79–80
    duty of, 46
    low-value, 105
    quality, quest for, 103–116, 114b
    standard of, 46–47
    technologies of, 17
Care Capacity Demand Programme (CCDM), 141
care delivery, changing models of, 328–329, 328t
care management, 328t
career
    in nursing, 1–8
    progression of, 335
CareKit, 205t
CareMonitor, 205t
caring
    competence in nursing, 83
    developing compassion in, 77
    emotional competence, 75–86
    in simulation, 275
'caring neutrality', 83
case management, 328t
case study, 311t
causation, 47
Centaur, 20–21
chemotherapy, 132f
Chief Nursing Officer (CNO), global health and, 366–367, 367b
child abuse and neglect (CAN), 231t
children, consent and, 50
Chinn, Teresa, 187
Chuzzlewit, Martin, 14
civil law, 46
Civil Liability Act 2002 (New South Wales), 47
classroom learning, 299
    clinical and theoretical knowledge in, 299–300
clients, 88
climate change
    environment and health services, 349–352, 352b

climate change *(Continued)*
    ethics in nursing, 39
    extreme weather events and, 343–345
    health and, 341–343, 342f, 343b
Climate Change Science 101, 343–345
climate crisis, 345–348, 347f
    health and, 348, 349f, 350f
climate impacts, 358
climate resilience development, 348
clinical and theoretical knowledge, 289–290
    in classroom learning, 299–300
    in clinical settings, 295–297, 296b, 297b, 297t
    reflection, 300b
clinical decision support systems (CDSS), 202t
clinical environment, 298
    simulated, 282
clinical experience, 297
clinical judgment, 290
clinical leader, 330–332
    attributes of, 330f, 331–332, 331f
    framework for being, 331f
    promoting, professional societies and organisations to, 333–334
clinical learning, theoretical learning and, connection to, 290–292, 292t
clinical nursing leaders, opportunities for, 326–327, 327b
clinical pathways, 328t
clinical placement, preparing for and making meaning of, 289–304
clinical practice, 298
    argument framework to, 125f
    critical thinking and, 124–125, 125f
    expert, significance of, 335
    reflection and, 158
clinical quality, digital health interventions for, 201–202, 202t
clinical reasoning
    as argument, phases of, 126–127
    definition of, 126–127
    development of, 273
    in simulation, 275
clinical settings
    clinical and theoretical knowledge in, 295–297, 296b, 297b, 297t
    students in, 295–296
clinical supervision, 162–163
CNO. *see* Chief Nursing Officer
Code of Conduct for Nurses, 146–147
Code of Ethics for Nurses, 36
Code of Ethics for Nurses in Australia, 144
coercive control, 233–235, 235b
cognitive behavioural therapy (CBT), 205t
collaboration
    authentic, 175
    in interprofessional learning, 169, 173
    reflection, 175b
collective political power, 140–143, 142t, 143b

College of Nursing, 18
colonisation, 63, 217–218
commitment, in interprofessional learning, 173
common law, 46
communication
    cultural safety and, 110
    digital, 179–180
    effective
        in integrated care, 174–175
        in nurses, 77
    enhanced, in interprofessional learning, 169
    skills, developing influence through, 142t
    therapeutic, 91
        skills, 95
community
    care in, 13–14
    empowered, 258
    nursing roles in, 259–264, 264b
    rural and remote
        ageing, 247
        health of, 246–247, 246b
        morbidity and mortality, 247
        population sparsity in, 245–246
        populations in, 244–245, 245b
        providing health services for, 247–249, 249b
        telehealth services for, 248, 252–253b
        tyranny of distance in, 245–246
community health, 258
compassion, 76–77b, 76–79, 77b, 78–79b
    barriers to, 80–81, 81b
    developing, 77
    emotional competence, 77–79
    enablers, 79–80
    fatigue
        preventing, 82, 82b
        understanding, 81–82
competence
    confidence and, 298
    in simulation, 275
complaints and notifications, 55–56
    health, 56
    performance, 55
    professional conduct, 55–56
complex environment, reflective practice and, 153–154
comprehensive account of the event, in root cause analysis, 112–113
conclusion, 121
conduct
    notification of, 55–56
    unethical, 35–41, 37b
        professional, 35–41, 37b
confidence
    competence and, 298
    in simulation, 275
confidentiality, in digital health, 208
consent
    capacity of, 50–51

consent *(Continued)*
    children and, 51
    informed, 49
    obtaining, 50
    patient, 48–50
    people with mental health issues, 51
consequential arguments, 92
constructivism, cultural, 63
consumers, 89
    interest of, critical thinking and, 125
contemplation, reflection and, 155–156
contemporary application, in nursing, 184–189
contemporary health systems, 335
contemporary healthcare settings, 324
contemporary nursing, 306
continuing professional development (CPD), 54, 187
continuous quality improvement (CQI), patient safety and, 111–112, 112t
continuum of engagement, 93t
contributory negligence, 48
convergent parallel research design, 312t
Corner, Sadie, 11, 11f
correctional nurses, 263–264, 264b
correlation study, 310t
CPD. *see* continuing professional development
creative expression, 162
criminal assault, 52
criminal law, 46
criminal negligence, 53–54
critical appraisal, in research, 314
critical friend, 160
critical incident analysis, 159, 161, 162b
critical qualitative research, 311
critical review, 313t
critical social theory, 158–159
critical thinker, becoming, 117–134, 118b, 133b
critical thinking, 118–119, 120b, 121b, 132, 133b
    argument and, 121–124, 122f
    characteristics of, 119–121, 121b
    clinical practice and, 124–125, 125f
    clinical reasoning and, 126–127
    development of, 131–132, 132b
    ethics of, 129–131, 131b
    habits of mind and, 119–120
    holistic definition of, 120–121, 120b, 121f
    in nursing, 124–129
    reflective practice and, 154–155
    research and, 127–129
    scepticism and, 119
    in simulation, 275
cultural awareness, 69
cultural constructivism, 63
cultural diversity, benefits of, in Australian immigration policy development, 67t
cultural safety, 63–64, 70f, 71, 110
    in nursing and midwifery, 61–74
    nursing care, 69–71, 70b

cultural sensitivity, 69–70
culturally responsive practice, 220t
culturally safe practice, 236–238, 238b
culture, 62
   concept of, 62–64
   dynamic, 62–63, 63b
   social determinants of health and, correlation between, 68–69
curiosity, critical thinking and, 120
curriculum, nursing, 292

D
damage, 47
data revolution, 361–363
death, due to negligence, 47
debriefing, 295–296
Debriefing Assessment for Simulation in Healthcare (DASH), 281
decision making
   clinical, 292
   ethical, 34, 131
defence
   allegation of negligence, 48–51
   allegation of trespass, 50
   against false imprisonment, 50
   of necessity, 50
defibrillators, 205t
deficit explanations, dispelling, 219t
definition
   of critical thinking, 118
   of cultural safety, 63–64
   of culture, 62
   of nursing, 1–2, 2b
   of power, 138–139
delivery models, care, 328–329, 328t
descriptive study, 310t
design, 308t
deteriorating patient, in simulation, 275
dichlorodiphenyltrichloroethane (DDT), in environment, 340–341
Dickens, Charles, 14
differential access, 217f
digital age, communication in, 174–175
digital health, 197–212
   ethics and, 207–208
   opportunities associated with, 200–201, 201b
digital health interventions, 198–199b, 203–204
   common, 205t
   technologies, 198
      barriers to, 206–207
      ethics and, 207–208
      patient engagement in, 204–206
      for patient safety and clinical quality, 201–202, 202t
digital health literacy, nursing and, 198–200, 199–200b, 206
digital nursing, 190–191
dignity, 92
discrimination, 216–217
dispositions, 120
distance, tyranny of, in rural and remote communities, 245–246
diversity, cultural, in Australia, 67t
documentation, of patient care, 112
domestic violence, 229
Donabedian's model of quality, 109t
drawing, 162
'duty to care', 232

E
EBP. *see* evidence-based practice
education, 187–189, 188b
   apprenticeship mode of, 22
   emotions and, 159
   global health and, 370–371, 371b
   history of nursing and, 22–23
   interprofessional, 168, 168b
   reflection and, 155
   specialisation and, 23
educationalists, reflection and, 157–158
EHR. *see* electronic health record
elder abuse, 230–231
electronic health records (EHRs), 202t, 204
embedded research design, 312t
Embrace2, 205t
emotional competence, 75–86
emotional safety, 282–283, 283b
emotions, education and, 159
empathy, 77–79, 78–79b, 91
employer requirements, social media and, 192–193, 193b
empowered people, 258
empowerment, 88–89
empowerment, of nursing, 140
energy, affordable and clean, 346f
enlightened views, of history of nursing, 10
enlightenment, 157
Ennis, Robert H, 118
entrapment, 231t, 233–235, 235b
environment
   clinical, 298
   complex, reflective practice and, 153–154
   health services and, 349–352, 352b
   nursing and, 339–356
      history of, 340–341
      role in, 353–354
   safe learning, 282–283
e-professionalism, 190–193
equity
   advocacy for, 145
   in health industry, 341–343
   in nursing, 213–228, 225b
ergonomic risks, occupational health nurses and, 262
errors, 34–35
   of healthcare, far-reaching impacts, 108
ethical argument, 92
ethical principlism, 35t

ethics
    of argument, 129, 130f
    character, 35t
    codes of, 129
    of critical thinking, 129–131, 131b
    decision making and, 34
    digital health and, 207–208
    everyday, 37–38, 38b
    future, challenges, 38–39
    human, 35t
    issues related to journalling, 160–161
    moral, 35t
    in nursing, 33–44, 40b
    in person-centred care and patient participation, 99–100, 100b
    professional, 34
    social media and, 190–193
    unethical professional conduct, ethical and, 35–41, 37b
    virtue, 35t
ethnography, 311t
European Journal of Cardiovascular Nursing (EJCN) Journal Club, 187
evaluation, 127f
evidence-based practice (EBP), 125
    leadership in, 334–335, 334b
    in research, 314, 315b
exemplary ethical professional conduct, 35
exercise, of power, 143–144
experiences, clinical, 297
experiential knowledge, 293
experimental study, 310t
expert clinical practice, significance of, 335
expressing agency, 143
extracurricular simulation, participation in, 272–274, 274b
extreme weather events, climate change and, 343–345
eye movement desensitisation reprocessing (EMDR), 205t

F
Facebook, 182
    for building online communities, 185–186
fairness, ethical principles of, 190–191
false imprisonment, 49
families, affected by violence, 230–232
    coercive control and entrapment, 233–235, 235b
    culturally safe and respectful practice, 236–238, 238b
    effects of, 232
    Indigenous and First Nations peoples, 236, 238b
    intrafamilial, 231t
    misconceptions of, 233, 233b, 234t
    social justice, intersectionality and rights, 232–233
    type of, 231t
fatigue, compassion
    preventing, 82, 82b
    understanding, 81–82
feedback
    for lifelong learning, 293–295, 295b
    in simulation, 275, 278–280, 281b

feminist research, 311t
FIFO services. *see* fly-in fly-out (FIFO) services
Finlayson, Jean, 26, 26f
First Nations peoples
    Australian, 64
    violence and, 236, 238b
first victims, of healthcare errors, 108
fly-in fly-out (FIFO) services, 247–248
fourth victims, of healthcare errors, 108
freedom
    movement, 46
    reflection and, 157
Freire, Paulo, 158
friend, 160
functional nursing, 328t
Fund's enduring message, 14
future ethical challenges, 38–39

G
Gamp, Sarah, 14
general practitioners, 261–262
glasshouse, greenhouse gases and, 343–344, 344f
Glasziou's triangle, 307f
global health, nursing and, 357–376
    associations in, 368b
    education in, 370–371, 371b
    ethical migration in, 358, 363–365, 365b
    global and regional priorities in, 363–365
    Global Strategic Directions for Nursing and Midwifery in, 358, 361–363, 362f, 363b
    governance in, 366–367, 367b, 372
    health policy in, 365
    health workforce in, 363, 364f, 366f
    human resources for health, 361–363
    Millennium Development Goals in, 358
    planning, 365–367, 366f
    policy and planning in, 361–363
    regulation in, 368–370, 370b, 372
    strategic partners in, 367–371, 368b
    strategies and policies for, 359–361, 360f, 361b
    sustainable development goals in, 361
    universal health coverage in, 361
Global Standards for the Initial Education of Professional Nurses and Midwives, 369
Global Strategic Directions for Nursing and Midwifery (SDNM), 358, 361–363, 362f, 363b
globalisation, 324, 358
Godden, Judith, 12
governance, global health and, 366–367, 367b, 372
government, politics and, 139–140
greenhouse gases (GHGs), 341, 345f
grey literature, in research, 316–317, 317b
GriefLine, 205t
grounded theory, 311t
grounds, 122
growth mindset, 294
guide, ethical, 129
guided reflective writing, 160

H

habits of mind, critical thinking and, 119–120
habitus, 39–40
HACS. *see* hospital-acquired complications
hair loss, 132f
Head to Health helpline, 205t
Headspace, 205t
health
   climate change and, 341–343, 342f, 343b
   climate crisis and, 348, 349f, 350f
   global, nursing and, 357–376
      associations in, 368b
      education in, 370–371, 371b
      ethical migration in, 358, 363–365, 365b
      global and regional priorities in, 363–365
      Global Strategic Directions for Nursing and Midwifery in, 358, 361–363, 362f, 363b
      governance in, 366–367, 367b, 372
      health policy in, 365
      health workforce in, 363, 364f
      human resources for health, 361–363
      Millennium Development Goals in, 358
      planning, 365–367, 366f
      policy and planning in, 361–363
      strategic partners in, 367–371, 368b
      strategies and policies for, 359–361, 360f, 361b
      sustainable development goals in, 361
      universal health coverage in, 361
   nurses on, 138
   practitioners, 56
   social determinants of. *see* social determinants of health
Health app, 205t
health disparities, in nursing, 214–216, 215b, 225b
   effects of, in healthcare, 218
   framing, within a social justice-rights-equity nexus, 215–216, 216b
   pathways to, 217f
   patient safety and, 105–106, 106b
   responding better to those belonging to groups commonly affected by, 219–225
      families affected by violence, 223–224, 223b, 225b
      Indigenous peoples, 219–221
      LGBTQI people, 222, 224b
      older people, 221–222
      youth, 223–225
health industry, equity in, 341–343
health interventions, digital, 198–199b, 203–204
   common, 205t
   technologies, 198
      barriers to, 206–207
      ethics and, 207–208
      patient engagement in, 204–206
      for patient safety and clinical quality, 201–202, 202t
health literacy, general practice nurses and, 261
Health Ombudsman Act 2013, 54
health promotion, 184–186, 185b
   in community, 259
health services
   access to, 64–65
   care of, 103
   environment and, 349–352, 352b
   integrated, 258
   for rural and remote communities, 247–249, 249b
health workforce, 363, 364f, 366f
healthcare, 248
   access to, 326
   care delivery models in, 328
   in context, 324–325b, 324–326, 325b, 326b
   effects of disparities in, 218
   primary, nursing and, 257–266, 258–259b, 264b
      in community, 259–264, 264b
      components of, 258
      definition of, 258–259
   professionals, 324
   reforms, 326
   settings, contemporary, 324
healthcare errors, far-reaching impacts of, 108
healthcare practices, encourage participation to shape, 92–99
   meso-level participation, 96–99, 97–98t, 99b
   micro-level participation, 94–96, 95t, 96b
   public participation, 96–99, 97–98t, 99b
healthcare providers, benefits of, in integrated working, 175
healthcare system
   advocacy in, 145
   climate crisis and, 348
healthy migrant effect, 69
Helmstadter, Carol, 12
historical trauma, 231t
history, of nursing, 2–3, 3b, 10–11
   Australia and, 12–13, 23–27
   community and, care in, 13–14
   developing education and, 22–23
   enlightened view of, 10–11
   identity and, 23–27
   institutional nurses and, 13
   midwifery and, 24–25
   modern nursing's antecedents, 11–12
   New Zealand and, 12–13, 23–27
   pre-modern, 12
   statutory regulation and, 18–19
   traditional views of, 10
   voluntary regulation and, 18
   war and, 19–22
home front, 21–22
homogeneous group, 224
hope, in health services, 352, 352b
horizontal integration, 171
hospital-acquired complications (HACS), 103–104
human resources
   for health, 361–363
   lack of, 80
human rights, 35t
humanistic nursing, 83

hydrochlorofluorocarbons (HCHCs), in environment, 340–341

I

ICM. *see* International Confederation of Midwives
ICN. *see* International Council of Nurses
idea, critical thinking and, 131
I-DECIDE, 205t
identity, and history, 23–27
immigration, of healthcare professionals, 366–367, 367b
immigration policy, Australian, 67t
impairment, 56
imprisonment, false, 49
inclinations, 120
inclusiveness, in Australian immigration policy development, 67t
incompetence, moral, 36
Indigenous communities, 250
Indigenous extended families (whānau), violence within, 231t
Indigenous peoples
    climate change and, 343
    health disparities and, 219–221
    healthcare needs of, 61–62
    violence and, 236, 238b
    working with, 66b
inequalities, 214
inequities, 214
influence, developing, 142t
    workplace strategies for, 140
information, literacy, 299
informed consent, 49
innovation, in interprofessional learning, 173
inquisitiveness, critical thinking and, 120
Instagram, 183
institutional nurses, 13
institutional training schemes, 15–17
institutions, history of nursing and, 13
insulin pumps, 205t
integrated care
    communication in, effective, 174–175
    definition of, 171
    domains of successful, 175
    mutual trust, foster, 174
    nurse
        as effective interprofessional team members, 173
        in interdisciplinary teamwork, 171–173, 173b
        in multidisciplinary teamwork, 171–173, 173b
        in transdisciplinary teamwork, 171–173, 173b
    provision of, 171
    reflection, 175b
    roles in, clearly defined, 174
integrated health services, 258
integration, in Australian immigration policy development, 67t
integrity, 190–191
interdisciplinary teamwork
    description of, 172
    nurse in, 171–173, 173b

interest, of consumers, critical thinking and, 125
intergenerational violence, 231t
internal cardiac monitoring, 205t
International Classification for Patient Safety (ICPS), conceptual framework for, 109t
International Confederation of Midwives (ICM), 368
International Council of Nurses (ICN), 4, 18, 368
    Code of Ethics for Nurses, 129
international recruitment, ethical migration and, 363–365, 367b
interpersonal relationship skills, critical thinking and, 131
interpersonal violence, 229
interprofessional education, 168, 168b
interprofessional learning, 167–178
    development of, in team practices, 174
    importance of, 168–169, 169b
interprofessional practice, 328t
interprofessional protocols, in effective communication, 175
interprofessional working, 167–171
    benefits of, 175–176
intersectionality, 218, 232–233
intimate partner violence (IPV), 230, 231t
intrafamilial family violence, 231t
introspection, 158
IPV. *see* intimate partner violence
iSAFE, 205t

J

journalling, 160
    challenges to, 160
    ethical issues related to, 160–161
    legal issues related to, 160–161
    for reflective practice, 159
    techniques for, 160b
justice
    in digital health, 208
    ethical principles of, 190–191

K

knowledge
    connecting clinical and theoretical learning and, 290–292, 292t
    developing influence through, 142t
    development of, 292–293
    power and, 138–139

L

large language models (LLMs), nursing and, 199
law
    civil, 46
    common, 46
    criminal, 46, 52
    patient safety and, 46–48, 47–48b
leader, clinical, 330–332
    attributes of, 330f, 331–332, 331f
    framework for being, 331f

leader, clinical *(Continued)*
   promoting, professional societies and organisations to, 333–334
leadership, 79, 321
   in action, 329–330
   in evidence-based practice, 334–335, 334b
   global health and, 366–367, 367b, 372
   in interprofessional learning, 173
   opportunities for, 326–327, 327b
   for patient safety, 111, 111t
   promoting
     in practice setting, 332–334
       professional societies and organisations in, 333–334
   servant, 330
learning
   classroom, 293
   clinical, 293
   cultural safety and, 110
   lifelong, 293
   process of, 292
   process skills for, 292
   resources for, 292
   simulation, 267–288
     benefits and challenges of, 274–277, 275b, 276b, 276t, 277b
     bridging theory and practice in, 268–269
     moving forward with, 283–286, 284–286b, 284b
     types of, 269–272, 270f, 271f
   technology for, 300
legal aspects, of nursing practice, 45–60
   civil law as, 46–51
     negligent advice, 46
     patient consent, 48–50
     patient freedom of movement, 46
     patient safety, 46–48, 47–48b
   common law as, 46
   complaints as, 55–56
   criminal law as
     assault, 52
     negligence, manslaughter, 53–54
   drug regulation as, 54–55
   nursing practice regulation as, 54–55
   patient information as, 53–54
   vicarious liability as, 51–52
legends, of nursing, 2–3, 3b
legislation, 46
   adjacent, social media and, 192
LGBTQI people, health disparities and, 222, 224b
liability, 47
Lifeline, 205t
lifelong learning, 4, 293
LinkedIn, 183
listening, in feedback, 279–280
literacy, information, 299
literature review, 312, 313t
litigation, incidence of, 125
low-value care, 105

M

machine learning (ML), nursing and, 199
macro-level participation, 96–99, 97–98t, 99b
mainstreaming, in Australian immigration policy development, 67t
malaria, climate change and, 341–343
Manage Medication, 205t
manikin simulations, 271, 271f, 284–286b
Manpower Directorate, 21–22
manslaughter, 53–54
Māori people, in New Zealand, 65
mapping review, 313t
marginalisation, 61–62
Mask-Ed™, 270–271, 270f
'material risks', 48
MedAdvisor, 205t
media
   healthcare services and, 351
   in whistleblowing, 146–147
medical practitioners, in WHO, 359
Medicines (Designated Prescribers: Nurse Practitioners) Regulations 2005, 141–142
Medicines (Designated Prescriber-Registered Nurses Practising in Diabetes Health) Regulations 2011, 141–142
Medicines (Designated Prescriber-Registered Nurses) Regulations 2016, 141–142
MedicineWise, 205t
Medisafe Pill Reminder, 205t
Medsafe codes, 192
Member of the British Empire (MBE), 26
membership, 39–40
mens rea, 52
mental health issues, people with, 51
mental health screening, 205t
mentoring, 335
meso-level participation, 96–99, 97–98t, 99b
meta-analysis, 313t
methodology, 308t
methods, 308t
miasmatic theory, 15
micro-level participation, 94–96, 95t, 96b
midwifery
   cultural safety in, 61–74
   identity of, 24–25
Midwifery Officer, global health and, 366–367, 367b
midwifery organisations, examples of, 334b
migration, of healthcare professionals, 358
military attacks, ethics in nursing, 39
Millennium Development Goals (MDGs), 358
MindSpot, 205t
missed nursing care, 107–108, 107b
mixed methods research, 311–312, 313t
   designs in, 312t
mobile health applications, 198
models, of care delivery, 328–329, 328t
modern healthcare, 184–189

moral delinquency, 36
moral distress, 153–154
moral impairment, 36
moral incompetence, 36
moral rights, 35t
moral turpitude, 36
moral values, 34
morbidity, in rural and remote communities, 247
mortality, in rural and remote communities, 247
motion monitoring, 205t
movement, freedom of, 46
multiculturalism, 65
   in Australian immigration policy development, 67t
multidisciplinary teamwork
   description of, 172
   nurse in, 171–173, 173b
Multi-Employer Collective Agreements, 141
multi-sectoral policies and actions, 258
Mutual Recognition Agreement, 19
mutual trust, foster, 174
My Asthma portal (MAP), 205t
My Fitness Plus, 205t
myPlan, 205t
myths, nursing, 2–3, 3b

N

National Competency Standards for the Midwife, 155
National Health and Medical Research Council (NHMRC)
   evidence hierarchy, 314
natural language processing (NLP), nursing and, 199
naturalistic paradigm, in research, 310t
NCDs. *see* non-communicable diseases
NCNZ. *see* Nursing Council of New Zealand
near misses, reporting of, 112
necessity, defence of, 50
negative societal attitudes, to older people, 221–222
negligence, 46–48, 47–48b
   advice and, 46
   contributory, 48
   criminal, 53–54
   manslaughter, 53–54
negligent advice, 46
Neil, Elizabeth Grace, 367
nested research design, 312t
neutrality, caring, 83
New Zealand
   correctional nurses in, 263
   Health and Disability Commission 2018, 145
   healthcare in early, 12–13
   history of, 66b
   Māori people in, 65
   multicultural, 68
   nursing, milestones in, 19–23
New Zealand Nurses Organisation (NZNO), 36
NGOs. *see* non-government organisations
NHMRC. *see* National Health and Medical Research Council

Nightingale, Florence, 10, 340–341
NMBA. *see* Nursing and Midwifery Board of Australia
NMC. *see* Nursing and Midwifery Council
no breach of duty, 48
no causation, 48
no duty of care, 48
non-communicable diseases (NCDs), 326
   globalisation and, 358
non-government organisations (NGOs), 359
non-maleficence, ethical principles of, 190–191
Notes on Nursing (1860), 340–341
notification
   mandatory, 56–57, 57b
   of notifiable conduct, 55–56
nurse-led model of practice, innovative, 333b
nurses, 6
   Aboriginal, 26–27
   climate change and, 351
   collective political power, 140–143, 142t, 143b
   correctional, 263–264, 264b
   effective communication, 77
   as effective interprofessional team members, 173
   institutional, 13
   in interdisciplinary teamwork, 171–173, 173b
   leader, 321–338, 323b
      opportunities for, 327b
   migration of, 358–359
   in multidisciplinary teamwork, 171–173, 173b
   occupational health, 262–263
   patient safety competencies for, 109
   power of, 138–139
   practice, general practitioners, 261–262
   public confidence in, 1
   religious, 25–27
   role of, 293
      in environmental health, 353–354
      to minimising low-value care, 105, 106t
   school health, 260–261
   shortage of, 324
   social media and, recommendations for, 193b
   in transdisciplinary teamwork, 171–173, 173b
   in WHO, 359
nursing
   as academic discipline, 306
   'back-blocks', 21
   barriers to compassion in, 80–81, 81b
   career in, 1–8
   choosing, 4–5
   compassion in, 76–77, 76–77b, 77b
   contemporary, 306
   critical thinking in, 124–129
   cultural safety in, 61–74
   culture in, 62–64
   definition of, 1–4, 2b, 4b
   digital health literacy and, 198–200, 199–200b, 206
   environment and, 339–356
      history of, 340–341

nursing *(Continued)*
   role in, 353–354
  ethics, 34–35, 35b, 35t
   everyday, 37–38, 38b
   role of, 39–41
  functional, 328t
  fundamental outcomes of, 77
  future of, 27–28
  global health and, 357–376
   associations in, 368b
   education in, 370–371, 371b
   ethical migration in, 358, 363–365, 365b
   global and regional priorities in, 363–365
   Global Strategic Directions for Nursing and Midwifery in, 358, 361–363, 362f, 363b
   governance in, 366–367, 367b, 372
   health policy in, 365
   health workforce in, 363, 364f
   human resources for health, 361–363
   Millennium Development Goals in, 358
   planning, 365–367, 366f
   policy and planning in, 361–363
   regulation in, 368–370, 370b, 372
   strategic partners in, 367–371, 368b
   strategies and policies for, 359–361, 360f, 361b
   sustainable development goals in, 361
   universal health coverage in, 361
  health disparities in, 214–216, 215b, 225b
   effects of, in healthcare, 218
   framing, within a social justice-rights-equity nexus, 215–216, 216b
   responding better to those belonging to groups commonly affected by, 219–225
  historical influences on, 17
  history of, 10–11
   Australia and, 12–13
   community and, care in, 13–14
   developing education and, 22–23
   enlightened views of, 10–11
   identity and, 24–25
   institutional nurses and, 13
   institutional training schemes, 15–17
   midwifery and, 24–25
   modern nursing's antecedents, 11–12
   New Zealand and, 12–13
   pre-modern, 12
   statutory regulation and, 18–19
   traditional views of, 10
   voluntary regulation and, 18
   war and, 19–22
  leaders, opportunities for, 326–327, 327b
  legends of, 2–3, 3b
  modern nursing's antecedents, 11–12
  myths, 2–3, 3b
  organisations, professional, examples of, 334b
  patient perspectives in, 87–102
  patient safety and, 103–116, 114b

nursing *(Continued)*
  competencies, 109
  continuous quality improvement and, 111–112, 112t
  definition of, 105
  frameworks and models in, 109, 109t
  importance of, 104–105, 104t
  leadership for, 111, 111t
  legal and ethical aspects of, 113, 113b
  to minimising low-value care, 106t
  responsibilities in, 108
  role of, 108
  person-centred care in, 87–102
   encourage participation to shape healthcare practices, 92–99
   theoretical debates to practice, 91–92, 92b
   who are we caring for?, 88–89, 89b
  politics and, 136–138, 137–138b
  pre-modern, 12
  primary, 328t
  primary healthcare and, 257–266, 258–259b, 264b
   in community, 259–264, 264b
   components of, 258
   definition of, 258–259
  professional regulation and conduct, 6–7, 6b, 7b
  reform, 14–17
  relevance to, 184–189
  research in, 305–320
   critical appraisal in, 314, 315t
   definition of, 306–307
   evidence-based practice in, 314
   mixed methods, 311–312, 312t
   nurses' involvement in, 307–309, 307f, 309b
   in nursing, 305–320
   process, 312–314, 312b
   qualitative, 310–311, 310t
   quantitative, 309, 310t
   terminology in, 308t
  roles of, in community, 259–264, 264b
  rural and remote, 243–256, 254b
   extended, advanced and solo, 250–251, 251b
   nature of, 249
   populations in, 244–245, 245b
   roles in, 250–251, 251b
   scope of practice, 249–250
   workforce, 251–253
  shortage in, 136
  simulation learning in, 267–288
   benefits and challenges of, 274–277, 275b, 276b, 276t, 277b
   bridging theory and practice in, 268–269
   moving forward with, 283–286, 284–286b, 284b
   types of, 269–272, 270f, 271f
  social media and, 179–196, 189b, 193b
   contemporary application in, 184–189
   e-professionalism and, 190–193
   ethics and, 190–193
   innovation in, 184f

nursing *(Continued)*
    introduction, 179–194
        modern healthcare, 184–189
        relevance to nursing and, 184–189
    stereotypes, 2–3, 3b, 136
    sustaining, 5–6, 6b
    team, 328t
    violence, 229–242
    visioning the future by knowing the past, 9–32, 29b
Nursing and Midwifery Board of Australia (NMBA), 54, 290
    competencies, 155
    Registered Nurse Standards for Practice, 297, 297b, 297t
Nursing and Midwifery Council (NMC), 146
nursing care, missed, 107–108, 107b
Nursing Council of New Zealand (NCNZ), 36, 155
nursing curriculum, 292
nursing ethics, 34–35, 35b, 35t
nursing misconduct, related to social media, 191f
nursing practice
    legal aspects of, 45–60
        civil law as, 46–51
        common law as, 46
        complaints as, 55–56
        criminal law as, 46, 52
        nursing practice regulation as, 54–55
        patient information as, 53–54
        vicarious liability as, 51–52
    policy frameworks for, 327, 327b
    power and politics in, 135–152, 148b
    regulation of, 54–55
nursing praxis, 156
NZNO. *see* New Zealand Nurses Organisation

O

Objective Structured Clinical Assessments (OSCA), 272
Objective Structured Clinical Examinations (OSCE), 272
occupational health nurses, 262–263
O'Donohue, Lowitja, 26–27
older people, health disparities and, 221–222
One Health approach, 352–353
online communities, 185
online counselling and theory, 205t
online portals, in research, 317
open-mindedness, critical thinking and, 120
organisational culture, 80
organisational values, 329
organisations
    benefits of, in integrated working, 176
    to promote clinical leadership, 333–334
Osburn, Lucy, 16, 16f

P

pacemakers, 205t
paradigm, 308t
parents, consent and, 50
parliamentary law, 46

participation
    in healthcare, 92–99
        meso-level participation, 96–99, 97–98t, 99b
        micro-level participation, 94–96, 95t, 96b
        public participation, 96–99, 97–98t, 99b
    in root cause analysis, 113
participatory action research, 311t
partnership, advocacy for, 144–147, 147b
part-task trainer simulations, 271, 271f
pathways, clinical, 328t
patient
    consent of, 48–50
    freedom of movement of, 46
    information, 53–54
    in integrated working, benefits of, 175
    safety of, 46–48, 47–48b, 103–116, 114b
        competencies, 109
        continuous quality improvement and, 111–112, 112t
        definition of, 105
        digital health interventions for, 201–202, 202t
        frameworks and models in, 109, 109t
        importance of, 104–105, 104t
        leadership for, 111, 111t
        legal and ethical aspects of, 113, 113b
        to minimising low-value care, 106t
        responsibilities in, 108
        role of, 108
        in simulation, 275
    simulated, 272
patient allocation, 328t
patient care
    coordinated, in interprofessional learning, 168–169
    documentation of, 112
    impact on, 81
patient outcomes, improved, in interprofessional learning, 168
patient portals, 202t
patient safety
    digital health interventions for, 201–202, 202t
    in simulation, 275
patient services, 186
patient support, 184–186, 185b
patient-centred care, to person-centred care, 90–91
PEARLS debriefing model, 281
peer-reviewed journals, in research, 316, 317b
people-centred care, 358
perseverance, critical thinking and, 120
personal attributes, 79
personal growth, in extracurricular simulations, 273–274
'personal resilience', concept of, 146–147
personal stress, 80
personal values, 329
person-centred care
    in integrated working, 170
    in nursing, 87–102
        encourage participation to shape healthcare practices, 92–99

person-centred care *(Continued)*
    theoretical debates to practice, 91–92, 92b
    who are we caring for?, 88–89, 89b
  patient-centred care to, 90–91
personhood, 90
phenomenology, 311t
photography, 162
physical hazards, occupational health nurses and, 262
physical safety, 282
Plato, 157
policy, 189, 190b
  in effective communication, 175
  frameworks, for nursing practice, 327, 327b
  immigration, Australian, 67t
political, economic, technological and sociocultural (PETS) factors, 290–292, 291f
political conflict, ethics in nursing, 39
political power, collective, 140–143, 142t, 143b
political theorists, reflection and, 157–158
politics
  government and, 139–140
  nursing and, 136–138, 137–138b
  power and, 139–140
  in practice of nursing, 135–152, 148b
population approach, whole of, interprofessional working and, 171
population sparsity, 245–246
populations, in rural and remote communities, 244–245, 245b
positivistic paradigm, in research, 310t
postmodernism, 158–159
post-structuralism, 158–159
post-traumatic stress disorder (PTSD), in refugees, 68
poverty, 218
power, 138–139, 139b
  collective political, 140–143, 142t, 143b
  definition of, 138–139
  exercise of, 143–144
  imbalance of, 144–145
  knowledge and, 138–139
  of nurse, 138–139
  politics and, 139–140
  in practice, 143–147, 144b
  of nursing, 135–152, 148b
practice
  evidence-based, leadership in, 334–335, 334b
  innovative nurse-led model of, 333b
  integration of, ability for, 290
  interprofessional, preparation for, 169
  reflective, 293
  setting, promoting leadership in, 332–334
  significance of, 335
  and theory
    bridging, 268–269
    linking of, 295–296
  transition to, clinical and theoretical knowledge and, 298–299, 299b

practice nurses, general practitioners, 261–262
pragmatism, 309
precedent, 46
predatory journals, 316
pre-modern nursing, 12
pre-reflection, 156
preventable harms, in healthcare errors, 103–104
Prig, Betsy, 14
primary healthcare, nursing and, 257–266, 258–259b, 264b
  in community, 259–264, 264b
  components of, 258
  definition of, 258–259
primary nursing, 328t
'principle-based' approach, 369
principles, 130
privacy, in digital health, 208
procedure, 189, 190b
professional codes, 191–192
professional conduct, 190–191
professional development, 82, 187–189, 188b
professional ethics, 34
professional growth, in extracurricular simulations, 273–274
professional networking, social media and, 186–187, 187b
professional nursing organisations, 141
  examples of, 334b
professional regulation, 18
  nursing, 6–7, 6b, 7b
professional socialisation, in interprofessional learning, 169
professional societies, to promote clinical leadership, 333–334
professional values, 329
professionalism, social media and, 190–191
prototypical ethical professional conduct, 35
psychological restraint, 49
psychology, reflection and, 158
PTSD. *see* post-traumatic stress disorder
public confidence, 1
public media, in whistleblowing, 146–147

Q

qualitative research, 310–311, 310t
qualitative systematic review, 313t
quality of care, 214
quantitative research, 309
quasi-experimental study, 310t

R

racism, 61–62, 218
rapid review, 313t
rationale, 132, 132f
realistic scenarios, immersion in, 273
reality, reflection and, 158
reality shock, 298
reason, sound argument and, 123

reasoning, critical thinking as, 119
records, patient information, 53–54
recruitment, social media and, 186–187, 187b
reflection, 154–155, 157b
  action and, 157, 158
  benefits of, 158–159
  clinical practice and, 158
  contemplation and, 155–156
  critical incident analysis and, 159, 161, 162b
  critical social theory and, 158–159
  criticisms of, 163–164
  definition of, 155–157
  education and, 155
  framework for, 161
  problems of, 163–164
  psychology and, 158
  responses on, 163–164
  strategies for, 159–163
  writing and, 159–161
reflection-in-action, 156
reflection-on-action, 156
reflections, 62
reflective conversations, in simulation, 278–281, 281b
reflective practice, 153–166, 293
  clinical supervision and, 162–163
  critical thinking and, 154–155
  engagement and, 161
  groups of, 163
  journalling and, 160
    challenges to, 160
    ethical issues related to, 160–161
    legal issues related to, 160–161
    for reflective practice, 159
    techniques for, 160b
  roots of, 157–158
  self-awareness and, 162–163
reforms
  healthcare, 326
  nursing, 14–17
refugees, 68
registered nurse (RN), 119
Registered Nurse Standards for Practice, 155
regulation
  global health and, 368–370, 370b, 372
  of nursing practice, 54–55
  professional, 18
  statutory, 18–19
  voluntary, 18
relevant, sound argument and, 122
religious nurses, 25–27
remote monitoring, 202t
  of blood glucose level, 205t
  of ECG and heart rate, 205t
repeated practice, in simulation, 275
reporting errors, cultural safety and, 110
research, 189, 190b
  argument as, 128f

research *(Continued)*
  critical appraisal in, 314, 315t
  critical thinking and, 127–129
  definition of, 306–307
  evidence-based practice in, 314
  mixed methods, 311–312, 312t
  nurses' involvement in, 307–309, 307f, 309b
  in nursing, 305–320
    approaches, 309–317
    paradigms of, 310t
  process, 312–314, 312b
  qualitative, 310–311, 310t
  quantitative, 309, 310t
  terminology in, 308t
resilience, 146–147
resources, for learning, 292
respect, 92
  in interprofessional learning, 173
respect for autonomy, ethical principles of, 190–191
respectful practice, 236–238, 238b
review, literature, 312, 313t
rights
  family violence and, 232–233
  human, 35t
risk, 48
RN. *see* registered nurse
role play, 271, 284–286b
roles
  clearly defined, in integrated care team, 174
  of nurses, 293
root cause analysis (RCA), 112–113
Royal College of Nursing Australia, 18
Royal Victorian College of Nursing (RVCN), 22
rural and remote communities
  ageing, 247
  health of, 246–247
  morbidity and mortality, 247
  population sparsity in, 245–246
  populations in, 244–245, 245b
  providing health services for, 247–249, 249b
  state of health in, 246b
  telehealth services for, 248, 252–253b
  tyranny of distance in, 245–246
rural and remote nursing, 243–256, 254b
  communities in, 246–247
  extended, advanced and solo, 250–251, 251b
  nature of, 249
  roles in, 250–251, 251b
  scope of practice, 249–250
  workforce, 251–253
RVCN. *see* Royal Victorian College of Nursing

S

safe learning environment, 282–283
Safe Patient Care Act 2015, 141
safety
  cultural, 63–64, 70f, 110

safety *(Continued)*
   in nursing and midwifery, 61–74
     emotional, 282–283, 283b
     of patient, 46–48, 47–48b, 103–116, 114b
     physical, 282
     in workplace, 262
Salvation Army, 26
Savage, Ellen, 20–21, 21f
scenarios, stereotypical, in simulation, 275
scepticism, 119
Schön, Donald, 156
scoping review, 313t
SDH. *see* social determinants of health
second victims, of healthcare errors, 108
Seer, 205t
self-assessment, 293–294, 294f
self-awareness, 162–163
self-care
   practices, 82
   understanding compassion fatigue in nursing and its prevention, 81–82
self-compassion
   practising, 82
   understanding compassion fatigue in nursing and its prevention, 81–82
self-consciousness, 118
self-management, 95
self-reflection, in simulation, 278–281, 281b
self-scrutiny, 164
sensitivity, cultural, 69–70
sequential explanatory research design, 312t
sequential exploratory research design, 312t
serious games, 271
service delivery level, advocacy at, 145
service users, 88
sexual violence, 231t
simulated patient, 272
simulation
   extracurricular, participation in, 272–274, 274b
     development of clinical reasoning skills, 273
     immersion in realistic scenarios, 273
     opportunity to practise without assessment, 273
     personal and professional growth, 273–274
     working with other disciplines, 273
   manikin, 271, 271f, 284–286b
   part-task trainer, 271, 271f
   tips to gain most out of, 277–278
   value of, 269b
   virtual, 272
   virtual reality, 272
simulation learning, 267–288
   benefits and challenges of, 274–277, 275b, 276b, 276t, 277b
   bridging theory and practice in, 268–269
   moving forward with, 283–286, 284–286b, 284b
   types of, 269–272, 270f, 271f
situation, 129–130

skills and knowledge, in simulation, 275
smart infusion pumps, 202t
SMP, 205t
social determinants of health (SDH), 216–218
   culture and, correlation between, 68–69
   good, climate crisis and, 348
social justice
   advocacy for, 144–147, 147b
   family violence and, 232–233
   in nursing, 213–228, 225b
     effects of, in healthcare, 218
     responding better to those belonging to groups commonly affected by, 219–225
     social determinants of health, 216–218
social justice-rights-equity nexus, framing disparities within, 215–216, 216b
social media
   characteristics and statistics of, 181f
   definition of, 180–184
   ethics, 190–193
   nursing and, 179–196, 189b, 193b
     contemporary application in, 184–189
     e-professionalism and, 190–193
     ethics and, 190–193
     innovation in, 184f
     introduction, 179–194
     modern healthcare, 184–189
     relevance to nursing and, 184–189
social media guidelines, for whistleblowing, 146–147
social networking, 180
socialisation, professional, in interprofessional learning, 169
societies, professional, to promote clinical leadership, 333–334
solidarity, 39–40
sound argument, 122–124, 124b
sound evidence, critical thinking and, 125
South Pacific Chief Nursing Midwifery Officers Alliance (SPCNMOA), 367
SPCNMOA. *see* South Pacific Chief Nursing Midwifery Officers Alliance
specialisation, streams of, 23
spectacles, pair of, 117–118
standards
   adoption of, in effective communication, 175
   of care, 46–47
state of health, in rural and remote communities, 246b
State of the World's Nursing (SOWN) report, 366–367
state violence, 231t
state-of-the-art review, 313t
statutory law, 46
statutory regulation, 18–19
stereotypes, 2–3, 3b
sTherapy, 205t
strategic partners, global health and, 367–371, 368b
stress
   occupational health nurses and, 262

stress *(Continued)*
  personal, 80
  workplace, 80
students, in clinical setting, 295–296
supervision, 162–163
support, seeking, 82
sustainable development goals (SDGs), 361
  in climate change, 341–343, 342f, 343b, 346f
Swiss cheese model, 109t
systematic map, 313t
systematic search, 313t
systematised review, 313t
Systems Engineering Initiative for Patient Safety (SEIPS) model 3.0, 109t

T

team nursing, 328t
teamwork
  cultural safety and, 110
  interdisciplinary
    description of, 172
    nurse in, 171–173, 173b
  multidisciplinary
    description of, 172
    nurse in, 171–173, 173b
  transdisciplinary
    description of, 172
    nurse in, 171–173, 173b
technology
  of care, 17
  for learning and development, 300
telehealth, 199–200b, 201, 202t, 328t
  for rural and remote communities, 248, 252–253b
TENS machine, 205t
test, 'but for', 47
The Nursing and Midwifery Board of Australia's Registered Nurse Standards of Practice (2016), 117–118
theoretical debates to practice, 91–92, 92b
theoretical learning, and clinical learning, connection to, 290–292, 292t
theorising, reflection and, 155–156
theory
  integration of, ability for, 290
  and practice
    bridging, 268–269
    linking of, 295–296
theory-practice gap, 298
therapeutic communication, 91
  skills, 95
Therapeutic Goods Association (TGA) codes, 192
thinking, reflection and, 155–156
third victims, of healthcare errors, 108
13YARN, 205t
TikTok, 183–184
time constraints, 80
'To err is human' landmark report, 104
Torres Strait Islanders, in Australia, 64–65
tort, 46, 49
total patient care, 328t
touching, 48
traditional views, of history of nursing, 10
transdisciplinary teamwork
  description of, 172
  nurse in, 171–173, 173b
transformational leadership, 330
transition period, from graduate to practitioner, 298–299, 299b
Trans-Tasman Mutual Recognition Act 1997, 19
trauma, 231t
  historical, 231t
Treaty of Waitangi, 65
'trespass to person', 48–50
trust, mutual, foster, 174
truthfulness, 190–191
tweetorials, 188–189
Twitter, 182
tyranny of distance, in rural and remote communities, 245–246

U

umbrella review, 313t
unethical conduct, 35–41, 37b
united in diversity, in Australian immigration policy development, 67t
United States, Institute of Medicine, 104, 104t
universal health coverage, 361
unsound argument, 124
utilitarianism, 35t

V

validity, sound argument and, 123
values, 130
vertical integration, 171
vicarious liability, 51–52
victim blaming, 218
violence
  families affected by, health disparities and, 223–224, 223b, 225b
  family, 230–232
    coercive control and entrapment, 233–235, 235b
    culturally safe and respectful practice, 236–238, 238b
    effects of, 232
    Indigenous and First Nations peoples, 236, 238b
    intrafamilial, 231t
    misconceptions of, 233, 233b, 234t
    social justice, intersectionality and rights, 232–233
    type of, 231t
  health consequences of, 232
  within Indigenous extended families (whānau), 231t
  nursing, 229–242
  sexual, 231t
  state, 231t
viral disease pandemics, ethics in nursing, 39
virtual care, 205t

virtual games, 271
virtual reality (VR), 272
virtual reality simulation (VRS), 272
virtual simulation (VS), 272
virtue ethics, 35t
Virtuli T, 270f
voluntary consent, 49
voluntary regulation, 18
vulnerability, patient safety and, 105–106, 106b
vulnerable populations, 348
Vyner Brooke, 20

W

war, 19–22
wearable health devices, 202t, 205t
wearable sensor technology, 204–206
'WeNurses' X page, 187
WHA. *see* World Health Assembly
whistleblowing, 146
    guidelines for, 146–147
    legal protection in, 147
WHO. *see* World Health Organization
WHO 'LIVES' approach to protecting victim-survivors of family violence, 237t
wildfires, health impacts of, 350f
work, safety and, 262
workforce, 186, 187b
    health, 363, 364f, 366f
    interventions, 187b
    rural and remote nursing, 251–253
working, with other disciplines, 273
workplace stress, 80
World Health Assembly (WHA), 359
World Health Organization (WHO), 359, 360f
    regional offices of, 365
    strategy of, in nursing, 137
World War I, 19–20
World War II, 19–20
writing, reflection and, 159–161

X

X, 182
X chat, 188–189

Y

Yammer, 186
youth, health disparities and, 223–225
YouTube, 182–183
    for health promotion, 186